INTERNATIONAL SERIES OF MONOGRAPHS IN PURE AND APPLIED BIOLOGY

Division: **ZOOLOGY**

General Editor: **G. A. Kerkut**

Volume 43

THE PHARMACOLOGY OF SYNAPSES

THE PHARMACOLOGY
OF SYNAPSES

BY

J. W. PHILLIS

*Department of Physiology, Monash University,
Clayton, Victoria, Australia*

1966

PERGAMON PRESS

*Oxford · London · Edinburgh · New York
Toronto · Sydney · Paris · Braunschweig*

Pergamon Press Ltd., Headington Hill Hall, Oxford
4 & 5 Fitzroy Square, London W.1
Pergamon Press (Scotland) Ltd., 2 & 3 Teviot Place, Edinburgh 1
Pergamon Press Inc., Maxwell House, Fairview Park, Elmsford, New York 10523
Pergamon of Canada Ltd., 207 Queen's Quay West, Toronto 1
Pergamon Press (Aust.) Pty. Ltd., 19a Boundary Street, Rushcutters Bay,
N.S.W. 2011, Australia
Pergamon Press S.A.R.L., 24 rue des Écoles, Paris 5ᵉ
Vieweg & Sohn GmbH, Burgplatz 1, Braunschweig

First edition 1970

Library of Congress Catalog Card No. 71–102093

PRINTED IN GREAT BRITAIN BY A. WHEATON & CO., EXETER
08 015558 8

FOR SIR JOHN C. ECCLES

CONTENTS

CONTENTS

PREFACE

THE invitation from Professor G. A. Kerkut to write this book came at a particularly opportune time. The recent development of fluorescent histochemical techniques for the detection of monoamines, and the rapid progress in neuropharmacology that has followed the development of microiontophoretic techniques of drug application, have contributed to the dramatic advances in our understanding of synaptic pharmacology. Indeed, the present decade may well rival in significance the previous major era of the 1930's, during which the foundations of chemical transmission were so brilliantly laid. It has been an exciting experience to observe, participate in and now to chronicle, the development of neuropharmacology during the past 10 years.

In this book I have attempted to analyse and record many of the remarkable developments that have occurred during the past decade. Reference is also made to earlier work which has retained its significance, such as the experiments which established that acetylcholine is a transmitter at neuromuscular and ganglionic synapses. In many instances I have been able, through the generosity of my colleagues, to quote new developments even before their final publication.

The compilation of this book has been greatly assisted by the appearance of a number of excellent reviews and symposia. Reference to these sources has usually been made at the beginning of the relevant sections, and I would like to acknowledge my debt to the reviewers who have previously brought the subject together.

It is assumed that the reader of this book will already have some understanding of the physiological properties of nerve and muscle cells. Further knowledge of the electrical properties of excitable cells can be gained from many sources. However, the accounts in *Synaptic Transmission* by Professor H. McLennan and *The Physiology of Synapses* by Sir John Eccles can be considered to be complementary to the present book.

During the writing of this book I have been greatly assisted by my colleagues I. McCance, A. K. Tebēcis, D. H. York, P. C. Vaughan, G. A.

Bentley and L. B. Geffen who have criticized chapters and contributed many valuable suggestions. I also wish to thank Miss D. Harrison and Miss S. Woolley for their assistance with the illustrations; Mrs. J. Baillie for her assistance with the bibliography; and Mrs. S. Browne, J. L. Deeker and Miss C. M. Kinnane for their work in the preparation of the manuscript.

J. W. PHILLIS

ACKNOWLEDGEMENTS

Grateful thanks are due to the following publishers and their editors for their generosity in giving permission for reproduction of figures:

Science; The Rockefeller University Press; The Anatomical Society of Great Britain and Ireland; *Acta Physiologica Scandinavica;* Macmillan (Journals) Ltd.; *Japanese Journal of Physiology;* S. Karger A.G.; The Williams & Wilkins Co.; Cambridge University Press; *The Journal of Physiology;* Elsevier Publishing Company; North-Holland Publishing Company; *American Journal of Physiology; Journal of Neurophysiology; Circulation Research.*

CHAPTER 1

INTRODUCTION

A. CONCEPTS

The concept that the nervous system is composed of discrete units or nerve cells was initially proposed by His and Forel and then independently by Cajal. After Waldeyer suggested the name "neurone" for nerve cells, the theory of the independence of nerve cells became known as the neurone theory. It was Cajal who, above all others, established that the functional connections between nerve cells are effected by close contacts, and not by continuity in a syncytial network, as proposed in the rival reticular theory of Gerlach and Golgi. The name "synapse" was given to these functional connections between nerve cells by Sherrington and it is with the details of operation of junctions between nerve cells and between nerve cells and effector cells that this book is concerned.

B. TRANSMISSION ACROSS THE SYNAPSE

The first speculations on the nature of transmission across junctional regions were put forward during the last century when DuBois-Reymond suggested that junctional transmission might be either chemical or electrical and thus initiated the two rival hypotheses of chemical and electrical transmission.

The next significant development occurred in 1904 when Elliott suggested that sympathetic nerve impulses liberate adrenaline at the junctional regions on smooth muscle, and a little later Dixon (1906) proposed that parasympathetic nerve impulses release a muscarine-like substance. In 1914, Dale commented on the fidelity with which acetylcholine reproduced the actions of parasympathetic stimulation, just as adrenaline did those of stimulation of the sympathetic system. Dale also noted and differentiated between the nicotinic and muscarinic actions of acetylcholine.

The experiments of Loewi (1921) demonstrated for the first time the

release of a chemical, "Vagustoff" (acetylcholine), during nerve stimulation and showed that the vagus inhibited the heart by means of this release.
Cannon and Bacq (1931) subsequently showed that stimulation of the
sympathetic nerves caused the release of an adrenaline-like substance
which accelerated the heart.

A series of classical investigations (Feldberg and Gaddum, 1934;
Feldberg and Vartiainen, 1934; Dale, Feldberg and Vogt, 1936; Brown,
Dale and Feldberg, 1936), which will be described in more detail in subsequent chapters, established that acetylcholine is the transmitter at skeletal
neuromuscular and ganglionic synapses. In 1935, Dale suggested an extension of the chemical transmitter hypothesis to account for excitation and
inhibition in the central nervous system.

Despite these findings the electrical hypothesis of synaptic transmission
in the central nervous system continued to have considerable support until
the advent of intracellular recording in 1951. However, the observations
made with this new technique were difficult to reconcile with the theories
of electrical transmission developed by Eccles and other scientists (see
Eccles, 1964), and the concept of chemical transmission at synaptic junctions was generally accepted.

However, since the discovery of a special type of electrically transmitting
synapse in crayfish (Furshpan and Potter, 1959), electrical transmission
has been described at several junctions. These include the giant motor
synapses of the crayfish (Furshpan and Potter, 1959), in which the synaptic
membrane is an efficient electrical rectifier, ensuring one-way transmission.
The septal junctions of the giant axons in the longitudinal nerve cord of
some forms of Annelidae and Crustaceae allow transmission in either
direction, as these low resistance membranes do not possess any rectifying
properties (Kao and Grundfest, 1957).

Both chemical and electrical transmission of excitation have been
demonstrated in the large calciform synapses in the ciliary ganglion of the
chick (Martin and Pilar, 1963a, b).

Electrotonic transmission of excitation between adjacent nerve cells has
been demonstrated in various species. These include the two giant cells in
the segmental ganglia of the leech (Hagiwara and Morita, 1962). An extensive study of electrotonic transmission between the spinal electromotor
neurones of Mormyrid electric fish has been reported by Bennett, Aljure,
Nakajima and Pappas (1963). In addition to the electrophysiological
evidence for electrical transmission, the authors noted that there was actual

fusion of the dendrites in their histological preparations and not the usual separation by a 200 Å cleft. At these presumed electrical transmitting areas there were none of the special features of chemically transmitting synapses, such as vesicles and mitochondria.

Washizu (1960) has presented another example of electrical transmission, that between motoneurones in the amphibian spinal cord. Recording intracellularly from an isolated toad spinal cord, he found that 20% of the motoneurones could be excited by stimulation of either of two adjacent ventral roots. The responses were not identical as there was always a latency difference of at least 0·6 msec between the two routes of excitation. As there was no prepotential associated with excitation from either ventral root, Washizu concluded that the later response was probably the result of ephaptic transmission through dendritic junctions between motoneurones. Although subsequent investigations have shown that the excitation is preceded by a graded depolarization (Kubota and Brookhart, 1962; Katz and Miledi, 1963; Grinnell, 1966), which led Kubota and Brookhart (1962) to attribute it to a synaptic excitatory action by motor-axon collateral onto motoneuronal dendrites, it seems that Washizu's original explanation is more probable (Grinnell, 1966).

An inhibitory synapse, which operates by electrical transmission, has been described in the Mauthner cells of fish (Furukawa and Furshpan, 1963). By a detailed study with intra- and extracellular recording from Mauthner cells it has been established that activation of the fine nerve fibres around the axon hillock region applies a hyperpolarizing current to the axon hillock, thus effecting an inhibition. It has been suggested that the intracellular hyperpolarization is a passive result of the generation of an external hyperpolarizing potential around the axon hillock. This extracellular potential has been attributed to the failure of the impulse to invade the terminal portions of axons which surround the axon hillock. These terminals become sources for extracellular current flow to the more proximal, excited, zones of these fibres.

C. IDENTIFICATION OF CHEMICALLY AND ELECTRICALLY TRANSMITTING SYNAPSES

A distinction between chemically and electrically transmitting synapses can be based on their morphological, physiological and pharmacological properties. Ideally, intracellular electrodes must be inserted into both pre-

and postsynaptic elements, as has been possible with the crayfish giant synapse (Furshpan and Potter, 1959) and chick ciliary ganglion (Martin and Pilar, 1963a, b). Where the presynaptic element is very small in relation to the postsynaptic structure, as at neuromuscular junctions, chemical transmission is obligatory. At amphibian neuromuscular junctions, the maximum current that could be provided by the presynaptic element would fail by a factor of hundreds to produce the transfer of charge of $2–4 \times 10^{-9}$ coulombs that Fatt and Katz (1951) calculate to occur across the uncurarized endplate membrane.

However at many junctions where it is technically not feasible to insert a microelectrode into the presynaptic element, it may be difficult to distinguish between the two types of transmission. In a recent paper, Rall, Burke, Smith, Nelson and Frank (1967) discuss the evidence for the generation of monosynaptic excitatory postsynaptic potentials in motoneurones by dorsal root afferents presented in a preceding series of papers (Smith, Wuerker and Frank, 1967; Nelson and Frank, 1967; Burke, 1967; Rall, 1967). They conclude that for distal dendritic input locations, the various types of synaptic mechanism are virtually indistinguishable, and that for somatic and proximal dendritic input locations, mechanisms involving either electrical transmission (through a low resistance electric coupling between the afferent fibres and the motoneurone) or chemical transmission would be consistent with their evidence.

The criteria for distinguishing chemical and electrical transmission have previously been reviewed by Eccles (1964) and will be discussed only to a limited extent in the present account.

1. *Chemical Synapses*

In the classical type of chemically transmitting synapse, the arrival of an impulse at the presynaptic terminal evokes a release of a chemical mediator which, after diffusion across the synaptic cleft, attaches to receptors on the postsynaptic membrane. At excitatory junctions, the transmitter increases the permeability of the postsynaptic membrane to sodium and potassium ions (Takeuchi and Takeuchi, 1960a), thereby causing a depolarization or excitatory junctional potential. At inhibitory synapses, the transmitter increases the permeability of the postsynaptic membrane to chloride and/or potassium ions, stabilizing and frequently hyperpolarizing the postsynaptic membrane. Hyperpolarizing potentials are designated as inhibitory junctional potentials.

The possibility of a different mechanism for the generation of inhibitory junctional potentials has recently been postulated by Koketsu and Nishi (1967) and Nishi and Koketsu (1967). Their evidence suggests that the slow inhibitory postsynaptic potential in bullfrog sympathetic ganglion cells is due to a sodium pump which removes sodium from the interior of the cell, causing a hyperpolarization. As the sodium pump may be activated by catecholamines, this system can be included as a chemically transmitting synapse. The criteria discussed below are applicable to identification of chemical synapses of the first type only.

Properties of Chemical Synapses

Morphological criteria for chemically transmitting synapses may include the presence of accumulations or aggregations of synaptic vesicles in the presynaptic element and the characteristically dense areas of membrane on either side of the synaptic cleft. Intracellular recording would be expected to reveal the occurrence of miniature postsynaptic potentials and the quantal nature of postsynaptic potentials. These have been demonstrable only at some synapses. Generation of the postsynaptic potential will occur after a variable synaptic delay and will not therefore be concurrent with the presynaptic spike potential. At some junctions, the transmitter may have a prolonged duration of action, possibly lasting for several minutes.

Alterations in the membrane potential of the postsynaptic cell will either increase or decrease the amplitude of chemically evoked post-synaptic potentials. Reversal of inhibitory junctional potentials by hyperpolarization and of excitatory junctional potentials by intense depolarization may be demonstrable. Liberation of the transmitter from activated presynaptic terminals may be demonstrable. Potentiation or antagonism of the postsynaptic actions of the transmitter by specific potentiators or antagonists will also aid in the identification of the transmitter.

2. *Properties of Electrical Synapses*

Electron micrographs reveal that the pre- and postsynaptic membranes are fused with no visible synaptic cleft. The synaptic delay is negligible for electrical synapses, postsynaptic potentials arising concurrently with the presynaptic spike potential. Electrical coupling between pre- and post-synaptic structures is necessarily large. An increase in the amplitude of depolarizing postsynaptic potentials during hyperpolarization of the postsynaptic membrane and a decrease during depolarization may occur on account of the rectifying properties of the synaptic membrane.

D. CRITERIA FOR IDENTIFICATION OF CHEMICAL TRANSMITTERS

In the subsequent chapters of this book, the pharmacology of various structures will be discussed, and the question of whether various drugs can be considered as transmitters at a particular synapse will frequently arise. A series of criteria have been developed from the classical studies on the peripheral nervous system which established acetylcholine as a transmitter at neuromuscular and ganglionic synapses. The criteria which must be satisfied by any drug which is postulated as a synaptic transmitter are listed below.

1. The substance must be present in those neurones from which it is released.
2. The neurone must possess the necessary enzymic mechanisms for the manufacture of the transmitter and for its release.
3. The presence of the various precursors and intermediaries in the synthetic pathway should be demonstrable.
4. There may be systems for the inactivation of the transmitter. These could include an enzyme system for the inactivation of the transmitter and a specific uptake mechanism for the reabsorption of transmitter into the pre- or postsynaptic structures.
5. During stimulation, the substance may be detectable in extracellular fluid collected from the region of the activated synapses.
6. When applied to the postsynaptic structure, the substance should mimic the action of the synaptically released transmitter.
7. Pharmacological agents which interact with the synaptically released transmitter should interact with the suspected transmitter in an identical manner.

This list of criteria may be useful in the assessment of the likelihood of any substance being a transmitter at a particular synaptic junction. The significance of each of these criteria has recently been discussed by Werman (1966), who stresses that criteria (6) and (7) are of fundamental importance. The actual employment of these criteria at specific synaptic junctions will be encountered during the subsequent chapters and for this reason the criteria will not be commented on at this stage.

The dendrites and somas of neurones in the central nervous system are densely covered with synapses and the axons receive synaptic contacts as well. It is more than likely that neurones in the central nervous system, and to a lesser extent those in ganglia, have several transmitters acting on their surfaces. For example, experiments have shown that at least three transmitters act on the Renshaw cell: two excitatory transmitters (one cholinergic and one non-cholinergic, Curtis, Phillis and Watkins, 1961) and an inhibitory transmitter (Biscoe and Curtis, 1966). Other experiments have shown that neurones in the cerebral cortex receive both cholinergic and non-cholinergic inhibitory inputs (Phillis and York, 1967a, 1968a, b). A further complication is provided by the evidence, described in Chapters 7, 8 and 10, that transmitters may have more than one action on the same cell. The increased complexity of pharmacological studies in the presence of multiple transmitters will be appreciated.

CONCLUSIONS

1. Evidence for both chemical and electrical transmission across synapses has been reviewed. Although the bulk of evidence supports the chemical transmission hypothesis, there is currently an increasing interest in the possibility that electrically transmitting junctions are present in the mammalian central nervous system.

2. The properties of the electrical and chemical types of junction are discussed.

3. A set of seven criteria for the identification of neurotransmitters is presented on page 6.

CHAPTER 2

THE METABOLISM
OF ACETYLCHOLINE

THE acetylcholine of vertebrate tissues is synthesized by a specific enzyme, choline acetyltransferase (Nachmansohn and Machado, 1943), present in cholinergic neurones and capable of transferring acetyl groups from coenzyme A (CoA) to choline (Feldberg and Mann, 1946; Lipmann and Kaplan; 1946; Nachmansohn and Berman, 1946). The presence of choline acetyltransferase in some non-neural and even non-conducting tissues, such as the placenta or corneal epithelium (Kato, 1960; Williams and Cooper, 1965), presents an interesting problem. The acetylcholine system in these tissues may have some role in the control of ion or water movements across cell membranes related to the function of such cells. In theory, acetylcholine can also be formed by a reversed action of acetylcholinesterase, the enzyme whose normal role is the hydrolytic destruction of acetylcholine, and whose cellular distribution is in many respects similar to that of choline acetyltransferase. The conditions which would favour such a reversal of the reaction probably never occur *in vivo*. Synthesis of acetylcholine requires the presence of various factors including choline, coenzyme A and active acetate. The chemical energy required for the acetylation of coenzyme A is usually supplied in the form of adenosine triphosphate.

A. ACETYLCHOLINE AND CHOLINE ACETYLTRANSFERASE IN THE NERVOUS SYSTEM

1. *Distribution*

The distribution of acetylcholine and choline acetyltransferase has been studied in detail in the mammalian nervous system. From the analysis of peripheral nerve trunks, two groups of neurones emerge: those which contain acetylcholine and choline acetyltransferase in relatively high concentrations and those which contain little or no ester or enzyme.

The ability to form and store acetylcholine in the peripheral nervous system appears to be confined to the cholinergic motor nerves innervating skeletal muscles, all autonomic preganglionic trunks and parasympathetic postganglionic fibres (Hebb, 1963). The evidence that postganglionic adrenergic nerves do not contain acetylcholine or the synthesizing enzyme has been derived mainly from experiments in which the superior cervical ganglion and the proximal part of its postganglionic fibres have been analysed after chronic preganglionic denervation (Hebb, 1963).

The normally high content of acetylcholine and choline acetyltransferase in autonomic ganglia is drastically reduced by preganglionic denervation, revealing that most of the enzyme is located presynaptically (Buckley, Consolo, Giacobini and Sjoqvist, 1967). Analyses conducted on isolated cells of the 7th lumbar ganglion of the cat have demonstrated that choline acetyltransferase is present in only about 13% of the cell bodies (Buckley *et al.*, 1967). These are probably the cells of origin of the cholinergic sweat secretory and vasodilator fibres which arise in this ganglion.

The evidence that little acetylcholine or choline acetyltransferase is present in peripheral sensory nerves is derived from analyses of nerves that are predominantly sensory in function (MacIntosh, 1941) and dorsal spinal roots (MacIntosh, 1941; Hebb and Silver, 1956; Cohen, 1956). The small amounts of choline acetyltransferase that are present in the dorsal roots of various animals suggest that there may be a limited number of cholinergic afferent fibres in peripheral nerves.

In the central nervous system, the levels of acetylcholine and choline acetyltransferase fluctuate extensively from one area to another (Table 1). In some parts of the brain, notably the caudate nucleus and olfactory trigone, the enzyme concentration may be higher than in most peripheral nerves and ganglia, whereas in other areas, such as the cerebellar cortex, the levels of acetylcholine and choline acetyltransferase are very low.

Feldberg and Vogt (1948) have proposed the interesting concept that cholinergic nerve cells may alternate with non-cholinergic neurones, somewhat as they do in sympathetic pathways. In support of this idea, they cited evidence showing that in two sensory pathways, auditory and visual, the second and fourth order neurones may be cholinergic (as indicated by their ability to synthesize acetylcholine), while the first and third order neurones are not. Unfortunately this elegantly single hypothesis has not been

TABLE 1.

ACETYLCHOLINE AND CHOLINE ACETYLTRANSFERASE IN SOME PERIPHERAL AND CENTRAL NERVOUS TISSUES

Tissue	Acetylcholine content[a]		Choline acetyltransferase[b]	
	μg/g fresh tissue	species	μg acetylcholine formed/g fresh tissue/hr	species
Ventral spinal roots	9–18	dog, cat	2500, 4000, 5000	goat, rabbit dog
Dorsal spinal roots	0–0·25	dog, cat	0–6	cat, dog
Sciatic nerve	4–6	cat	300–680, 1120	goat, rabbit
Superior cervical ganglion	18–44	cat	1600–2000	sheep
Spinal cord, ventral horn	1·5	dog	500	goat
Spinal cord, dorsal horn	2·5	dog	—	
Medulla	1–2·7	cat	—	
Pons	1·4–5·0	cat	—	
Cerebellar cortex	0·1–0·3	cat	50	cat
Superior colliculus	4·5	cat	400	cat
Lateral geniculate nucleus	3·3	cat	520	dog
Hippocampus	—		520	dog
Hypothalamus	1·6–2·1	cat	50,400	cat, dog
Thalamus	2–4	cat	340	cat
Basal ganglia	7	cat	1400–2200	cat
Cerebral cortex	2·2–4·5	cat	175–270	cat
Olfactory bulb	1·3	cat	440	cat

[a] Values for acetylcholine content are from MacIntosh (1941), Feldberg (1945) and Deffenu, Bertaccini and Pepeu (1967).

[b] Values are from Hebb and Silver (1956) and Hebb (1963). Where necessary, values for choline acetyltransferase for fresh tissue have been calculated on the assumption that 1 g acetone powder is equivalent to 5 g fresh tissue.

substantiated by later pharmacological analyses and does not appear to have a tenable basis.

It has been suggested by some workers that much of the acetylcholine-like activity of brain extracts is due to other substances (Holz and Schumann, 1954; Hosein, Proulx and Ara, 1962; Hosein and Orzeck, 1964). However, the application of a variety of pharmacological and chromatographic techniques to brain extracts from a number of different species has failed to provide any evidence for the presence of other compounds resembling acetylcholine (Whittaker, 1963). Similar conclusions have been reached by McLennan, Curry and Walker (1963), Pepeu, Schmidt and Giarman, (1963) and Ryall (1963). The compounds observed by Holtz and Schumann (1954) and by Hosein and his colleagues have not been adequately characterized chemically and may be either paper-chromatographic artifacts or autolysis products (Whittaker, 1965).

2. *Synthesis and Storage of Acetylcholine*

The investigations of Birks and MacIntosh (1957, 1961) have given a comprehensive picture of the cellular mechanisms involved in the manufacture and release of acetylcholine in ganglia. Essentially their technique involved accurate measurements of the acetylcholine content and output of the superior cervical ganglion. Perfused ganglia were studied under resting conditions or during prolonged activation by maximal preganglionic volleys over a wide range of frequencies. An analysis of the metabolic pathways was made possible by the use of hemicholinium-3 (HC-3) which has been shown to inhibit acetylcholine synthesis (MacIntosh, Birks and Sastry, 1956; MacIntosh, 1961) and by the suppression of acetylcholinesterase activity with anticholinesterases, such as eserine and tetraethylpyrophosphate.

The synthesis of acetylcholine is dependent on a continuing supply of choline and of glucose. When this is ensured, it has been shown by direct estimation that acetylcholine synthesis in the superior cervical ganglion, can be depressed to a negligible level by HC-3 (Birks and MacIntosh, 1957, 1961). As would be expected, there is then a profound depression of the release of acetylcholine during prolonged periods of stimulation and an associated block of transmission through the ganglion. The block is not due to a curarizing action of HC-3 as it only develops during prolonged stimulation, and a period of rest restores transmission, as also does an intravenous injection of choline (Birks and MacIntosh, 1961). The concepts developed by Birks and MacIntosh are summarized in the hypothetical model presented in Fig. 2.1. It is postulated that the acetylcholine of the cat superior cervical ganglion is contained in three main compartments. There

is, firstly, about 40 mμg of acetylcholine in a compartment where it cannot
be depleted by prolonged stimulation of the presynaptic fibres to a ganglion
in which synthesis of acetylcholine has been blocked by HC-3, and where
it is inaccessible to the acetylcholinesterase of the ganglion. This so-called
"stationary acetylcholine" is for the most part located in the extrasynaptic
portions of the preganglionic axons within the ganglion.

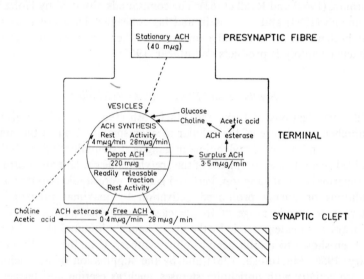

FIG. 2.1. Schematic representation of the metabolism of acetylcholine in
presynaptic terminals of the cat superior cervical ganglion. Based on description of Birks and MacIntosh (1961). Full description in text.

In a ganglion whose cholinesterase remains active, the whole of the
acetylcholine not included in the stationary fraction is available for release
by nerve impulses, as is shown by its disappearance from active ganglia in
which synthesis has been prevented by HC-3. This fraction has been called
"depot acetylcholine" and must be located in the presynaptic terminals
since the preganglionic axons are not depleted of their acetylcholine by
stimulation in the presence of HC-3. In an average ganglion, the depot
acetylcholine amounts to 220 mμg or about 85% of the extractable total.
Depot acetylcholine is composed of two subfractions, one of which is
smaller and more readily liberated than the other. Birks and MacIntosh
suggest that acetylcholine from the larger, more stable, subfraction may

have to pass into the smaller before it can be discharged. Since depot acetylcholine is present in terminals which have not been treated with cholinesterase inhibitors, it has been assumed that it is on some way protected from acetylcholinesterase, possibly by inclusion in synaptic vesicles.

A third store of intracellular acetylcholine has been described in ganglia whose cholinesterase has been inactivated. This has been called "surplus acetylcholine" and although it is formed rather slowly, it may rise to a level above that of depot acetylcholine. Since it quickly disappears when cholinesterase is reactivated, it must be located in a compartment where it would have been destroyed in the presence of the active enzyme. Surplus acetylcholine cannot make an important contribution to the acetylcholine release during stimulation since the volley output from an eserinized ganglion remains constant whilst surplus acetylcholine is accumulating. It also provides an explanation for the paradox that during activation of a ganglion perfused with eserinized Ringer Locke, there is a progressive decline in the release of acetylcholine despite a well-maintained content of acetylcholine in the ganglion (Brown and Feldberg, 1936; Kahlson and MacIntosh, 1939).

The idea that presynaptic acetylcholine is released from a particulate store has also been reached by neurophysiological investigators studying the mechanics of synaptic transmission. The small fluctuations in membrane potential recorded at the neuromuscular junction by Katz and his colleagues (Fatt and Katz, 1952; del Castillo and Katz, 1956) were attributed to a spontaneous release of "packets" or "quanta" of acetylcholine. At about the same time, electron microscopists were discovering that the neuromuscular junction and other, presumably chemical, transmitting synapses were characterized by small spherical bodies, the so-called synaptic vesicles (De Robertis and Bennett; 1955, Robertson, 1956), adjacent to the synaptic cleft on the presynaptic side. Quantal release became equated with vesicle packaging (De Robertis and Bennett, 1955; del Castillo and Katz, 1955b, 1956; Palay, 1956) although the evidence to support this assumption was meagre. At the neuromuscular junction, the results of experiments on degeneration and regeneration of nerve terminals are in accord with the hypothesis, since spontaneous release of quanta ceases and vesicles disappear at about the same time (Reger, 1957; Birks, Katz and Miledi, 1960). Attempts to produce an experimental alteration in vesicle numbers at the neuromuscular junction, in conjunction with an alteration in quantal release, though originally unsuccessful (Birks,

Huxley and Katz, 1960), have recently yielded promising results (Hubbard and Kwanbunbumpen, 1968). The latter authors were able to demonstrate that nerve stimulation and hemicholinium caused a significant fall in vesicle volume and numbers.

At other junctional sites, it has been possible to isolate vesicles, some of which have been found to contain and to take up acetylcholine (De Robertis, 1964; Whittaker, 1965; Marchbanks, 1968). Alterations in vesicle numbers accompanying various experimental procedures of physiological interest have also been claimed. Thus De Robertis and his colleagues found changes in vesicle numbers after dark adaptation in rabbit retina (De Robertis and Franchi, 1956) and striking alterations in vesicle numbers at adrenal medullary synapses after splanchnic nerve stimulation (De Robertis and Ferreira, 1957).

As mentioned above, it has been possible to isolate presynaptic nerve terminals or "synaptosomes" and synaptic vesicles by the use of the technique of subcellular fractionation of brain samples. This technique has been described in detail elsewhere (De Robertis, 1964; Whittaker, 1965) and is now widely employed as a method for studying the distribution of various substances in biological tissues. Hebb and Smallman (1956) were originally able to demonstrate that 70–90 % of the choline acetyltransferase and acetylcholine in homogenised brain tissue is attached to the particulate, cell structure, fraction, with the balance in the soluble cytoplasmic component. When the particulate fraction is analysed by centrifugation over a density gradient column of sucrose solutions, the bulk of the acetylcholine and choline acetyltransferase is found in the "synaptosome" or nerve terminal fraction. Electron microscopy has revealed that this fraction contains broken-off nerve terminals consisting of clusters of vesicles with cytoplasm and occasional mitochondria, surrounded by a thin external membrane, to which segments of the thickened postsynaptic membrane frequently remain attached (Gray and Whittaker, 1962). Whittaker has suggested that the homogenization process does not rupture the nerve endings, but merely shears them away from their axons and postsynaptic attachments. The external membrane of the nerve ending seals up at the site of the break, and the entire ending then behaves as a subcellular particle with sedimentation properties broadly similar to those of mitochondria.

Suspension of "synaptosomes" in a hypotonic medium has the effect of causing them to swell and burst, releasing a proportion of the synaptic vesicles and mitochondria. Density gradient fractionation of the disrupted material enables the partially damaged synaptosomes, the released mitochondria and vesicles, and the stable cytoplasmic components to be separated out in different fractions (Whittaker, Michaelson and Kirkland, 1964; Whittaker and Sheridan, 1965). Acetylcholine can be recovered partly in the fraction of partially disrupted synaptosomes and partly in the fraction of isolated vesicles. Vesicular acetylcholine can be released by incubation, acid or ultrasonic treatment.

Choline acetyltransferase is localized mainly in the synaptosome fraction of guinea-pig brain, from which it can readily be released by hypo-osmotic treatment (Whittaker et al., 1964). It then behaves like a soluble cytoplasmic component, reflecting the small molecular weight of the enzyme (67,000 for rabbit brain enzyme; Bull, Feinstein and Morris, 1964). Whittaker and his colleagues interpret this difference in the distribution of acetylcholine and choline acetyltransferase after hypo-osmotic treatment as an indication that the synaptic vesicles are not complete storage factories for the manufacture of acetylcholine, but storage granules, which take up acetylcholine from the nerve ending cytoplasm. These opinions are in contrast to the views of De Robertis (McCaman, Arnaiz and De Robertis, 1965; De Robertis et al., 1963), who consider that synaptic vesicles from rat brain contain choline acetyltransferase as well as acetylcholine.

Tuček (1966) has recently demonstrated that hypo-osmotic shock fails to release the choline acetyltransferase of several mammalian species, other than the guinea-pig. Moreover, the enzyme remains bound to the particulate structural components of the nerve endings under conditions where most of their acetylcholine is released, suggesting that the choline acetyltransferase is not localized within the synaptic vesicles with acetylcholine.

Differential centrifugation of ventral spinal roots or sciatic nerve homogenates has provided evidence that their choline acetyltransferase activity is associated with the microsomal or small granule fraction (Hebb, 1963). Axonic acetylcholine, on the other hand, appears to be in a "free" form and its distribution is not restricted to the microsomal or small granule fraction (Carlini and Green, 1963a; Hebb, 1963). There is evidence that choline acetyltransferase is distributed throughout the length of cholinergic neurones and is conveyed from the cell soma by axonal flow (Hebb and Silver, 1963). It is possible that acetylcholine is formed continuously by the enzyme and is normally destroyed by cholinesterase, which is also believed to be distributed throughout the neurone (Koenig and Koelle, 1961; Clouet and Waelsch, 1961). The synaptic vesicles may constitute a device to raise the steady state concentration of acetylcholine in the nerve terminals by protecting it from hydrolysis by cholinesterase.

Comparisons of the subcellular distribution of acetylcholine in the caudate nucleus and spinal cord provide an interesting illustration of the packaging of acetylcholine in nerve terminals. In the caudate nucleus, where cholinergic neurones are largely represented by their terminals, inclusion of the cholinesterase inhibitor in the initial suspension medium increases the total acetylcholine content by no more than 10% and very little free acetylcholine is recovered in the supernatant (Laverty, Michaelson, Sharman and Whittaker, 1963). By contrast, in the spinal cord, where the motoneurone somata probably constitute a major source of acetylcholine, the presence of eserine has a marked effect, about 90% of the acetylcholine in eserinized homogenates being in a "free" form in the supernatant.

3. Axonic Acetylcholine and Choline Acetyltransferase

Two explanations have been suggested to account for the presence of acetylcholine and choline acetyltransferase in nerve cell axons. The first explanation, that acetylcholine has a function in the conduction of nerve impulses (Nachmansohn, 1959), has not been generally accepted by neurophysiologists. There is as yet no critical evidence to substantiate this theory, and the apparent absence of acetylcholine and choline acetyltransferase in many nerves makes it unlikely that conduction is dependent on a cholinergic mechanism.

A second explanation is based on the theory of axoplasmic flow described by Weiss and Hiscoe (1948). In his first experiments, Weiss (1947) showed that ligation of nerves causes them to swell up on the side proximal to the ligature, whilst distally the diameter of the fibres is reduced. Upon release of the ligature, the dammed-up material advances distally at about 1 mm or more per day. From these and subsequent experiments, it was concluded that the growth of a nerve fibre depends on the production of new axoplasm by the perikaryon, which then migrates into the axon. The cell body, then, acts as a source of supply for the axon and its terminals.

In 1948, Feldberg and Vogt suggested that the presence of choline acetyltransferase in the axon could be accounted for in terms of this hypothesis by assuming that it is in transit between the cell body, where it is manufactured, and the nerve ending where it has its function. Subsequently, Hebb and Waites (1956) verified this idea experimentally when they showed that ligation or section of cervical sympathetic nerves causes choline acetyltransferase to accumulate on the proximal side and to decrease on the distal side of the ligature or section. On the distal side, almost all of the enzyme disappears in 3 to 4 weeks and its presence therefore, appears to be dependent on continuity of the axon with the cell body.

This evidence implicates the cell body as a major site of choline acetyltransferase synthesis within the neuron. Hebb (1963) has suggested that the enzyme is attached to some part of the axon structure, such as the endoplasmic reticulum, and is kept in transit by the growth of this structure. It may be surmised that as it reaches the nerve terminals, the enzyme-carrying membrane breaks up or is budded off to form vesicles.

4. *Release of Acetylcholine*

It seems likely that the quantum hypothesis of transmitter release originally proposed by del Castillo and Katz (1954a) for transmission at the neuromuscular junction of the frog is applicable to chemical transmission at all synapses. The theory, which has recently been reviewed in detail (Martin, 1966; Martin and Veale, 1967), assumes that there are a large number of "quanta" or packages of transmitter stored in the nerve terminal, each with a finite probability of release following a nerve stimulus. The hypothesis implies that the number of quanta released by a series of nerve impulses will fluctuate in a predictable way, the quantum contents being distributed according to the binomial distribution, or if the probability is small enough, by the Poisson distribution. This prediction has been confirmed at several nerve–muscle synaptic junctions.

In addition to being released by stimulation, individual quanta are released from the terminal spontaneously, producing "miniature end-plate potentials". At the neuromuscular junction, the number of quanta available for immediate release is probably of the order of 1000 and the total number of quanta available for release in the absence of synthesis may be of the order of 500,000 (Thies, 1965; Elmqvist and Quastel, 1965). The fraction available for immediate release at the neuromuscular synapse therefore seems to be much less than 1% of the total population. In the mammalian ganglion, however, this figure appears to be closer to 20%

(Birks and MacIntosh, 1961). A probability of release for quanta in frog muscle of the order of $0 \cdot 1$ and in mammalian muscle of $0 \cdot 3$ can be deduced from estimates that 100 and 300 quanta per nerve impulse are released at the amphibian and mammalian neuromuscular junctions respectively (Martin, 1955; Boyd and Martin, 1956; Liley, 1956).

The exact nature of the coupling between the nerve terminal action potential and the release of transmitter has remained obscure. The coupling depends on the level of calcium in the bathing fluid and magnesium blocks transmitter release, presumably by competing with calcium. The importance of sodium ions has been stressed by Birks and Cohen (1965), who found that a reduction of calcium, in sodium depleted solutions, resulted in a marked increase in the quantum content of endplate potentials. It was also shown that agents which inhibit the sodium pump, and thereby presumably increase the internal sodium concentration, also produce an increase in the release of acetylcholine. The authors have explained these findings by postulating that sodium and calcium interact and compete for sites on the inner surface of the membrane.

5. *Uptake of Acetylcholine*

In contrast to the studies on uptake mechanisms for noradrenaline in sympathetic nerves, relatively little interest has been devoted to a study of the mechanisms of inactivation of acetylcholine, other than its hydrolysis by cholinesterase. The ability of brain tissue to accumulate exogenous acetylcholine has been studied by a number of investigators with varying results. In minced brain tissue and cortical slices, Mann, Tennenbaum and Quastel (1938) and Elliott and Henderson (1951) found only a small uptake of acetylcholine in the presence of eserine. On the other hand, Polak and Meeuws (1966) demonstrated that when Soman (pinacolyl methylphosphonofluoridate) was used for the prevention of acetylcholine hydrolysis, acetylcholine was taken up against a concentration gradient. When eserine was substituted for Soman, the uptake of acetylcholine was strongly inhibited.

The effects of various substances which interfere with cholinergic transmission on the uptake of acetylcholine in cortex slices of the mouse brain have recently been described by Schuberth and Sundwall (1967). The uptake was shown to be an active process in that it occurred against a concentration gradient, required oxygen and was inhibited by dinitrophenol.

The acetylcholine precursor, choline, is also taken up by brain cortex slices by an active process. Comparisons showed that the maximal rate of uptake of acetylcholine was some 40% slower than that of choline. The transport of choline and acetylcholine also differed with respect to their susceptibility towards certain drugs. Thus hemicholinium-3 was about ten times stronger as an inhibitor of acetylcholine transport than of choline transport. Choline transport was unaffected by eserine, atropine, oxo-tremorine and morphine, which, in concentrations of 2×10^{-5}M, depressed acetylcholine uptake. By contrast, sodium pentobarbitone, pentamethylene tetrazole and adrenaline were without effect on acetylcholine transport in concentrations of 10^{-4}M.

It is tempting to speculate that drugs which inhibit acetylcholine transport *in vitro* in low concentrations, might have similar effects *in vivo*, this being related to their pharmacological actions. Atropine has been shown to cause a fall in brain acetylcholine (Giarman and Pepeu, 1964) and an increase in the rate of release of acetylcholine from the cerebral cortical surface (Mitchell, 1963; Szerb, 1964; Phillis, 1968) which suggests that it may occupy receptor sites and prevent the reabsorption of released acetylcholine. Atropine also prevents the uptake of labelled carbachol of isolated brain slices (Creese and Taylor, 1965). Release of acetylcholine from the eserinized cerebral cortex (Phillis, 1968) may be similarly facilitated by a block of the uptake mechanisms. Studies on the effects of acetylcholine potentiators and antagonists on uptake mechanisms are still in their infancy, but a comparison with the analogous situation at adrenergic synapses suggests that this may be an important factor in their mode of action.

6. *The Acetylcholine Receptor Substance*

There have been many attempts to characterize the acetylcholine receptor; that macromolecular constituent of postsynaptic membranes with which acetylcholine reacts in such a specific manner. Some have identified the receptor substance with acetylcholinesterase, which Župančič (1953) called "receptive cholinesterase". Nachmansohn (1963), on the other hand, has dissociated the effect of the enzymes involved in the acetylcholine system from the "receptor substance". He described this receptor as a protein which changes its shape under the influence of acetylcholine, producing a change in ionic permeability. Ariëns and Simonis (1962) have also described the receptor as a protein.

The antagonism of acetylcholine by curare at the neuromuscular junction has been explained as a competitive interaction between these two substances, which are thought to combine with the same receptor. As the competition between acetylcholine and curare can be attributed to their chemical similarity, curare or curare-like compounds have been used to characterize the acetylcholine receptor, with which they form stable combinations.

The first attempts to isolate the acetylcholine receptor substance were made by Chagas *et al.* (1956) using extracts from the electric organ of the eel, *Electrophorus electricus*. They used a labelled synthetic curare-like compound, gallamine, to measure the affinity of a quaternary ammonium ion to the fractional extracts. Ehrenpreis (1960) also tried to isolate acetylcholine receptor protein from extracts of electric organ and measured the interaction of labelled *d*-tubocurarine with fractionated extracts. The receptor protein was isolated by precipitating it with curare, added to different fractions of the electric organ obtained by ammonium sulphate fractionation.

More recently, Ehrenpreis (1962) has described this protein as a drug-binding one, with non-specific properties for the binding of acetylcholine. This has been confirmed by Beychock (1965), who came to the conclusion that Ehrenpreis's acetylcholine receptor protein could not be regarded as the specific acetylcholine receptor.

A mucopolysaccharide analogue of hyaluronic acid which interacts preferentially with labelled curare and gallamine has been extracted from electric organ extracts (Hassón and Chagas, 1959; Hassón, 1962). However, the binding between this compound and gallamine or curare is readily reversible in comparison with that exhibited *in vivo* by the acetylcholine receptor and it is also, therefore, unlikely to be a specific receptor.

The sialoprotein extracted by Trams and Lauter (1964) from electric organ extracts and described by them as the receptor substance has proven to be an even weaker receptor than the mucopolysaccharide described above (Hassón-Voloch, 1968).

The tendency of the acidic groups of macromolecules to react non-specifically with the strongly basic ammonium ions of substances like curare and gallamine apparently accounts for the properties of the various compounds that have been extracted from electric organs. A new approach to the identification of the specific acetylcholine receptor may, consequently, have to be found.

B. CHOLINESTERASES

Interest in the nature and distribution of cholinesterases in the nervous system stems from the likelihood that they are involved in cholinergic synaptic transmission. The stability of cholinesterases and their amenability to demonstration by histochemical procedures has spurred the efforts of many investigators interested in cholinergic transmission.

Although the significance of cholinesterase at the skeletal neuromuscular junction is well established, the question of whether any reliance can be placed on the presence of cholinesterase at other synaptic junctions as an indicator of cholinergic transmission has yet to be resolved. It must be stressed that the current interest in cholinesterase distribution may fade when satisfactory histochemical techniques for the localization of acetylcholine or choline acetyltransferase are developed. A technique for revealing choline acetyltransferase may well be developed from the new fluorescent immunochemical methods within the near future.

1. *Various Types of Cholinesterase*

There is a good deal of controversy, particularly in the early literature, about the nomenclature for cholinesterases. Stedman, Stedman and Easson (1932) prepared an enzyme from horse serum, which they called *cholinesterase*. This enzyme was considered to be a specific esterase for acetylcholine and other choline esters. However, it splits butyrylcholine and proprionylcholine at a higher rate than acetylcholine. Nachmansohn and Rothenburg (1945) later demonstrated that the cholinesterase in erythrocytes, nerves and muscle tissue, in contrast to the serum esterase, has a high affinity for acetylcholine and acetyl-β-methylcholine, but splits butyrylcholine at a very low rate. Enzyme of this type was called *acetylcholinesterase* (Angustinsson and Nachmansohn, 1949).

The Enzyme Commission (1964) has recommended that the name *acetylcholinesterase* should be applied to erythrocyte and brain cholinesterases of the type previously designated as true, specific, aceto- or Type I cholinesterase. The commission further recommended that the name *cholinesterase* should be applied to serum and other cholinesterases that had been previously been known as pseudo, non-specific, unspecific, butyro- or Type II cholinesterase. However, to avoid confusion this enzyme will be referred to as pseudocholinesterase.

2. Acetylcholinesterase in Nervous Tissue

(a) Subcellular distribution

The subcellular distribution of brain enzyme was studied by Aldridge and Johnson (1959) and Toschi (1959). These workers agree that the enzyme is bound to membrane fragments, which are recovered mainly in the microsome fraction. In Whittaker's (1965) experiments the activity was not sharply localized in any one fraction, as considerable amounts of cholinesterase were recovered in the mitochondrial and synaptosomal fractions. The highest activity was again in the microsomal fraction.

By contrast, De Robertis (1964; De Robertis, Iraldi, Arnaiz and Salganicoff, 1962) claim that the enzyme is localized primarily in their "cholinergic fraction" of synaptosomes. On hypotonic rupture of the fraction, the greater part (72%) of the cholinesterase was recovered in the coarse particulate debris, but the remainder was found in a small particulate fraction, which was thought to consist of synaptic vesicles mixed with some postsynaptic membranes (De Robertis et al., 1963). Evidence has been presented (Whittaker et al., 1964), that the synaptic vesicle fraction of De Robertis et al. is contaminated with partially disrupted synaptosomes and membrane fragments, and that these are the source of the enzyme in this fraction.

(b) Histochemical and biochemical studies

The publication, by Koelle and Friedenwald (1949), of a histochemical technique for the localization of cholinesterase has stimulated an enormous volume of literature on this subject. The original technique has since undergone various modifications, including adaptation to electron microscopy and it would be impossible to describe the many results that have been obtained in a limited section of this book. For this reason the following discussion will be restricted to cholinesterase at the skeletal neuromuscular junction, in autonomic ganglia and in certain areas of the central nervous system. A comprehensive account of acetylcholinesterase distribution at the light microscope level has been prepared by Koelle (1963).

In the original histochemical techniques for cholinesterases (Gomori, 1948), the substrates, long chain fatty acid esters of choline, were insufficiently specific to distinguish between cholinesterase and non-specific esterase activity. The thiocholine technique developed by Koelle and

Friedenwald (1949) employs acetylthiocholine and butyrylthiocholine as substrates. Acetylthiocholine is hydrolysed by both acetylcholinesterase and pseudocholinesterase, whereas butyrylthiocholine is split predominantly, though not exclusively, by pseudocholinesterase. The use of selective inhibitors for acetyl- or pseudocholinesterase enables a clear distinction to be made concerning the nature of the enzyme under investigation. Non-specific esterases can be distinguished from cholinesterases by their greater resistance to inhibition by anticholinesterases such as eserine or diisopropylphosphofluoridate (DFP).

(i) *Skeletal neuromuscular junction.* This synapse has been intensively studied with respect to both the localization of acetylcholinesterase and the pharmacological actions of the anticholinesterases. Prior to the development of histochemical and ultramicroanalytical techniques for acetylcholinesterase, Marnay and Nachmansohn (1938) obtained indirect evidence that the acetylcholinesterase of skeletal muscle was concentrated in the areas of termination of the motor nerves. This has been confirmed by later, more direct, approaches. Selective localization of acetylcholinesterase at the endplate region has been unequivocally demonstrated by the ultramicroanalytical determinations of Giacobini and Holmstedt (1960). The activity per unit volume of single endplates, isolated by microdissection, was found to be at least fifty times as high as samples taken from other regions of the muscle.

The most precise histochemical results with the light microscope are those of Couteaux (1958) who has published an account of his own findings and those of many other investigators (including Koelle, 1950; Couteaux and Taxi, 1952; Coers, 1953; Gerebtzoff, Philippot and Dallemagne, 1954) in relationship to the detailed structure of the motor endplate revealed by electron microscopy.

The highest concentration of acetylcholinesterase, which accounts for most of the cholinesterase at neuromuscular junctions (Denz, 1953), appears to be localized postsynaptically at the surface and infoldings of the subneural apparatus (Fig. 2.2). The axonal terminals contain relatively little enzyme.

Most of the conclusions drawn from histochemical studies at the level of the light microscope have received confirmation in the subsequent electron microscope investigations. Lehrer and Ornstein (1959) used the α-naphthylacetate hexazotinized pararosaniline technique on mouse intercostal muscle. Deposits of the reaction product were present within the cleft between the axoplasmic and sarcoplasmic membranes and between the axoplasmic membrane and its supporting cells.

Barrnett (1962) employing a modification of the thiolacetic acid technique (Crevier and Bélanger, 1955) adapted for electron microscopy, observed the reaction product at four sites, including the plasma membrane of the muscle covering the junctional folds, in the primary and secondary synaptic clefts, the prejunctional axoplasmic membrane and in vesicular structures in the presynaptic nerve terminals. Basically similar results were obtained by Davis and Koelle (1967) using gold thiocholine and thiolacetic acid methods (Fig. 2.3).

The reported effects of sectioning the motor nerve on the acetylcholinesterase of motor endplates have been extremely variable. In the earlier literature, reviewed by Brooks and Myers (1952), the acetylcholinesterase of skeletal muscle was reported to fall, remain unchanged or rise in various investigations. Brooks and Meyers (1952) reported no change in the acetylcholinesterase of the guinea pig serratus anterior muscle five weeks after section of the motor nerve. Brzin and Zajicek (1958), using a technique of ultramicro-analysis of single endplates of mouse gastrocnemius, found that a high proportion of acetylcholinesterase was present 75 days after section of the sciatic nerve.

Histochemical investigations have tended to confirm that at least some acetylcholinesterase persists at the myoneural junction, after denervation (Sawyer, Davenport and Alexander, 1950; Coers, 1955; Savay and Csillik, 1956; Schwarzacher, 1957) although Snell and McIntyre (1956) reported a complete disappearance of acetylcholinesterase from the endplates of guinea-pig gastrocnemius muscles 45 days after denervation.

Quantitative changes in cholinesterase activity of denervated muscle fibres and sole plates have been evaluated in the sternomastoid muscle with an ultramicro-analytical technique (Guth, Albers and Brown 1964). Following denervation, the endplate and non-endplate activity in this muscle decreased rapidly, reaching approximately 50% of normal within 1 week. A very small additional loss in activity occurred during the subsequent 7 weeks. The total protein content of the muscle declined more slowly, reaching 50% of normal after 3 weeks. By contrast, after tenotomy, there was a more marked decrease in the total protein content than of the cholinesterase activity, suggesting that the neural influence on cholinesterase is fairly specific. During reinnervation, endplate and non-endplate cholinesterase reappeared at a comparable rate (Guth and Brown, 1965).

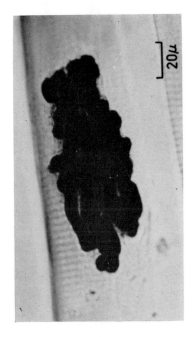

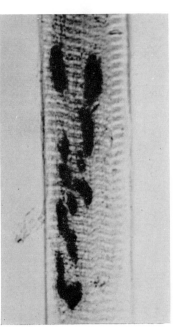

FIG. 2.2 Examples of acetylcholinesterase stained "en grappe" (left) and "en plaque" (right) neuromuscular junctions on single muscle fibres of the scalenus muscle of the lizard, *Tiliqua nigrolutea*. Acetylthiocholine incubation medium. The magnification is the same for both micrographs. (U. Proske, unpublished observations).

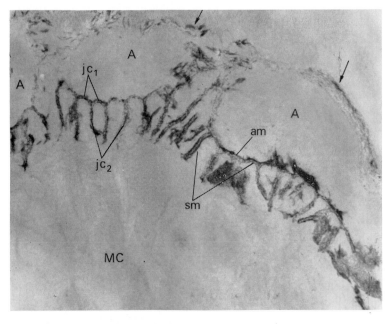

Fig. 2.3. Electron micrograph showing sections of motor endplate of mouse intercostal muscle stained for acetylcholinesterase by gold-thiocholine method, followed by brief fixation in osmium tetroxide. Three portions of the axonal terminal (A) make junctional contact with the muscle cell (MC). Enzymatic reaction product is present principally at the prejunctional axonal membrane (am) and postjunctional sarcoplasmic membrane (sm) of the muscle cell. Moderate amounts of deposit are also in the primary (jc_1) and secondary (jc_2) junctional clefts. Deposit at the external surface (arrows) of the axonal terminal is less well localized, but probably represents axon-to-Schwann cell-to-Schwann cell apposition × 31,000. (Davis and Koelle, 1967).

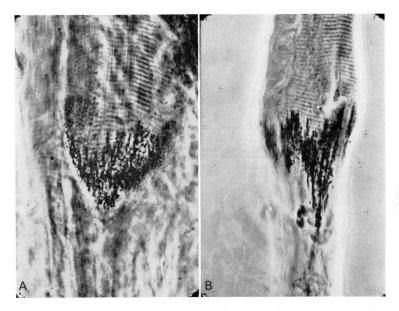

Fig. 2.4. A. Whole mount of the myo-tendinous junction of a single muscle fibre, M. opponens digiti minimi, man, stained for acetylcholinesterase by incubation en bloc, isolation of the single muscle fibre with its myotendinous junction under the dissecting microscope. Phase contrast: magnification × 720. B. Isolated muscle fibre end, M. soleus, rat, stained for acetylcholinesterase following fixation in 10% formol for 20 min. and pH = 5·6 of the incubation medium. Phase contrast: same magnification (Schwarzacher, 1961).

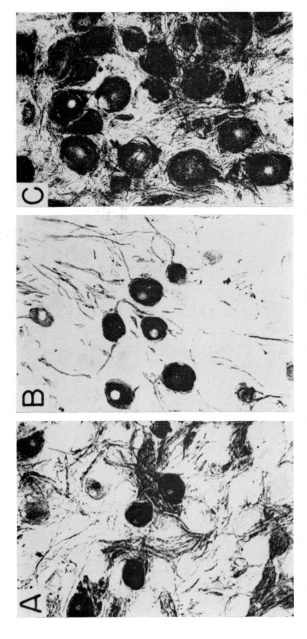

FIG. 2.5. Autonomic ganglia from the cat, stained for acetylcholinesterase activity. Section (10μ) incubated 80 min in acetylthiocholine medium following selective inhibition of pseudocholinesterase with diisopropylfluorophosphate. Magnification × 200. A. Stellate ganglion, normal. B. Stellate ganglion, preganglionically denervated. C. Ciliary ganglion (Koelle, 1963).

(ii) *Musculotendinous junctions.* The localization of acetylcholinesterase at the musculotendinous junction of individual striated muscle fibres of the frog and mouse was described by Couteaux (1953) and has since been confirmed in other species. Schwarzacher (1961) has shown, both manometrically and histochemically, that the myotendinous enzyme consists entirely of acetylcholinesterase, and appears to be bound to the fibre surface membrane, forming at the fibre tip, deep infoldings into which collagenous fibres of the tendon are inserted (Fig. 2.4). In mammals, neither motor nor sensory nerve endings are found at these sites. Sectioning of the nerve in adult mammals did not affect the intensity of acetylcholinesterase staining at muscle–tendon junctions, even after prolonged periods of muscle denervation (Gerebtzoff, 1957).

Lubinska and Zelená (1967) have shown in rats, that denervation of muscles performed at birth or before the tenth postnatal day results in the disappearance of acetylcholinesterase from the myotendinous junctions, whereas in older animals it persists after nerve section. In muscles reinnervated after crushing the nerve at birth, the enzyme gradually reappears at the myotendinous junctions. The effects of denervation and reinnervation in neonatal animals suggest that the motor nerve fibres exert some influence on the development and maintenance of the myotendinous cholinesterase.

(iii) *Autonomic ganglia.* Analyses of homogenates of the superior cervical and other sympathetic ganglia have shown that they contain high concentrations of both acetyl and pseudo-cholinesterase. The marked fall in the former which follows preganglionic denervation suggests that much of the acetylcholinesterase is localized in the terminals of the preganglionic fibres (Sawyer and Hollinshead, 1945). These findings have been confirmed and extended by subsequent ultramicro-analytical and histochemical investigations.

The acetylcholinesterase in autonomic ganglia of the cat is confined to the neuronal elements. Pseudocholinesterase is restricted to the glial cells (Koelle and Koelle, 1959). In the stellate ganglion (Fig. 2.5A), high acetylcholinesterase activity is present in the entering preganglionic axons, their terminals on the ganglion cells and in some of the ganglion cells. All the ganglion cells are surrounded by a dense network of acetylcholinesterase-stained fibres which terminate as fine fibrils or expanded bulbs. A few stained fibres leave the ganglion with the postganglionic trunks, but the majority of postganglionic fibres are practically unstained. Identification of most of the stained fibres as preganglionic is confirmed by their absence in ganglia which have been denervated (Fig. 2.5B).

The stellate ganglion cells can be divided into three classes with respect to acetylcholinesterase activity. A small number are heavily stained, a comparable number are moderately stained and the majority are unstained or only minimally reactive (Koelle, 1955; Holmstedt and Sjöqvist, 1959). In the ciliary ganglion, which gives rise exclusively to cholinergic postganglionic fibres, all the neurones contain high concentrations of acetylcholinesterase (Fig. 2.5C).

Electron microscopic localization of acetylcholinesterase in ganglia has been attempted by Koelle and Foroglou-Kerameos (1965) and Kása and Csernovsky (1967). Cells in the superior cervical ganglion of the rat were divisible into three types. Some cells were lacking in enzyme activity, in others which reacted weakly, the end-product was associated with ribosomes and in the third group which exhibited marked activity, the reaction product was associated with the endoplasmic reticulum. The synaptic membranes of axosomatic synapses were inactive. In the pre- and postganglionic axons, the axon tubules exhibited acetylcholinesterase activity.

The effects of denervation and axotomy on the cholinesterase content of sympathetic ganglia have been extensively documented. Sawyer and Hollinshead (1945) reported an 80% decrease in the acetylcholinesterase activity of cat superior cervical ganglia 10 to 15 days after preganglionic section. The acetylcholinesterase activity of the same ganglion in the rat was reduced to 57% of its control value two weeks after preganglionic section, and to 52% three weeks after axotomy (Dhar, 1958). A comparable reduction following denervation has also been observed in the seventh lumbar ganglion of the cat (Buckley et al., 1967). Gromadzki and Koelle (1965) showed a loss of approximately 75% in the enzyme content of the superior cervical ganglion of the cat after denervation, in contrast to a loss of only 6% after axotomy. Härkönen (1964) has reported histochemical findings of an almost complete disappearance of both pre- and postsynaptic acetylcholinesterase in the superior cervical ganglion of the rat following axotomy. The marked losses of acetylcholinesterase found after axotomy of the superior cervical ganglion of the rat can be accounted for by the presence of moderate to high concentrations of the enzyme in essentially all the sympathetic ganglion cells of this species (Koelle, 1954; Eränkö, 1966).

In an important series of experiments, in which histochemical and ultramicro-analytical procedures were combined, it has been shown that less than 13 % of the cell bodies in the 7th lumbar ganglion of the cat have a high acetylcholinesterase activity (Sjöqvist, 1963; Giacobini, Palmborg and Sjöqvist, 1967). The remaining cells show only traces of the enzyme. These densely staining cells do not contain noradrenaline, which is found in approximately 88 % of the cells in this ganglion, and are thought to be identical with the 13 % of cells which contain choline acetyltransferase (Buckley *et al.*, 1967). The percentage of cells with choline acetyltransferase activity remains the same after preganglionic denervation, even though the choline acetyltransferase content of the ganglion decreases by about 98 %. These cells are considered to be the source of the cholinergic (sweat secretory and vasodilator) fibres which arise in this ganglion.

The presence of moderate amounts of acetylcholinesterase activity in ganglionic neurones, which contain noradrenaline, but not choline acetyltransferase, makes it questionable whether the presence of this enzyme in a neurone can be considered as evidence for a cholinergic function. It is more likely that the acetylcholine and choline acetyltransferase content of its cell body, rather than the acetylcholinesterase activity reflect the cholinergic nature of a neurone.

From a comparison of the effects produced by several anticholinesterase compounds of varying lipid-solubility, Koelle and his colleagues concluded that the acetylcholinesterase in ganglia is separable into internal and external fractions with respect to the relationship of its active sites to the cell membrane (McIsaac and Koelle, 1959). Characteristic effects of anticholinesterases on ganglionic transmission were obtained by inhibition only of the external fraction, which was termed "functional acetylcholinesterase"; the internal fraction could be inactivated selectively without immediately apparent effects and was called "reserve acetylcholinesterase". In order to determine whether the "functional" enzyme is distributed on the pre- or postsynaptic membrane, Koelle and Koelle (1959) compared the effects of various inhibitors on normal and denervated ganglia. The results showed that in the stellate and superior cervical ganglia, essentially all the enzyme was presynaptic. In the ciliary ganglion it was located both pre- and postsynaptically.

Koelle (1962, 1963) has discussed the general problem of the physiological function of acetylcholinesterase at synapses. He argues that if acetylcholinesterase were solely involved in the hydrolysis of acetylcholine, after its liberation from the terminal and subsequent production of a postsynaptic potential, then the enzyme would be concentrated in a post synaptic location. The presence of acetylcholinesterase presynaptically may be related to a protection of the terminal from an excessive depolarizing action of its own acetylcholine. Koelle (1962, 1963) has proposed that the immediate action of acetylcholine released by a nerve impulse is on the presynaptic terminal, causing it to release additional quanta of acetylcholine in order to facilitate transmission across the synaptic cleft. In effect, this would serve as an amplification mechanism, and presynaptic acetylcholinesterase would prevent the perpetuation of this process of self-re-excitation. Participation of acetylcholine in the release of other humoral transmitters has been envisaged by both Koelle (1962, 1963) and Burn and Rand (1965).

The results of electrophysiological studies on the action of acetylcholine on presynaptic terminals at the skeletal neuromuscular junction are discussed in detail in Chapter 4. Although the findings do not support the "amplifier" hypothesis proposed by Koelle, they are not altogether incompatible with this concept. The hypothesis of a cholinergic link in the sympathetic postganglionic adrenergic transmission has stimulated a great deal of investigation. Despite the plausibility of much of the evidence, the hypothesis has not been generally accepted and until more information is available, it will be difficult to come to a definite conclusion. The arguments for and against the cholinergic link hypothesis have been discussed in detail in several recent reviews (Burn and Rand, 1965; Ferry, 1966; Iversen, 1967).

(iv) *Central nervous system.* The distribution of acetylcholinesterase in the central nervous system has been intensively studied by a number of investigators employing both histochemical and biochemical techniques (see reviews by Gerebtzoff, 1959; Koelle, 1963; Silver, 1967). The significance of acetylcholinesterase distribution as an indicator of cholinergic pathways has been evaluated in a limited number of situations either by studying the correlation between the relative levels of choline acetyltransferase and acetylcholinesterase (Lewis, Shute and Silver, 1967; Goldberg and McCaman, 1967) or by a pharmacological analysis of the synaptic effects of stimulation of enzyme-containing pathways (McCance, Phillis and Westerman, 1968; McCance and Phillis, 1968).

Shute and Lewis (1961, 1965) have emphasized that acetylcholinesterase may be present in the cell bodies of neurones which are unlikely to be cholinergic and regard the presence of the enzyme in the axon and pre-synaptic terminals as an essential criterion. However, the demonstration of acetylcholinesterase in noradrenaline-containing nerve fibres in sym-pathetically innervated organs (Jacobowitz, 1965; Jacobowitz and Koelle, 1965; Eränkö, 1966) throws considerable doubt into the validity of this assumption. It is difficult to escape the conclusion that, whilst the presence of a high level of acetylcholinesterase activity in the soma and axonal processes of a neurone may be an indication of its cholinergic nature, this is not necessarily so. The complications involved in the acceptance of the hypothesis that the presence of histochemically demonstrable acetyl-cholinesterase at synaptic junctions is indicative of cholinergic transmission can be illustrated by recent studies on the cerebellar cortex.

The widespread presence of the enzyme at synapses in the guinea-pig cerebellar cortex has led Kása and Csillik (1962; 1966; Csillik and Kása 1966) to conclude that acetylcholine is the universal transmitter in this structure; a finding that is difficult to reconcile with the low levels of choline acetyltransferase in the cerebellar cortex of this species (Goldberg and McCaman, 1967) and currently available knowledge of cerebellar pharma-cology. There is, moreover, no apparent correlation between the levels of choline acetyltransferase and acetylcholinesterase in the various strata of the cerebellar cortices of different species (Goldberg and McCaman, 1967).

At synapses in the central nervous system where acetylcholine is a transmitter, acetylcholinesterase presumably has a similar role to that at the skeletal neuromuscular junction. Cholinesterases and acetylcholine have also been implicated in the control of passive permeability and active transport of structures such as erythrocytes, skin capillaries and the placenta (Koelle, 1963). Evidence has been based largely on the demon-stration of the presence of acetylcholine or cholinesterase in membranous structures and on the effects of cholinesterase inhibitors in the partitioning of various ions, and is not, as yet, conclusive. An involvement in functions of this type may explain the presence of acetylcholinesterase in neurones that are apparently non-cholinergic. Koelle (1955, 1963) has speculated whether the presence of acetylcholinesterase in non-cholinergic neurones might be "vestigial" in the ontogenetic sense; a result of incomplete differentiation during the course of embryonic development. This sugges-tion was advanced by Mendel and his associates (Mendel et al., 1953) with regard to the aliesterases, since their prolonged inhibition has no demon-strable effect on rats, but interferes with the growth of bacteria and seeds and cultures of malignant cells. In the course of ontogenesis, acetyl-cholinesterase may be synthesized at certain sites, where its function is evanescent or only potential. An example of this may be the appearance of acetylcholinesterase in developing Purkinje cells of the cerebellum.

By combining histochemistry with operative procedures, Shute and Lewis (1961) developed a method for determining the polarity of cholin-esterase-containing fibres in the central nervous system. When such fibres are transected, the intensity of the acetylcholinesterase reaction increases in the terminal portion of axons still connected to their cells of origin, whereas fibres separated from their cell bodies lose activity. An extensive survey of the presence and polarity of acetylcholinesterase-containing fibres has enabled these authors to trace two major ascending cholinergic pathways from the reticular and tegmental nuclei of the brain stem of the rat. The pathways, which project to virtually all cortical and subcortical structures, have been designated the "dorsal" and "ventral tegmental pathways" (Figs. 2.6 and 2.7) (Shute and Lewis, 1963, 1965, 1967; Lewis and Shute, 1967).

Krnjević and Silver (1965) using similar methods, have demonstrated a system of cholinergic tracts linking various areas of the cerebral cortex (Fig. 2.8). These fibres form a predominantly tangential system beneath the cortex, with ascending branches which form a complex network in the deeper half of the cortex, with rather diffuse endings, especially in relation to the pyramidal cells of layer V. The main subcortical connections of this system can be traced to the corpus striatum and the septal area and may be comparable to the ascending fibres described by Shute and Lewis.

Although no cerebral cortical cells in the cat show strong acetylcholin-esterase activity, comparable with that of known cholinergic neurones, some spindle cells of the deepest layer of the cortex often have relatively large amounts of intracellular enzyme (Fig. 2.9B) and may therefore be the cholinergic cells whose axons constitute the system described above. Many large pyramidal cells in layer V of the cortex consistently showed moderate acetylcholinesterase activity (Fig. 2.9A) and often formed a relatively well-defined layer at the depth where acetylcholine-excited cells are found.

Studies on the development of acetylcholinesterase staining in embryos have shown that the primary cortical elements of the cat are devoid of the enzyme (Krnjević and Silver, 1966). In the primitive forebrain acetyl-cholinesterase is found only in the developing lenticular nucleus and in the

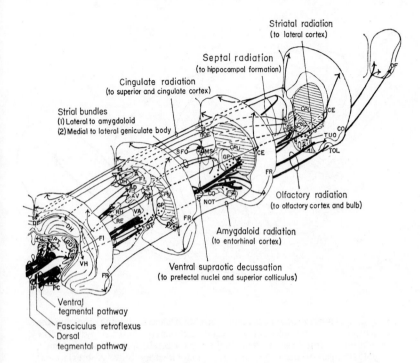

FIG. 2.6. Exploded diagram of rat forebrain, showing cholinesterase-containing pathways. Asterisks indicate distribution of acetylcholinesterase-containing cells. Areas of dense neuropil are hatched. Natural spacing of sections increased 5 times. Abbreviations: A, alveus; ACB, nucleus accumbens; AD, anterodorsal thalamic nucleus; AL, lateral amygdaloid nucleus pars ventralis; AV, anteroventral thalamic nucleus; CE, external capsule; CO, optic chiasma; CPU, caudate-putamen; DB, diagonal band; DF, dorsal fornix; DH, dorsal hippocampus; FI, fimbria; FR, rhinal fissure; GP, globus pallidus; H, habenular nuclei; IP, interpeduncular nucleus; LGD, dorsal nucleus of lateral geniculate body; LGV, ventral nucleus of lateral geniculate body; MS, medial septal nucleus; NOT, nucleus of lateral olfactory tract; OT, optic tract; PC, cerebral peduncle; PF, parafascicular-centromedian nucleus; PT, pretectal nuclei; RE, reticular thalamic nucleus; SFO, subfornical organ (Shute and Lewis, 1963).

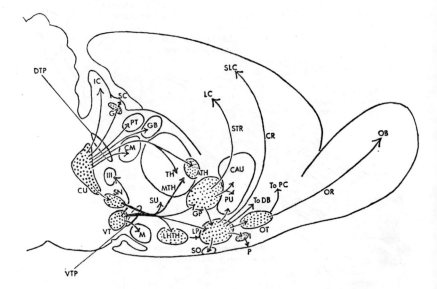

FIG. 2.7. Diagram, based on results of cholinesterase-staining, showing the constituent nuclei (stippled) of the ascending cholinergic reticular system in the mid-brain and fore-brain, with projections to the cerebellum, tectum, thalamus, hypothalamus, striatum, lateral cortex and olfactory bulb. Abbreviations: ATH, antero-ventral and antero-dorsal thalamic nuclei; CAU, caudate; CM, centromedian (parafascicular) nucleus; CR, cingulate radiation; CU, nucleus cuneiformis; DB, diagonal band; DTP, dorsal tegmental pathway; G, stratum griseum intermediale of superior colliculus; GB, medial and lateral geniculate bodies; GP, globus pallidus and entopeduncular nucleus; I, islets of Calleja; IC, inferior colliculus; III, oculomotor nucleus; LC. lateral cortex; LHTH, lateral hypothalamic area; LP, lateral preoptic area; M, mammillary body; MTH, mammillo-thalamic tract; OB, olfactory bulb; OR, olfactory radiation; OT, olfactory tubercule; P, plexiform layer of olfactory tubercule; PC, precallosal cells; PT, pretectal nuclei; PU, putamen; SC, superior colliculus; SLC, supero-lateral cortex; SN, substantia nigra pars compacta; SO, supraoptic nucleus; STR, striatal radiation; SU, subthalamus; TH, thalamus; TP, nucleus reticularis tegmenti pontis (of Bechterew); VT, ventral tegmental area and nucleus of basal optic root; VTP, ventral tegmental pathway (Shute and Lewis, 1967).

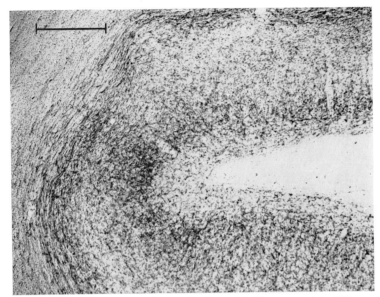

FIG. 2.8. Low power photomicrograph of acetylcholinesterase-stained fibres around the posterior cruciate sulcus of the feline cerebal cortex. Scale: 0·5 mm (Krnjević and Silver, 1965).

A   B

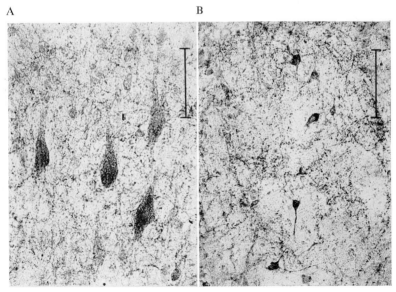

FIG. 2.9. Acetylcholinesterase activity associated with (A) pyramidal cells of layer V in the anterior sigmoid gyrus and (B) small polymorph cells in layer VI on the posterior sigmoid gyrus of the feline cerebral cortex. Strong enzyme activity extends into the neuronal processes of the polymorph cells, but not the pyramidal cells. Scale: 100μm (Krnjević and Silver, 1965).

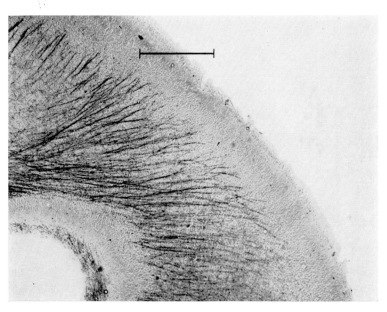

Fig. 2.10. Acetylcholinesterase-containing fibres from the lenticular nucleus invading the lateral wall of primitive forebrain. Note absence of staining in cortical lamina. Cat embryo at about 40 days. Scale: 0·5 mm (Krnjević, 1965b).

septum, both of which probably arise from the striatal ependyma. Acetyl-cholinesterase containing fibres spread out from these regions and invade the rest of the hemisphere (Fig. 2.10) but do not penetrate the neocortical areas much before birth. It is interesting to note that acetylcholine has no clearly detectable action on cortical neurones of the cat until the third week of post-natal life (Krnjević, Randić and Straughan, 1964).

The cerebella of many, but not all, mammalian species are particularly rich in acetylcholinesterase (Fig. 2.11) (Austin and Phillis, 1965). By contrast, its content of acetylcholine and choline acetyltransferase is amongst

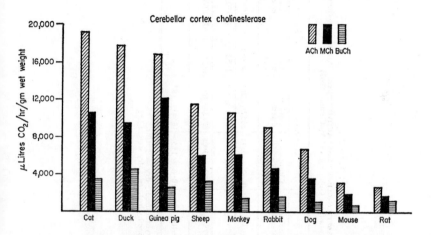

FIG. 2.11. Rates of hydrolysis of acetylcholine (ACh), acetyl-β-methylcholine (MCh) and butyrylcholine (BuCh) by cerebellar cholinesterases from several species of animal. Figures expressed in terms of wet weight of tissue used. Manometric estimations. (Austin and Phillis, 1965).

the lowest of the entire brain. However, acetylcholine in the cerebellar cortex is known to be located in synaptosomes (Isräel and Whittaker, 1965), and can be released by electrical stimulation of the cerebellar surface (Phillis and Chong, 1965).

The stratification of the cerebellar cortex makes it particularly suitable for ultramicro-analytical studies of the enzyme contents of its various layers. Goldberg and McCaman (1967) have compared the cholinesterase and choline acetyltransferase contents of molecular and granular layers and underlying white matter of the cerebella of five species, but were

TABLE 2.

CHOLINE ACETYLTRANSFERASE[a] AND ACETYLCHOLINESTERASE[b] ACTIVITY IN THE CEREBELLA OF SEVERAL SPECIES
(Data from Goldberg and McCaman, 1967)

	Rat		Pigeon		Guinea-pig		Rabbit		Cat	
	Choline acetyl-transferase	Cholin-esterase	Choline acetyl-transferase	Cholin-esterase	Choline acetyl-transferase	Choline esterase	Choline acetyl-transferase	Choline esterase	Choline acetyl-transferase	Choline esterase
Molecular layer	0·98 ± 0·27	1000 ± 123	1·55 ± 0·30	4293 ± 316	0·62 ± 0·15	3757 ± 285	< 0·1	2087 ± 216	0·71 ± 0·19	2330 ± 288
Granular layer	1·92 ± 0·37	1472 ± 89	1·36 ± 0·19	2399 ± 190	1·60 ± 0·22	2390 ± 131	1·52 ± 0·14	3702 ± 643	1·23 ± 0·18	3694 ± 282
White matter	2·75 ± 0·48	1620 ± 223	1·38 ± 0·22	775 ± 132	2·60 ± 0·08	1192 ± 69	1·23 ± 0·10	1270 ± 126	0·44 ± 0·10	1193 ± 211
Deep nuclei	6·90 ± 0·51	1525 ± 232	10·5 ± 1·5	610 ± 58	10·6 ± 1·5	1354 ± 189			3·78 ± 1·08	1790 ± 276

[a] The activity is expressed as μmoles of acetylcholine synthesized/g dry weight/hr.
[b] The activity is expressed as μmoles of acetylthiocholine hydrolyzed/g dry weight/hr.
Each value represents the mean ± standard error.

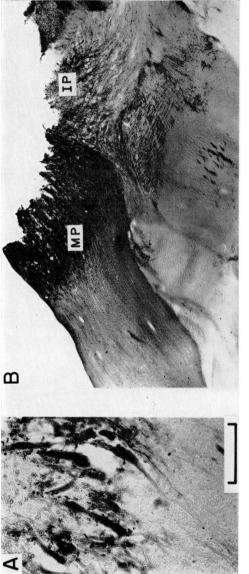

FIG. 2.12. A. High power photomicrograph of distended acetylcholinesterase containing axons on brain-stem side of severed middle cerebellar peduncle. Calibration —10μ. B. Acetylcholinesterase accumulation in severed middle peduncle (MP) and to a lesser extent in the inferior peduncle (IP). Incubation time inacetyl-thiocholine medium of 4 hr. (Phillis, 1968a).

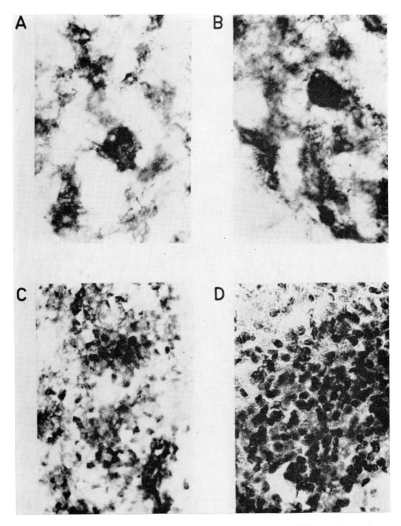

Fig. 2.13. Medium power photomicrographs of granule cell layers from the same section at different depths of the cerebellar cortex. A. At surface of cortex and B. 2mm below the surface. Note dense acetylcholinesterase reaction in cerebellar islands and surrounding unreactive cells. C. 4 mm and D. 6 mm below cortical surface many granule layer cells also contain the enzyme. Section incubated in acetylthiocholine medium for 4 hr. Calibration -30μ. (Phillis, 1968a).

unable to demonstrate a correlation between the levels of the two enzymes (Table 2). Histochemical studies on the feline cerebellum, carried out in this laboratory (Phillis, 1965, 1968a), have shown that cholinesterase-containing fibres entering the cerebellum in the middle peduncle, and to a lesser extent in the superior and inferior peduncles (Fig. 2.12), terminate as mossy afferent fibres in the granular layer. Related pharmacological investigations have confirmed that some mossy afferent fibres may be cholinergic (McCance and Phillis, 1968). Many of the cells within the granular layer contain acetylcholinesterase (Fig. 2.13), which persists after isolation of the cortex or peduncular transection and is not, therefore, likely to be associated with the mossy afferent terminals. The significance of these enzyme-containing granular neurones and the high content of the enzyme in the molecular layer has still to be determined, as pharmacological studies indicate that granule cell to Purkinje cell transmission is mediated by a non-cholinergic transmitter (Crawford, Curtis, Voorhoeve and Wilson, 1966; McCance and Phillis, 1968).

Many cells in the cerebellar deep nuclei, which contain rather higher levels of choline acetyltransferase, are excited by acetylcholine (Chapman and McCance, 1967). The large, multipolar neurons in these nuclei exhibit two patterns of response to acetylcholinesterase staining. Surface membranes on the soma and dendritic trunks stain on the majority of these cells, although the intensity of reaction varies. A cytoplasmic reaction for acetylcholinesterase is also discernible in some of the large deep nuclear cells, especially in the lateral part of the interpositus and dentate nuclei. Cholinesterase-containing axons leaving the cerebellum in the superior peduncle probably originate from these enzyme-containing cells, and collateral branches may be partially responsible for the acetylcholine sensitivity of other deep nuclear neurones. Pharmacological evidence for a cholinergic component in the cerebellar projection to the thalamus will be discussed in Chapter 7.

Purkinje cells, which normally do not stain for acetylcholinesterase in the adult cat, undergo a striking change after cortical isolation or peduncular transection. Four to eight days after such an operation, Purkinje cells in the isolated area stain for the enzyme. Purkinje cells exhibit a strong acetylcholinesterase activity in the entire cerebellar cortex of the cat during the first few weeks of postnatal life, and it appears that isolation causes a reactivation or reappearance of the enzyme.

A similar finding has been described in the isolated archicerebellum of the rat, which is the only area of the cerebellum of this species in which the Purkinje cells contain acetylcholinesterase in the immediately postnatal period of life (Kása, Csillik, Jóo and Knyihár, 1966).

3. *Pseudocholinesterase*

Pseudocholinesterase is widely distributed in tissues, including the nervous system, but its role has yet to be evaluated. Many suggestions have been made about its possible function (see Svensmark, 1965) including theories that it is involved in ion transport (Koblick, 1958; Fourman, 1966); in the assimilation of food (Gerebtzoff, 1959); in certain metabolic processes, such as the destruction of butyrylcholine, which might be produced as undesirable by-products of metabolism (Clitherow, Mitchard and Harper, 1963); in the regulation of choline metabolism (Zeller and Bissegger, 1943) or in the control of the level of choline in the plasma (Funnell and Oliver, 1965).

The pseudocholinesterase in glial cells may be involved in the control of activity in adjacent neurons (Desmedt and La Grutta, 1955), by influencing the permeability of glial cells to various ions or by protecting the neurons from exogenously released acetylcholine. Pseudocholinesterase is also present in some neurons (Abrahams and Edery, 1964; Shute and Lewis, 1963; Utley, 1966), where it may have a similar role to acetylcholinesterase.

CONCLUSIONS

1. This chapter is concerned with the three important members of the cholinergic system: acetylcholine, choline acetyltransferase and acetylcholinesterase.

2. The levels of acetylcholine and choline acetyltransferase vary extensively from one area of the nervous system to another. High levels are probably indicative of the presence of cholinergic neurones and fibre tracts, and lower levels may denote the presence of cholinergic nerve terminals.

3. The acetylcholine in nerve cell bodies and axons appears to be in a "free" form and is normally destroyed by cholinesterase. In the nerve terminals, it is apparently incorporated into packages or vesicles, in which it is protected from cholinesterase. Release from nerve terminals in "packets" or "quanta" may occur spontaneously or during depolarization of the nerve terminal, for instance, by an action potential.

4. The choline acetyltransferase of most mammalian species that have been investigated is not localized within the synaptic vesicles with acetylcholine, as it remains bound to particulate structural components of the nerve endings under conditions when acetylcholine is released.

5. Choline acetyltransferase appears to be synthesized in the nerve cell body and is transported to the terminals by axoplasmic flow.

6. Various substances, such as atropine and eserine, inhibit the uptake of acetylchline by nervous tissues. This action may be related to their pharmacological effects.

7. Acetylcholinesterase, a stable enzyme which is amenable to both biochemical and histochemical analysis, has been extensively investigated as an indicator of cholinergic cells and synapses. However, recent studies on the autonomic nervous system cast some doubt on the reliability of this assumption.

8. The presence of acetylcholinesterase in synaptic junctions in skeletal muscles, sympathetic ganglia and in areas of the central nervous system is largely dependent on the integrity of the afferent nervous pathways. The enzyme appears to be synthesized in the cell soma and transported to the nerve terminals.

9. Studies on the distribution of acetylcholinesterase in the brain (the cerebral and cerebellar cortices in particular) have provided evidence to support the hypothesis of cholinergic transmission in the central nervous system. However, no correlation between the levels of choline acetyltransferase and acetylcholinesterase in the cerebella of several mammalian species was observed.

CHAPTER 3

MONOAMINES IN THE
CENTRAL NERVOUS SYSTEM

A. CATECHOLAMINE METABOLISM

The uneven regional distribution of noradrenaline in the mammalian brain, and the effects on its concentration of certain drugs that effect behaviour, described by Vogt (1954), have stimulated a great deal of interest in the metabolism of central catecholamines. Several reviews on this subject have recently been published, including those of Himwich and Himwich (1964), Marley (1964), Hornykiewicz (1966), Glowinski and Baldessarini (1966), Iversen, (1967), Axelrod (1967), Bloom and Giarman (1968).

1. *Distribution*

The presence of an adrenergic substance "sympathin" in extracts of mammalian brain was first described by von Euler (1946). A few years later, Holtz (1950) confirmed this observation in brain and spinal cord and showed that the noradrenaline concentrations far exceed those of adrenaline. The presence of dopamine in brain was demonstrated by Weil-Malherbe and Bone (1957) and confirmed by Carlsson, Lindqvist, Magnusson and Waldeck (1958).

The pattern of distribution of noradrenaline first described by Vogt (1954) for the dog and cat brain is generally similar in other species. The highest concentrations are in the hypothalamus (Table 3), with a range of 1 to 3 μg/g in rat (Glowinski and Iversen, 1966a), cat (Bertler and Rosengren, 1959; McGeer, McGeer and Wada, 1963), monkey (Pscheidt and Himwich, 1963) and man (Bertler, 1961). Other regions can be ranked as follows: midbrain and pons, medulla oblongata and striatum, with low concentrations in the hippocampus, cerebral cortex, cerebellum and spinal cord. In the corpus striatum and the caudate nucleus, where the nor-

38

TABLE 3.

DISTRIBUTION OF NORADRENALINE AND DOPAMINE IN THE CENTRAL
NERVOUS SYSTEM[a]

Tissue	Noradrenaline		Dopamine	
	μg/g tissue	species	μg/g tissue	species
Spinal cord	0·18, 0·34	dog, cat	0–0·45	cat
Medulla	0·37, 0·39	dog, cat	0·13, 0·08	dog, cat
Pons	0·20, 0·20– 0·52	dog, cat	0·10, 0·11	dog, cat
Cerebellum	0·06, 0·13	dog, cat	0·03, 0·02	dog, cat
Inferior colliculus	0·11 } 0·40	dog, cat	} 1·59	cat
Superior colliculus	0·16	dog,		
Medial geniculate nucleus	0·13	dog		
Lateral geniculate nucleus	0·07	dog		
Midbrain	0·50	cat	0·53	cat
Hippocampus	0·14, 0·17	dog, cat	0·70	cat
Hypothalamus	1·03, 2·05	dog, cat	0·26, 0·75	dog, cat
Thalamus	0·08, 0·22	dog, cat	0·05, 0·05– 0·50	dog, cat
Basal ganglia	0·10, 0·22	dog, cat	5·90, 8·00	dog, cat
Cerebral cortex	0·12, 0·11– 0·28	dog, cat	0·01, 0·07	dog, cat
Olfactory bulb	0·05	dog,		

[a] Values in this table are taken from papers by Bertler and Rosengren (1959), Carlsson (1959), Holzbauer and Vogt (1956), Vogt (1954), Laverty and Sharman (1965), McGeer, McGeer and Wada (1963). It must be emphasized that there is often a considerable disparity between the results of different groups.

adrenaline concentration is relatively low (Sharman and Vogt, 1965), dopamine is found in very high concentrations (3 to 8μg/g) (Bertler and Rosengren, 1959; Hornykiewicz, 1966). There is generally more noradrenaline in gray than in white matter.

Since 1962, fluorescence microscopy has been used to study the localization of catecholamines at the cellular level. This technique is based on the formation of specific fluorescent derivatives of biogenic amines in the presence of formaldehyde. Monoamine-containing neurones in brain tissue were first described by Carlsson, Falck and Hillarp (1962) and Carlsson, Falck, Hillarp and Torp (1962). The distinction between catecholamines and serotonin has been based on differences in the colours of their fluorescent products (Falck and Owman, 1965). In the presence of formaldehyde, noradrenaline and dopamine are converted to isoquinolines with very similar fluorescence spectra. Prior to the recent development of microspectrofluorimetric techniques, complex pharmacological methods were used to differentiate between the various amines. For example, after treatment of animals with α-methyl-*m*-tyrosine neurones that contain mainly dopamine recover their fluorescence faster than noradrenaline-containing neurones. This appears to be due to the persistence of non-fluorescent metaraminol, formed by decarboxylation and β-hydroxylation of α-methyl-*m*-tyrosine in noradrenaline-containing neurones (Andén, 1964; Fuxe, 1965a). After treatment with the tyrosine analogue, meta-tyrosine, fluorescence disappears selectively from catecholamine neurones, but not from serotonin-containing neurones (Fuxe, 1965a). Treatment with α-methyldopa, followed by reserpine, leads to a disappearance of the fluorescent α-methyldopamine from dopamine-containing neurones, but in noradrenaline-containing neurones fluorescence does not disappear because the α-methylnoradrenaline formed is relatively resistant to depletion by reserpine (Carlsson, Dahlström, Fuxe and Hillarp, 1965).

In many areas of the brain, fine nerve fibres with extensive terminal arborizations and "varicosities" containing large amounts of catechol-amines or serotonin have been demonstrated with these techniques. These fibres resemble sympathetic nerve fibres of the periphery. Noradrenergic terminals are widely distributed, but are most abundant in the hypo-thalamus (Carlsson *et al.*, 1962), olfactory bulb (Dahlström, Fuxe, Olson and Ungerstedt, 1965), median eminence (Fuxe, 1964), limbic system and many nuclei of the cranial nerves (Dahlström and Fuxe, 1964, 1965). The distribution of these fibres in the spinal cord has also been described (Carlsson, Falck, Fuxe and Hillarp, 1964: Dahlström and Fuxe, 1965). Dopaminergic terminals are found mainly in the neostriatum, olfactory tuberculum, and nucleus acumbens (Andén *et al.*, 1966). Noradrenaline containing cell bodies tend to be concentrated in the ventral brain stem (Fig. 3.1) (Dahlström and Fuxe, 1964a).

Several kinds of evidence support the conclusion that amines are con-tained within specific neurones of the central nervous system. The experi-mental approaches used include axotomy, inhibition of the catabolism of amines, and the creation of lesions. After axotomy, catecholamines accumulate on the side of the transection proximal to the cell body, particularly after the use of monoamine oxidase inhibitors (Dahlström and Fuxe, 1964b). This phenomenon has been useful in mapping the distribution of noradrenergic and dopaminergic pathways. The findings are summarized in Fig. 3.2.

Further evidence for the existence of these pathways has come from analyses of the catecholamine content of various regions of the brain after specific lesions. Gross mesencephalic or specific hypothalamic lesions lead to a fall in the catecholamine content of the brain (Heller and Moore, 1965; Heller, Seiden and Moore, 1966; Andén *et al.*, 1966). Lesions have

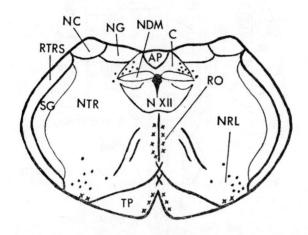

Fig. 3.1. Distribution of fluorescent monoamine-containing neurones in the rat brain stem. Schematic drawing of a transverse section of the medulla oblongata at the level of the area postrema. The CA cell bodies are indicated by dots, the 5-HT cell bodies by crosses. NG = nucleus gracilis; NC = nucleus cuneatus; NDM = nucleus motorius dorsalis n. vagi; AP = area postrema; N XII = nucleus hypoglossus; RO = nucleus raphé obscurus; NRL = nucleus reticularis lateralis; TP = tractus pyramidalis; NTR = nucleus tractus spinalis n. trigemini; SG = substantia gelatinosa; RTRS = radix tractus spinalis n. trigemini; C = nucleus commissuralis (Dahlström and Fuxe, 1965).

been used to demonstrate a nigro-striatal system of dopamine-containing neurones (Andén, Dahlström, Fuxe and Larsson, 1965; Poirier and Sourkes, 1965; Andén, Fuxe, Hamberger and Hökfelt, 1966). Thoracic cord section was found to decrease spinal cord noradrenaline (Magnusson and Rosengren, 1963) and several noradrenaline-containing bulbospinal

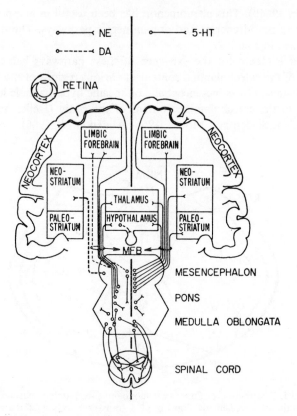

Fig. 3.2. Schematic drawing showing, in highly simplified form, the main monoamine neuron projection systems in the central nervous system (Andén *et al.*, 1966).

systems have subsequently been described (Dahlström and Fuxe, 1965). In addition, ascending systems containing noradrenergic neurones extend from the brain stem to the hypothalamus, preoptic area, limbic system and cerebral cortex. Precisely localized lesions in the median forebrain bundle of the lateral hypothalamus and in the dorsomedial brain stem tegmentum significantly decreased the noradrenaline and 5-hydroxytryptamine in the forebrain, whereas lesions in the ventrolateral tegmentum decreased noradrenaline only (Heller and Moore, 1965). Medial forebrain bundle lesions in the cat reduced noradrenaline concentrations, mainly in the telencephalon (Heller, Seiden and Moore, 1966). A noradrenergic innervation of the cerebellum has also been described (Andén, Fuxe and Ungerstedt, 1967).

Biochemical (Glowinski and Axelrod, 1966; Glowinski and Iversen, 1966a) and electron microscopic autoradiographic (Aghajanian and Bloom, 1967a) evidence indicates that radioactive noradrenaline or dopa, administered intraventricularly, label the endogenous stores of catecholamines. The localization of carbon-14 by autoradiography after the intraventricular administration of C^{14}-noradrenaline has been used to study the distribution of catecholamine-containing structures in the brain (Reivich and Glowinski, 1966). Catecholamine-containing systems are localised in the brain stem, hypothalamus, limbic system, and other subcortical structures, in general agreement with the conclusions of previous chemical and histochemical studies.

2. *Subcellular Distribution*

The intracellular localization of noradrenaline and dopamine has been studied by differential centrifugation and electron microscopy. A particulate fraction rich in noradrenaline was isolated from brain homogenates by Weil-Malherbe and Bone (1959). This finding was confirmed by Green and Sawyer (1960). In rat brain stem (Levi and Maynert, 1964) and bovine hypothalamus (Maynert and Kuriyama, 1964), 60% of the total noradrenaline was in a cell fraction containing synaptosomes and mitochondria. After further purification, 50% of the noradrenaline in this fraction was confined to synaptosomes. Regions of the rat brain with high concentrations of endogenous noradrenaline such as the hypothalamus and medulla oblongata, have a relatively higher proportion of this amine localized in particulate fractions than structures with low concentrations of endogeneous noradrenaline, such as the cerebellum and cerebral cortex (Glowinski and Iversen, 1966b). Rat brain synaptosomes can be disrupted by osmotic or sonic shock to liberate free vesicles which contain noradrenaline in amounts which vary with the vigour of the disruption procedure (Maynert, Levi and De Lorenzo, 1964). These liberated vesicles resemble the synaptic vesicles seen in intact tissues by electron microscopy; although they do not exhibit the sedimentation characteristics of splenic nerve particle preparations (Maynert *et al.*, 1964). "Dense core" vesicles, somewhat larger than those found in peripheral adrenergic nerve endings, are found in the anterior hypothalamus of the rat (Iraldi, Duggan and De Robertis, 1963), but these granulated vesicles are rare compared to the simple type of vesicle commonly found in the brain.

Histochemical findings indicate that noradrenaline is highly localized at axonal varicosities (Carlsson et al., 1962), which probably correspond to the synaptosomes containing noradrenaline that are obtained by sub-cellular fractionation. Normally there is relatively little noradrenaline in the cell bodies and proximal axons, although the amount varies from cell to cell and region to region. The origin of the noradrenaline found in the soluble subcellular fraction of brain homogenates and its functional significance as a site of storage of the amine are still subjects of controversy. The existence of an unbound form of intraneuronal noradrenaline is not yet clear.

Early studies on the subcellular distribution of dopamine indicated that it was equally distributed between the particulate and supernatant fractions of rabbit brain homogenates (Weil-Malherbe and Bone, 1959). Later studies have shown that the percentage of particle bound dopamine may only be 20 to 30% of the total amine, the bulk of the dopamine being recovered in the supernatant (Bertler, Hillarp and Rosengren, 1960; Weil-Malherbe, Posner and Bowles, 1961; Laverty et al., 1963).

It is interesting to note that the distribution of noradrenaline in the caudate nucleus of rats is different to that of its precursor, dopamine. This has been deduced from the observation that after the uptake of H^3-dopamine from the lateral ventricle, the ratio of "particle bound amine to amine in the supernatant" in the caudate nucleus was higher for the newly formed H^3-noradrenaline than for H^3-dopamine (Horny-kiewicz, 1966). The possibility exists therefore, that the noradrenaline containing structures in the caudate nucleus are different to those containing dopamine. The actual concentration of noradrenaline in this area is very low (Table 3). However, fluorescence microscopic evidence for the existence of a very labile store of noradrenaline has been presented (Csillik and Erulkar, 1964).

When the fluorescence microscopy evidence that dopamine in the striatum is concentrated in nerve terminals is considered, the fact that so little of the dopamine in this area is particle-bound is surprising. The possibility has to be considered that striatal dopamine terminals have different subcellular characteristics to those of other terminals.

3. *Synthesis*

Precursors and enzymes for dopamine and noradrenaline synthesis, (summarized in Fig. 3.3), first shown in the peripheral sympathetic system, are present in the brain. Phenylalanine and tyrosine are normal constituents of brain, present in a free form in low concentrations (Tallan, Moore and Stein, 1954), Dihydroxyphenylalanine (dopa) is readily decarboxylated to dopamine and it has been difficult to measure its concentration in brain tissue (Carlsson and Hillarp, 1962; Anton and Sayre, 1964). Peripherally administered tyrosine and dopa enter the brain (Chirigos, Greengard and Udenfriend, 1960; Carlsson and Hillarp,

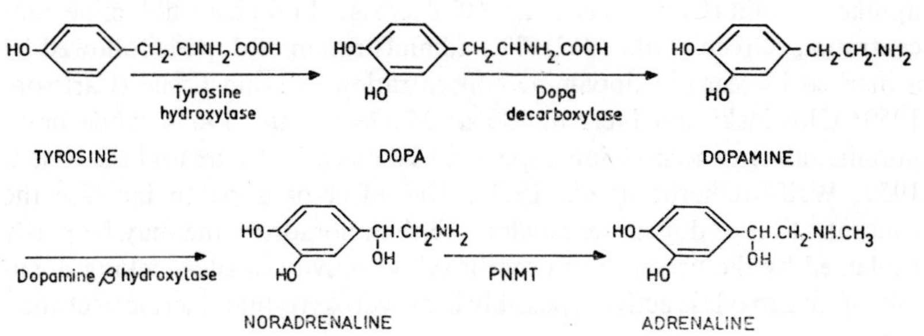

FIG. 3.3. Metabolic pathway for the biosynthesis of noradrenaline and adrenaline. PNMT is an abbreviation for the enzyme phenylethanolamine N-methyltransferase.

1962). These precursors are actively concentrated by brain slices *in vitro* (Guroff, King and Udenfriend, 1961; Yoshida, Namba, Kaniike and Imaizumi, 1963).

The enzymes necessary to convert tyrosine to noradrenaline are present in the central nervous system. Tyrosine hydroxylase activity has recently been measured in homogenates of brain stem and caudate nucleus (Nagatsu, Levitt and Udenfriend, 1964; Bagchi and McGeer, 1964). The conversion of tyrosine to dopa is the rate limiting step in the synthesis of noradrenaline in the peripheral sympathetic system, and is likely to be rate-limiting in the brain as well (Levitt, Spector, Sjoerdsma and Udenfriend, 1965). In addition, non-specific decarboxylation by which dopamine is formed from dopa occurs throughout the brain and the regional distribution of the decarboxylase involved is comparable to that of the cate-cholamines (Bogdanski, Weissbach and Udenfriend, 1957; Kuntzman, Shore, Bogdanski and Brodie, 1961). The hydroxylation of dopamine is the last step in the synthesis of noradrenaline and several other phenylethyl-amine derivatives appear to be hydroxylated by this enzyme, dopamine-β-hydroxylase (Creveling, Daly, Witkop and Udenfriend, 1962). Dopamine β-hydroxylase activity has been detected in the hypothalamus and, sur-prisingly, in the caudate nucleus, where very little noradrenaline is found (Udenfriend and Creveling, 1959).

The peripheral administration of catecholamine precursors can influ-ence the formation and concentration of dopamine and noradrenaline in the brain. Administration of amino acids that compete with tyrosine for uptake in brain (Chirigos et al., 1960) decreases brain catecholamine con-centration (Green et al., 1962). The administration of dopa is followed by a marked increase in dopamine concentration in brain tissue (Carlsson, 1959; Glowinski and Iversen, 1966a; McGeer et al., 1963), while brain noradrenaline concentration appears to be much less increased (Carlsson, 1959; Weil-Malherbe et al., 1961). The effect of dopa to increase the concentration of dopamine much more than noradrenaline may be partly explained by the presence of decarboxylase activity in sites lacking dopa-mine-β-hydroxylase activity, possibly in 5-hydroxytryptaminergic neurones, for example.

More direct demonstration of the formation of catecholamines from their precursors in brain tissue has been achieved by the use of labelled precursors. Thus radioactive dopamine and noradrenaline have been found in slices of specific areas of the brain after incubation with C^{14}-tyrosine (Masuoka, Schott and Petriello, 1963). Labelled dopa, dopamine and noradrenaline have been found in the brain after introduction of C^{14}-tyrosine into the lateral ventricle of rat brain (Glowinski, Iversen and Axelrod, 1966).

Thus a pathway for the synthesis of noradrenaline from tyrosine, similar to that present in the peripheral sympathetic system has been demonstrated in the brain. The presence of adrenaline in mammalian brain tissue is uncertain, and activity of the methyltransferase necessary for its formation from noradrenaline has been difficult to detect in brain tissues *in vitro* (Axelrod, 1962). However, there is some evidence that small amounts of labelled adrenaline, and its O-methylated derivative, metanephrine, can be synthesized *in vivo* (Milhaud and Glowinski, 1962).

After depletion with reserpine or α-methyl-*m*-tyrosine, catecholamine fluorescence reappears first in the cell body (Dahlström *et al.*, 1965), and after axotomy it accumulates proximally within cell bodies and axons (Dahlström and Fuxe, 1964). These observations have been taken to indicate that noradrenaline is synthesized in cell bodies and may be transported in a particle-bound form to the nerve endings. Two of the enzymes needed for noradrenaline synthesis, tyrosine hydroxylase and dopamine-β-hydroxylase have been found highly localized in a crude subcellular fraction that contains synaptosomes and mitochondria (Udenfriend and Creveling, 1959; Bagchi and McGeer, 1964; Nagatsu *et al.*, 1964). Tyrosine hydroxylase activity and the activity of nonspecific amino acid decarboxylase were retained in a purified brain synaptosomal subfraction that apparently contains the synaptosomes (McGeer, Bagchi and McGeer, 1965; Arnaiz and De Robertis, 1964). These enzymes also appear to synthesize noradrenaline at nerve terminals, since labelled dopamine and noradrenaline were present in a purified synaptosomal fraction of rat hypothalamus homogenised after an intraventricular introduction of labelled dopa (Glowinski and Iversen, 1966b).

4. *Drugs which Interfere with Catecholamine Synthesis*

(a) *Inhibition of synthetic enzymes.* Several compounds lower brain noradrenaline concentrations by interfering with enzymatic synthesis. Inhibitors of tyrosine hydroxylase are the most effective in lowering brain noradrenaline levels, probably because this step is rate-limiting in noradrenaline synthesis. The tyrosine hydroxylase inhibitor, α-methyltyrosine, produces a profound and rapid fall in brain noradrenaline (Spector, Sjoerdsma and Udenfriend, 1965). Its action appears to be limited to a reversible and competitive inhibition of tyrosine hydroxylase (Spector *et al.*, 1965). Repeated doses reduce brain noradrenaline to undetectable levels, but have no effect on 5-hydroxytryptamine levels. Signs of mild sedation or stimulation may occur. Since the metabolites, α-methyldopamine and α-methylnoradrenaline are detectable in brain tissue after the administration of α-methyltryosine, displacement by amine analogs may contribute to the depletion of noradrenaline (Maître, 1965).

α-Methyldopa (α-methyl-3, 4-dihydroxyphenylalanine) is a competitive inhibitor of dopa decarboxylase. Brain catecholamines are depleted after administration of α-methyldopa, to some extent as a result of decarboxylase inhibition, but, more importantly by displacement of noradrenaline

by the α-methylnoradrenaline formed from the metabolism of α-methyldopa (Sourkes, 1965; Stone and Porter, 1967). The concentrations of
5-hydroxytryptamine and histamine in brain are also decreased as a result
of the inhibition of the non-specific decarboxylating enzyme by α-methyldopa (Smith, 1960; Werle, 1961).

Other classes of decarboxylase inhibitors are known, including the
chalcones (Clark, 1959) and agents such as semicarbazide and other
hydrazine derivatives which affect pyridoxal phosphate, the coenzyme of
dopa decarboxylase (Porter et al., 1962).

(b) "*Formation of false transmitters*". Although noradrenaline is
normally the only adrenergic transmitter in mammals, it is now clear that
several other structurally related amines can be released from sympathetic
nerve terminals by nerve stimulation (Kopin, 1968). Such compounds,
which can be stored in place of noradrenaline in adrenergic nerve terminals
and released by nerve stimulation have been called "false transmitters". If
the false transmitter has reduced physiological activity, there may be a
failure of transmission at affected synaptic junctions.

The false transmitter formed from α-methyldopa is α-methylnoradrenaline and the first evidence of a release of α-methylnoradrenaline
from the rabbit heart by nerve stimulation was provided by Muscholl and
Maître (1963). In peripheral sympathetically innervated tissues of animals
pretreated with a monoamine oxidase inhibitor, there is an increase of
endogenous tyramine and its hydroxylated derivative, octopamine. The
latter amine accumulates in nerve endings and is released by nerve stimulation, acting as a false transmitter in competition with noradrenaline
(Kopin, Fisher, Musacchio and Horst, 1964). Similarly after monoamine
oxidase inhibition, endogenous octopamine and H^3-octopamine (Kakimoto
and Armstrong, 1962; Snyder, Glowinski and Axelrod, 1965), synthesized
from tyramine accumulate in the brain. The localization of labelled octopamine in a synaptosomal subcellular fraction suggests that this noradrenaline analog may act as a false transmitter in the brain.

Dopa decarboxylase decarboxylates a variety of aromatic L-amino
acids, including 5-hydroxytryptophan and histidine (Lovenberg, Weissbach and Udenfriend, 1962). Decarboxylation of these precursor amino
acids may occur non-specifically in neurones that possess the requisite
uptake mechanisms and decarboxylating enzyme (Gessa, Costa, Kuntzman and Brodie, 1962). Uptake of 5-hydroxytryptophan and its conversion
to 5-hydroxytryptamine by dopaminergic neurones have been demon-

strated in the visceral and parietal ganglia of the snail brain (Kerkut, Sedden and Walker, 1967b). These authors suggest that dopamine and 5-hydroxytryptamine may, in fact, normally occur concurrently in such neurones. Release of the amines synthesized from the exogenous precursors has still to be demonstrated but this appears to be conceivable. 5-hydroxytryptamine might then appear as a "false transmitter" released by noradrenergic or histaminergic neurones. It is not clear therefore, whether the behavioural effects produced by these precursors are due to the elevation of amine concentrations in specific neurone systems, or throughout all decarboxylase-containing neurone systems.

5. *Uptake and Storage*

Exogenous catecholamines accumulate in catecholamine-containing neurones by a relatively specific but complex phenomenon called "uptake" which involves at least two stages including transport across the neural membrane and ultimately retention in the intraneural storage granules. Accumulation of exogenous noradrenaline administered into the blood stream occurs only to a small extent in the brain, and only in areas where the blood–brain barrier for catecholamines is minimal, as in the area postrema and parts of the hypothalamus (Weil-Malherbe, Whitby and Axelrod, 1961). This problem has been circumvented by using *in vitro* studies or by direct introduction of catecholamines into the brain.

Brain slices accumulate tritiated noradrenaline to levels up to five times those in the incubating medium if the concentration of the amine in the medium is low (Dengler, Michaelson, Spiegel and Titus, 1962). The uptake is inhibited by ouabain or metabolic inhibitors indicating that it is an active process. Incubation of minced brain with labelled noradrenaline, followed by homogenization and subcellular fractionation in a sucrose density gradient has shown an accumulation of the radioactive amine in a synaptosomal fraction (Potter and Axelrod, 1963a). The subcellular distribution of the labelled amine paralleled that of endogenous noradrenaline. Dopamine is also concentrated by particulate fractions of brain (Itoh *et al.*, 1965).

Studies have shown that radioactive catecholamines introduced directly into the cerebrospinal fluid (Mannarino, Kirshner and Nashold, 1963; Milhaud and Glowinski, 1963), or lateral ventricle (Glowinski, Kopin and Axelrod, 1965; Glowinski and Iversen, 1966a) accumulate in brain. After intraventricular injection of H^3-noradrenaline or H^3-dopamine, the amines accumulated largely in the synaptosomal fraction (Glowinski and Iversen, 1966a; Glowinski, Snyder and Axelrod, 1966).

6. *Mechanisms of Release*

Very little is known about the mechanisms by which nerve impulses cause a release of noradrenaline from adrenergic nerves. In the adrenal medulla, the acetylcholine-mediated release of catecholamines involves an entry of calcium ions into the medullary cells. The amounts of catecholamine released from perfused adrenals in response to acetylcholine are dependent on the calcium content of the perfusing medium (Douglas and Rubin, 1961). Recent findings from studies on the adrenal medulla suggest that the release involves a discharge of intracellular storage particules or at least their contents. Secretion of catecholamines from the adrenal medulla is accompanied by a release of adenine nucleotides, which are known to be contained in the medullary catecholamine storage particles (Douglas, 1966). The release of medullary catecholamines is also accompanied by the release of a specific intravesicular protein, which can be isolated from the medullary storage particles (Kirshner, Sage, Smith and Kirshner, 1966; Kirshner, Sage and Smith, 1967). These authors suggest that medullary catecholamines may be released by a process of reversed pinocytosis. Evidence that noradrenaline is released in quantal packets at synapses in sympathetically innervated smooth muscle cells has been presented by Burnstock and Holman (1966). These findings, which are discussed in greater detail in Chapter 5, indicate that the mechanism of noradrenaline release may prove to be similar to that suggested for acetylcholine.

7. *Catabolism*

Oxidative deamination and O-methylation, the two enzymatic pathways of catecholamine metabolism in the peripheral sympathetic system also occur in the central nervous system (Fig. 3.4) (Mannarino *et al.*, 1963; Matsuoka, 1964; Glowinski *et al.*, 1965). Monamine oxidase activity in brain is widely and rather evenly distributed, with somewhat greater activity in the hypothalamus (Bogdanski *et al.*, 1957). Catechol-O-methyltransferase is also widely distributed in brain tissue and its cofactor, S-adenosylmethionine, is formed in the brain (Axelrod, Albers and

Clements, 1959; Baldessarini and Kopin, 1966). Monoamine oxidase is present in mitochondria, mainly at synaptic nerve endings (Arnaiz and De Robertis, 1962). The precise localization of catechol-O-methyl transferase, a soluble enzyme, at synapses has not been determined.

The noradrenaline metabolites, 3,4-dihydroxymandelic acid and normetanephrine (3-methoxy-4-hydroxyphenylethanolamine) (Matsuoka, Yoshida and Imaizumi, 1964) have been detected in brain. Several metabolites, which occur in the peripheral sympathetic system, have also been found in brain after the introduction of labelled noradrenaline into the

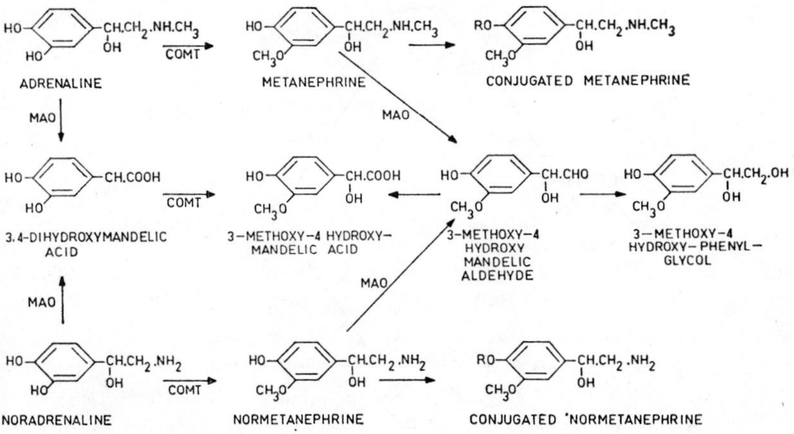

FIG. 3.4. Pathways for the metabolism of noradrenaline and adrenaline. MAO, monoamine oxidase, COMT, catechol-O-methyltransferase.

cerebrospinal fluid. They include normetanephrine, 3,4-dihydroxymandelic acid, 3,4-dihydroxyphenylglycol, 3-methoxy-4-hydroxymandelic acid and 3-methoxy-4-hydroxyphenylglycol (Mannarino et al., 1963; Glowinski et al., 1965). Regional differences in the relative concentrations of endogenous normetanephrine and dihydroxymandelic acid have been found in the rabbit brain (Matsuoka et al., 1964), suggesting that there are regional differences in the importance of monoamine oxidase and catechol-O-methyltransferase. However, tracer studies have failed to reveal any major regional differences in the relative amounts of methylated and deaminated radioactive metabolites formed from labelled noradrenaline in rat brain (Glowinski and Iversen, 1966a.)

Since monoamine oxidase is localized in mitochondria, and as inhibition of this enzyme leads to a marked rise in noradrenaline concentration (Spector, Prockop, Shore and Brodie, 1958; Green and Erickson, 1960) and fluorescence in central neurones, it is likely that it is involved in the intraneuronal metabolism of noradrenaline in the brain. There is some evidence that catechol-O-methyltransferase is very effective in metabolizing extraneuronal noradrenaline (Glowinski *et al.*, 1966).

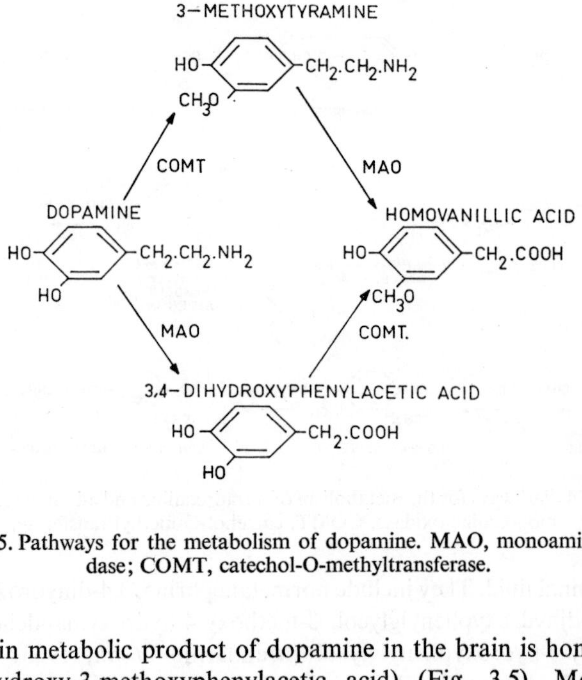

FIG. 3.5. Pathways for the metabolism of dopamine. MAO, monoamine oxidase; COMT, catechol-O-methyltransferase.

The main metabolic product of dopamine in the brain is homovanillic acid (4-hydroxy-3-methoxyphenylacetic acid) (Fig. 3.5). Monoamine oxidase and catechol-O-methyltransferase are involved in this reaction. Evidence has been presented that, in the brain, most of the dopamine formed from exogenous dopa is deaminated to form 3,4-dihydroxyphenylacetic acid, which is then O-methylated to homovanillic acid (Carlsson and Hillarp, 1962). Small amounts of brain dopamine may undergo O-methylation before oxidative metabolism as 3-methoxytyramine has been isolated from brain (Carlsson and Waldeck, 1964).

8. Inhibitors of Monoamine Oxidase and Cathechol-O-Methyl Transferase

(a) *Monoamine oxidase*. Since the discovery of iproniazid, many drugs have been used as monoamine oxidase inhibitors (Fig. 3.6) (Zeller, 1959; Pletscher, 1961). These compounds are now widely used for the treatment of psychic depression, angina pectoris and hypertension. They can be divided into compounds which produce a long-lasting inhibition by an

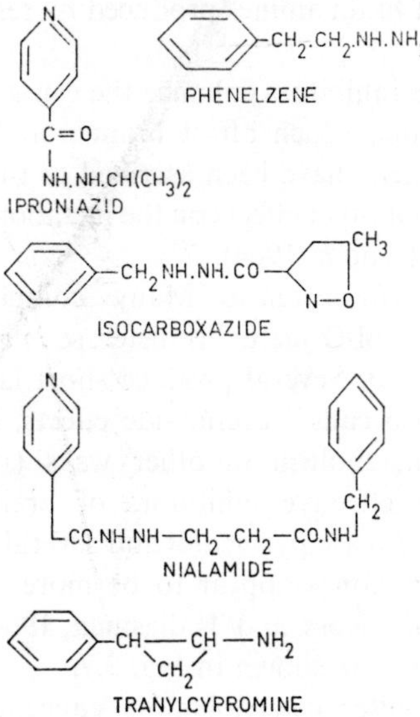

FIG. 3.6. Some inhibitors of monoamine oxidase.

irreversible, non-competitive, inhibition of the enzyme *in vitro* and *in vivo* (this group includes many hydrazine derivatives related to iproniazid), and those which produce a short-lasting, reversible, competitive inhibition of the enzyme, such as the harmala alkaloids, harmine and harmaline.

Noradrenaline concentrations in the brains of some animals are increased by monoamine oxidase inhibitors (Glowinski and Baldessarini, 1966). These increases are usually paralleled by increases in the concentrations of normetanephrine, dopamine and 5-hydroxytryptamine, although in the cat brain, 5-hydroxytryptamine concentrations increase whilst the noradrenaline levels remain unchanged (Glowinski and Baldessarini, 1966). The marked increase of normetanephrine, which follows monoamine oxidase inhibition in some species, indicates the importance of the extra-neuronal catechol-O-methyltransferase pathway in disposing of nor-adrenaline.

Monoamine oxidase inhibition enhances the central stimulation and elevations of brain catecholamine concentrations produced by precursors (Weil-Malherbe *et al.*, 1961). They reverse the central depression and reduce the depleting effects of brain amines produced by reserpine (Spector *et al.*, 1960).

Monoamine oxidase inhibitors enhance the central stimulant actions of drugs like amphetamine, which affect brain noradrenaline metabolism. Some of these phenomena have been ascribed to the inhibition of mono-amine oxidase alone, but other effects on the metabolism of catecholamines may also be involved (Kopin, 1964).

(b) *Catechol-O-methyltransferase.* Many compounds, with various structures, inhibit catechol-O-methyl transferase *in vitro*, but only a few of these are effective *in vivo*. Several produce short lasting effects on brain O-methylation, but also cause several side effects, including interference with noradrenaline metabolism in other ways (Ross and Haljasmaa, 1964a, b). The most effective inhibitors of brain catechol-O-methyl-transferase activity *in vivo* are pyrogallol and several dopacetamide deriva-tives, whereas the tropolones appear to be more effective in peripheral tissues (Carlsson, 1963; Ross and Haljasmaa, 1964b). The structures of some of these inhibitors are shown in Fig. 3.7.

Pyrogallol fails to alter catecholamine concentrations in the brain (Weil-Malherbe *et al.*, 1961), except after direct administration into the lateral ventricle of the rabbit brain (Matsuoka *et al.*, 1962). Dopacetamide derivatives have been reported to decrease the amount of normetane-phrine and 3-methoxytryamine in mouse brain (Carlsson, Corrodi and Waldeck, 1963). A tropolone-acetamide which did not affect the accumu-lation of exogenous noradrenaline in rat brain, markedly reduced the formation of normetanephrine (Glowinski and Axelrod, 1965). The dopacetamides increase the accumulation of dopamine and noradrenaline in the brain after administration of catecholamine precursors and potentiate their central excitant effects (Carlsson, 1964).

After the administration of dopa, pyrogallol enhances the accumulation of brain dopamine, but has no effect on the accumulation of noradrenaline (Weil-Malherbe *et al.*, 1961).

9. *Effect of Adrenergic Drugs on Presynaptic Noradrenaline*

Drugs that affect the adrenergic nervous system may exert their actions by interfering with the uptake across the neuronal membrane, the storage

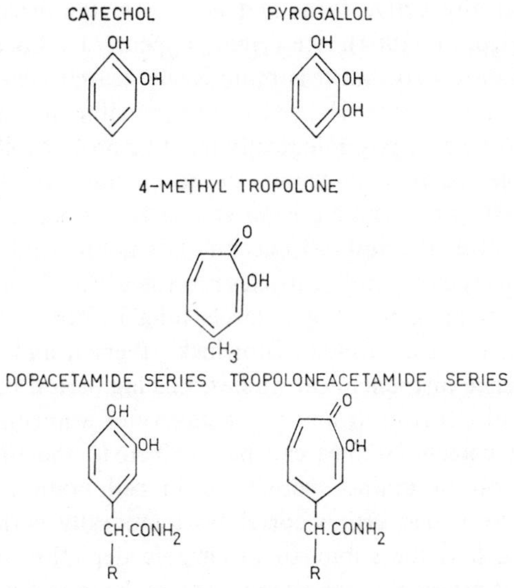

CATECHOL

PYROGALLOL

4-METHYL TROPOLONE

DOPACETAMIDE SERIES   TROPOLONEACETAMIDE SERIES

3.7. Some inhibitors of catechol-O-methyltransferase.

in the vesicles within the neurone, or the release of noradrenaline. Drugs such as cocaine, imipramine and sympathomimetic amines prevent the entry of noradrenaline into the noradrenergic neurone (Hertting, Axelrod and Whitby, 1961). Thus, these drugs increase the response to exogenous catecholamines by interfering with their inactivation by uptake into terminals, allowing more of the agent to react with the postsynaptic receptors. The supersensitivity resulting from chronic denervation of sympathetic nerves may be explained in part by the same mechanism.

Sympathomimetic amines, such as tyramine and amphetamine, release bound noradrenaline from the storage vesicles (Potter and Axelrod, 1963). Certain drugs, such as reserpine and tetrabenazine abolish the ability of the storage vesicle to bind noradrenaline (Holzbauer and Vogt, 1956; Pletscher, Brossi and Gey, 1962), resulting in a marked depletion of the stores of noradrenaline in the tissues. Though both sympathomimetic amines and reserpine reduce the content of catecholamines in tissues, they appear to do so by different mechanisms. The sympathomimetic amine, tyramine, rapidly releases noradrenaline so that it leaves the nerve terminal in a physiologically active form and is then metabolized mainly by O-methylation (Kopin, 1964). Reserpine appears to liberate the stored noradrenaline slowly so that it is more easily deaminated by monoamine oxidase within the neurone. Hence the noradrenaline released by reserpine leaves the neurone as a physiologically inactive product. Reserpine causes a marked depletion of endogenous noradrenaline in the brain. Studies with H^3 labelled noradrenaline have shown that uptake is depressed by reserpine. However, the ability to accumulate noradrenaline administered by injection into the cerebral ventricles returns within 24 hr after reserpine treatment and is back to normal levels long before endogenous amine levels have been re-established (Glowinski, Iversen and Axelrod, 1966). From fluorescence histochemical studies, this lag period between recovery from behavioral depression and the recovery of a normal intraneuronal distribution of catecholamines can be ascribed to the time required for axonal migration of amine, synthesized in cell bodies. The reserpine-induced behavioral depression correlates temporally with this period of reduced uptake and the submaximal chronic depletion of brain amines with reserpine is relatively asymptomatic after the initial effect (Häggendal and Lindqvist, 1964).

The storage vesicles bind not only noradrenaline, but other related compounds as well. For example, adrenaline, octopamine (β-hydroxylated tyramine) and several β-hydroxylated phenylethylamine derivatives can displace noradrenaline in the storage granules. Nerve stimulation can liberate these compounds so that they serve as false neurotransmitters (Rosell, Axelrod and Kopin, 1964; Kopin et al., 1965; Kopin, 1968). Certain drugs may also prevent the release of noradrenaline from the nerve. Examples of these compounds are guanethidine and bretylium (Hertting, Axelrod and Patrick, 1962).

Drugs used clinically as antidepressant substances, such as imipramine, desmethylimipramine and amitriptyline, interfere with the uptake of noradrenaline across the central adrenergic neural membrane (Glowinski and Axelrod, 1966). The antidepressant drugs may act clinically by preventing the re-uptake of released neurotransmitter, with a consequent increase in the amount of noradrenaline available to react with the adrenergic receptors. Imipramine and chlorpromazine have also been found to slow the spontaneous release of noradrenaline by neurones in the brain (Glowinski and Axelrod, 1966). Amphetamine has many actions on noradrenaline in the brain. Like imipramine, it blocks the uptake of noradrenaline across the neuronal membrane. It also releases bound noradrenaline in a physiologically active form and has been shown to inhibit monoamine oxidase in the brain (Glowinski, Axelrod and Iversen, 1966). Neither amphetamine nor imipramine have any effect on the uptake of dopamine by central adrenergic neurones (Glowinski et al., 1966).

The possible sites of action of drugs which interfere with transmission at adrenergic nerve terminals are summarized in Fig. 3.8.

B. DISTRIBUTION, BIOSYNTHESIS AND METABOLISM OF 5-HYDROXYTRYPTAMINE

Interest in the distribution and biochemistry of 5-hydroxytryptamine has been stimulated by the expectation that it may function as a synaptic transmitter in the central nervous system. This suggestion was originally based on the presence of 5-hydroxytryptamine in the brain (Amin, Crawford and Gaddum, 1954), and on the ability of several compounds, which are structurally related to 5-hydroxytryptamine and which block its action on smooth muscle, to influence mental activity (Gaddum, 1957; Woolley and Shaw, 1957). The ability of certain tranquillizing drugs to reduce the amounts of the amine in brain also suggested an involvement in neural processes (Pletscher, Shore and Brodie, 1956).

1. Distribution

The occurrence of 5-hydroxytryptamine in the central nervous system was first demonstrated by Tawarog and Page (1953) and Amin et al. (1954) and has since been confirmed by numerous researchers. The highest concentrations occur in the hypothalamus and amygdala, with progressively lower levels in the midbrain, pyriform cortex, hippocampus, thalamus,

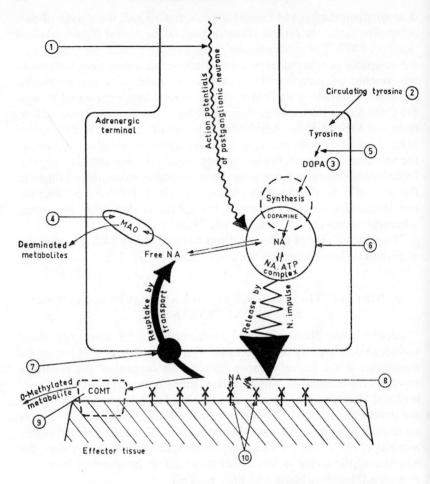

Fig. 3.8. A schematic representation of the sequence of events leading to noradrenaline release from a sympathetic nerve terminal and the ways in which various drugs can interfere with this sequence. Possible sites of action of drugs interfering with adrenergic mechanisms.

(1) Action potentials propagate to the terminals of sympathetic post-ganglionic neurones. Propagation in terminal regions may be blocked by adrenergic neurone-blocking drugs such as bretylium and guanethidine. Propagation may also be blocked at the synapse between pre- and postganglionic neurones by ganglion blocking drugs such as pempidine and chlorisondamine.

(2) Circulating tyrosine is the probable precursor used by adrenergic terminals for the biosynthesis of noradrenaline, circulating tyrosine enters the

brain stem, caudate nucleus (Table 4). Lower concentrations occur in the cerebral cortex, cerebellum and spinal cord.

The distribution of 5-hydroxytryptamine has been studied at the cellular level with fluorescence microscopy. By means of pretreatment of animals with monoamine oxidase inhibitors, it has been possible to establish the existence of ascending 5-hydroxytryptamine-containing fibres to the diencephalon and telencephalon (Dahlström and Fuxe, 1964). These fibres emanate mainly from the amine-containing nerve cells in the brain stem (nucleus raphé dorsalis and nucleus raphé medianus of the mesencephalon) and probably also from the amine-containing cells of the mesencephalic reticular formation (Fig. 3.1). In the rat, most of these fibres enter the medial forebrain bundle and terminate in the diencephalon and telencephalon (Fig. 3.2).

The techniques of axotomy, lesioning and drug-induced alterations in

---

adrenergic terminal possibly by a carrier-mediated transport process (?) Structurally related drugs such a α-methyl-*m*-tyrosine can take the place of tyrosine and be converted by the biosynthetic process into false adrenergic neurotransmitters.

(3) False neurotransmitters can also be synthesized from drugs which are related to other intermediates in noradrenaline biosynthesis, for instance α-methyl DOPA can take the place of DOPA.

(4) Free noradrenaline in the axoplasm is destroyed by monoamine oxidase, situated in intraneuronal mitochondria. This enzyme can be inhibited by a wide range of MAO inhibitors such as pheniprazine, nialamide or iproniazid.

(5) The rate-limiting step in noradrenaline biosynthesis, tyrosine hydroxlase, can be inhibited by drugs such as α-methyl-*p*-tyrosine or 3-iodotyrosine.

(6) The storage of noradrenaline in intraneuronal storage particles is prevented by drugs such as reserpine.

(7) The re-uptake of noradrenaline released by nerve impulses is effected by a membrane transport process which can be inhibited by many drugs, including cocaine, desipramine and many sympathomimetic amines.

(8) Many drugs can also be taken up into the adrenergic neurone by acting as substrates for this transport process. Once inside the neurone, drugs may displace noradrenaline from intraneuronal stores (indirect acting sympathomimetics), and may further take the place of noradrenaline by acting as false neurotransmitters (metaraminol, octopamine, α-methyl noradrenaline).

(9) The extraneuronal metabolism of noradrenaline by catechol-O-methyl transferase can be inhibited by pyrogallol and tropolones.

(10) The interaction of noradrenaline with α- and β-adrenergic receptors blocked by receptor blocking drugs such as phenoxybenzamine, phentolamine, DCI and pronethalol. The actions of noradrenaline on adrenergic receptors can be mimicked by direct-acting sympathomimetic amines such as adrenaline or synephrine (Iversen, 1967).

monoamine metabolism, described in the preceding section on catecholamines, have been extensively employed in these investigations into the distribution of 5-hydroxytryptaminergic pathways. After removal of large areas of the neocortex, the non-terminal parts of the fluorescent axons innervating the neocortex can be visualized and traced back to the medial forebrain bundle (Andén *et al.*, 1966). Lesions of the medial forebrain bundle of the rat (Heller, Harvey and Moore, 1962; Heller and Moore, 1965; Andén *et al.*, 1966) or in the lateral hypothalamus of the cat (Moore, Wong and Heller, 1965) cause a reduction of the 5-hydroxytryptamine content of the neocortex with an associated reduction in the level of non-specific decarboxylase (Andén *et al.*, 1966; Heller, Seiden, Porcher and Moore, 1966). Brain stem lesions in the ventromedial tegmental area of the upper pons and midbrain may cause a complete depletion of 5-hydroxytryptamine (and dopamine) in the corresponding striatum of the cat and monkey (Pourier *et al.*, 1967; Pourier and Sourkes, 1965).

TABLE 4.

DISTRIBUTION OF 5-HYDROXYTRYPTAMINE IN THE CENTRAL NERVOUS SYSTEM

Tissue	5-Hydroxytryptamine content (μg/g fresh tissue)	
	Dog[a]	Cat[b]
Spinal cord	0·26	0·37–0·82
Medulla	0·55–0·62	0·55–1·2
Pons	0·38–0·42	0·33–0·7
Cerebellum	0·07–0·09	0·2–0·3
Inferior colliculus		0·76
Midbrain	0·97–1·0	1·23–1·7
Hippocampus	0·25–0·64	0·71
Thalamus	0·65	0·43–1·09
Hypothalamus	0·37–1·75	1·78–2·49
Caudate nucleus	0·27–0·72	1·6–2·50
Cerebral cortex	0·17	0·21–0·69
Olfactory bulb	0·38	—

[a] Figures from Bogdanski, Weissbach and Udenfriend (1957); Paasonen, Maclean and Giarman (1957).

[b] Figures from Anderson and Cudia (1962); Bogdanski, Weissbach and Udenfriend (1957); Kuntzman, Shore, Bogdanski and Brodie (1961); McGeer, McGeer and Wada (1963).

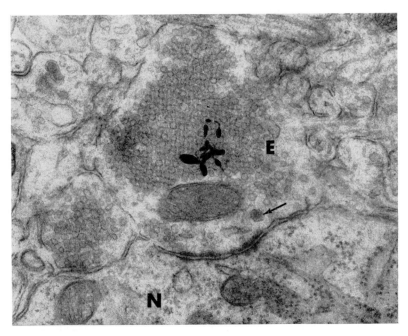

FIG. 3.9. Autoradiographic localization of tritiated 5-hydroxytryptamine in a nerve ending in the rat hypothalamus ($\times$ 50,000). The nerve ending shown forms a synaptic junction with a neuron cell body (N). A large dense-core vesicle (arrow) is seen near the synapse. The grains of silver produced by *beta* particles from the tritium are over a centrally situated clump of vesicles (Aghajanian and Bloom, 1967).

Few monoamine-containing nerve cell bodies have been detected in or rostral to the medial forebrain bundle in the rat, even after treatment with monoamine oxidase inhibitors or monoamine precursors (Andén et al., 1966).

Light and electron microscopic autoradiographic studies have been used to investigate the distribution and intracellular localization of intraventricularly administered tritiated 5-hydroxytryptamine (Aghajanian and Bloom, 1967b). Among the paraventricular regions examined (caudate nucleus, septum, amygdala, hypothalamus and midbrain central gray), the central gray was found to have the most intense autoradiographic activity after intraventricular administration of H^3-5-hydroxytryptamine. The activity in this area was predominantly in nerve endings and unmyelinated axons (Fig. 3.9).

In the spinal cord, 5-hydroxytryptamine is found in the gray matter, with much lower concentrations in white matter (Carlsson et al., 1963; Andén, 1965; Anderson and Holgerson, 1966). Histochemical and degeneration studies indicate that the amine is localized in descending nerve fibres from the brain stem reticular formation (Carlsson, Magnusson and Rosengren, 1963; Carlsson, Falck, Fuxe and Hillarp, 1964; Andén, Häggendal, Magnusson and Rosengren, 1964; Dahlström and Fuxe, 1965).

2. Sub-cellular Distribution

The intracellular localization of 5-hydroxytryptamine has been studied by differential centrifugation. The initial experiments (Whittaker, 1958) showed that 5-hydroxytryptamine was present in the synaptosome particulate fraction of the guinea-pig brain. The binding of 5-hydroxytryptamine appeared to be particularly labile, as a relatively high percentage of the amine was recovered in the supernatant fraction. Later experiments (Potter and Axelrod, 1962; Michaelson and Whittaker, 1963) confirmed the lability of the binding of this amine. Subcellular distributions similar to those reported for the guinea-pig brain have been found for dog caudate nucleus and hypothalamus (Laverty et al., 1963), rat brain stem (Levi and Maynert, 1964). Whittaker's experiments have been criticized by Kataoka (1962) and Inouye, Kataoka and Shinagawa (1963) on the grounds that the extraction technique did not eliminate substance P or other active polypeptides. The assay system (rat fundus strip) employed by Whittaker, is, however, insensitive to substance P.

Some workers (Zieher and De Robertis, 1963; Carlini and Green, 1963b; Ryall, 1964) have claimed that the microsomal fraction contains considerable amounts of 5-hydroxytryptamine. Whittaker (1965) attributes this result to contamination of the microsomal fraction by synaptosomes. Attempts have been made to separate the 5-hydroxytryptamine-containing particles from those containing acetylcholine by means of density gradients (Michaelson and Whittaker, 1963; Zieher and De Robertis, 1963). Although some evidence of separation was obtained, the overlap between the two types of particle was complete.

3. Synthesis

The steps in the synthesis of 5-hydroxytryptamine from tryptophan are presented in Fig. 3.10. The precursors and enzymes required for 5-hydroxytryptamine are present in the brain. Tryptophan is normally present in the brain (Tallan *et al.*, 1954). Until 1965, little was known of the enzyme that catalyzes the hydroxylation of tryptophan in normal mammalian tissues. Renson, Weissbach and Udenfriend (1962) had suggested that, although the phenylalanine hydroxylase of liver is capable of hydroxylating tryptophan, this enzyme is not responsible for the bulk of 5-hydroxyindoles produced *in vivo*. Grahame-Smith (1964) reported that tryptophan hydroxylase occurred in brain but at a low level of activity and Gal, Morgan, Chatterje and Marshall (1964) suggested that the rate of tryptophan hydroxylation in brain is too low to account for its 5-hydroxytryptamine content. However, with more sensitive methods of assaying enzymic activity, Jéquier, Lovenberg and Sjoerdsma (1967) were able to show a sufficiently high level of activity in rat brain stem to account for the 5-hydroxytryptamine levels in the brain. Conversion of tryptophan to 5-hydroxytryptophan appears to be the rate-limiting step in the synthesis of 5-hydroxytryptamine in the brain (Jéquier *et al.*, 1967). These authors concluded that the inhibition of tryptophan hydroxylase by *p*-chlorophenylalanine can be correlated with and is responsible for the depletion of brain 5-hydroxytryptamine that follows the administration of this compound. These findings extended those of Koe and Weissman (1966) who showed that *p*-chlorophenylalanine is a specific depletor of brain 5-hydroxytryptophan in mice, rats and dogs. However, although *p*-chlorophenylalanine does not affect 5-hydroxytryptophan decarboxylase activity, it reduces the increase in brain 5-hydroxytryptamine after 5-

hydroxytryptophan administration, suggesting that it may also suppress access of the precursor to its metabolic site (Koe and Weissmann, 1966).

5-hydroxytryptophan is readily decarboxylated to 5-hydroxytryptamine and has been difficult to detect in tissues (Hagen and Cohen, 1966), unless a prior administration of exogenous 5-hydroxytryptophan is given (Udenfriend, Weissbach and Bogdanski, 1957). Decarboxylation of 5-hydroxytryptophan to 5-hydroxytryptamine occurs throughout the brain.

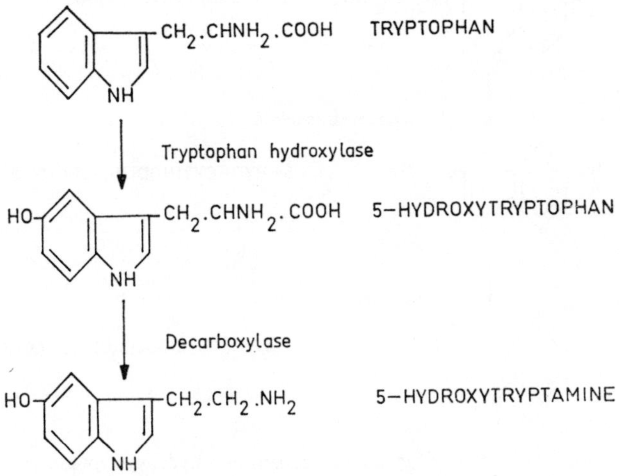

FIG. 3.10. Biosynthetic pathway for 5-hydroxytryptamine.

5-Hydroxytryptophan decarboxylase, discovered by Udenfriend, Clark and Titus in 1953, has since been shown to be identical with dopa decarboxylase, which catalyzes the conversion of dopa into dopamine (Hagen and Cohen, 1966). Its distribution and intracellular localization have been discussed in the preceding section.

4. *Metabolism*

Oxidative deamination by monoamine oxidase is the main pathway of 5-hydroxytryptamine breakdown in both nervous and non-nervous tissues (Blaschko and Levine, 1966). The two stages in this reaction are presented in Fig. 3.11. 5-Hydroxyindoleacetic acid is excreted in the urine.

Not all 5-hydroxytryptamine is destroyed by oxidation. For example, in the pineal gland 5-hydroxytryptamine is N-acetylated and O-methylated to melatonin (Axelrod and Weissbach, 1960, 1961). Studies on intact mice have shown that, although monoamine oxidase inhibition prevents the formation of 5-hydroxyindoleacetic acid, 5-hydroxytryptamine is metabolized to form 5-hydroxytryptamine-O-glucuronide (Weissbach, Lovenberg,

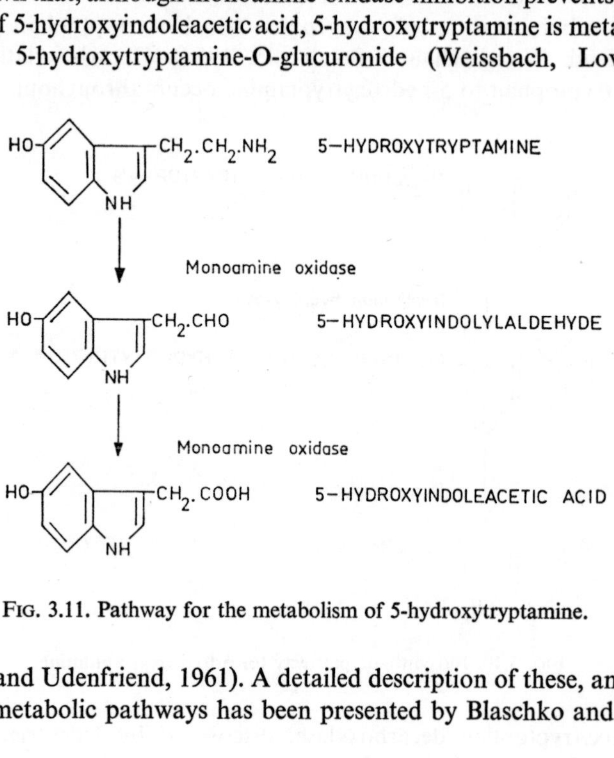

HO—⟨indole⟩—$CH_2.CH_2.NH_2$ 5—HYDROXYTRYPTAMINE

↓ Monoamine oxidase

HO—⟨indole⟩—$CH_2.CHO$ 5—HYDROXYINDOLYLALDEHYDE

↓ Monoamine oxidase

HO—⟨indole⟩—$CH_2.COOH$ 5—HYDROXYINDOLEACETIC ACID

FIG. 3.11. Pathway for the metabolism of 5-hydroxytryptamine.

Redfield and Udenfriend, 1961). A detailed description of these, and other possible metabolic pathways has been presented by Blaschko and Levine (1966).

5. *Uptake*

Uptake of labelled 5-hydroxytryptamine by the rat brain after intraventricular injection has been studied by Palaič, Page and Khairallah (1967). The exogenous amine was found to have a comparable distribution to endogenous amine, with 35% in the supernatant and 65% in the particulate fraction after high speed centrifugation of brain homogenate. Ouabain, noradrenaline and reserpine, but not desmethylimipramine, significantly decreased 5-hydroxytryptamine uptake, suggesting the presence of an active transport process. Noradrenaline may interfere with the storage and metabolism of 5-hydroxytryptamine by occupying similar uptake and storage sites.

Some studies have indicated that uptake and storage of biogenic amines are not highly specific processes, but are common to many amines (Jonasson, Rosengren and Waldeck, 1964; Musacchio, Kopin and Weise, 1965). According to Giachetti and Shore (1966), a dual uptake mechanism exists for a variety of amines. Firstly, a non-specific mechanism at the cell membrane which can be blocked by several drugs (cocaine, ouabain, imipramine) and secondly, a highly specific mechanism, probably localized at the level of synaptic vesicles, which is blocked by reserpine.

6. *Reserpine and 5-Hydroxytryptamine*

The way in which the tranquilizing drug, reserpine, produces sedation is still in dispute. Most investigators believe that the sedation is in some way connected with the release of brain amines by the drug, but they disagree on which amine is the most critical. The view presently in greater favour is that reserpine acts by depleting dopamine and noradrenaline.

However, Brodie and his colleagues (Brodie *et al.*, 1960; Brodie, Comer, Costa and Dlabac, 1966) have concluded that reserpine's action depends primarily on its release of 5-hydroxytryptamine from storage granules in brain neurones. According to this view, reserpine causes newly-synthesized 5-hydroxytryptamine to persist in a free form; this free amine then stimulates postsynaptic sites which serve parasympathetic and behavioural depressant functions. However in *p*-chlorophenylalanine treated animals, which lack the ability to synthesize 5-hydroxytryptamine, reserpine continues to have a sedative action (Koe and Weissman, 1966). It is therefore unlikely that the primary effect of reserpine is on 5-hydroxytryptamine.

As well as its action on catecholamines and 5-hydroxytryptamine, reserpine has been found to produce decreases in γ-aminobutyric acid and histamine and an increase in brain acetylcholine (Carlsson, 1966).

Tetrabenazine and certain other benzoquinolizines also cause a reserpine-like sedation and depress 5-hydroxytryptamine and noradrenaline levels in brain (Pletscher *et al.*, 1962).

C. HISTAMINE IN THE BRAIN

In comparison with the catecholamines and 5-hydroxytryptamine, relatively little exploration of histamine in the nervous system has been done, but the available evidence tends to show that there are several similarities between all these substances as regards their distribution and general pattern of metabolism in the brain. Recent reviews on histamine include those of Green (1964) and Kahlson and Rosengren (1965). *The Handbook of Experimental Pharmacology* series, volume 18, is devoted to histamine and anti-histaminics.

1. *Distribution in the Central Nervous System*

The presence of histamine in various areas of the feline central nervous system was initially described by Kwiatkowski (1943) and most of these original findings have been confirmed by subsequent investigators (Harris, Jacobson and Kahlson, 1952; Crossland, 1960; Adam, 1961; McGeer, 1964; White 1966). The detailed investigations of Adam (1961) and McGeer (1964) in the canine, feline and human brains have expanded the original findings and clarified the distribution of histamine in the brain (Table 5). Histamine is concentrated in some regions of the brain stem, including the hypothalamus and median eminence. In contrast to Kwiatowski (1943), Harris *et al.* (1952) and Crossland (1961) were unable to detect histamine in the cerebellum.

Non-neural structures in the brain such as the posterior lobe and stalk of the hypophysis, area postrema, choroid plexus (Adam, 1961) and pineal body (Giarman and Day, 1958) contain histamine, but in some of these structures the histamine may be confined to mast cells (Adam, 1961). Neural tissue in the brain does not contain mast cells (Riley, 1959; Adam, 1961).

Reports on the subcellular distribution of histamine in brain tissue agree that most of the histamine is particle-bound, but the reports are at variance regarding the kind of particle with which the histamine is associated (Carlini and Green, 1963b, c; Michaelson and Dowe, 1963). Bioassay of histamine in subcellular fractions showed that most of the particle-bound histamine was in the small particle fraction (Carlini and Green, 1963b), whereas the fluorimetric technique demonstrated that most of the histamine was in the larger nuclear and mitochondrial fractions (Michaelson and Dowe, 1963). This conflict has been resolved in more recent reports on the subcellular distribution of histamine in which it has been demonstrated that the amine is present in the nerve terminal and synaptic vesicle fractions of homogenates of dog thalamus and hypothalamus (Michaelson and

TABLE 5.

DISTRIBUTION OF HISTAMINE IN THE CENTRAL NERVOUS SYSTEM

Tissue	Histamine content (μg/g fresh tissue)	
	Dog[a]	Cat[b]
Spinal cord	0·04	0·3
Medulla	0·015–0·04	0·5
Pons	<0·1	0·4
Cerebellum	0·05	0·2
Inferior colliculus	0·2	}0·3
Superior colliculus	0·22	
Midbrain	0·22	0·6
Lateral geniculate nucleus	0·14	—
Medial geniculate nucleus	0·27	—
Hippocampus	0·08	—
Thalamus	0·24	0·5
Hypothalamus	0·46–0·90	1·25
Caudate nucleus	0·14	0·5
Cerebral cortex	0·07	0·3–0·4
Olfactory bulb	0·05	—

[a] Figures from Adam (1961).
[b] Figures from McGeer (1964).

Coffman, 1967) and rat brain and cerebral cortex (Snyder, Glowinski and Axelrod, 1966; Katoaka and De Robertis, 1967).

The retention of H[3]-histamine in rat brain after intraventricular administration has been studied by Snyder et al. (1966). Histamine disappeared from the rat brain in a multiphasic fashion, with a half-life of 1·6 hr during the first 6 hr and a half-life of 11 hr from 6 to 24 hr. By contrast, 40 min after intraventricular perfusion of the feline brain by C[14]-histamine, only 0·5% of the perfused amine had been retained (White, 1960).

The effects of psychotropic drugs on brain histamine levels have been studied by several groups (Green and Erickson, 1964; Adam and Hye, 1964, 1966; Snyder et al., 1966; White, 1966). Adam and Hye (1964, 1966) have reported on the effects of reserpine, the compound 48/80 and chlorpromazine on brain histamine in cats. They showed that 48/80 lowered the histamine concentration in the pituitary and hypophyseal stalk (where the amine is present in mast cells) but not in the hypothalamus and thalamus. Reserpine lowered the histamine content in the hypothalamus and thalamus, but not in the pituitary. High doses of chlorpromazine raise the concentration of histamine in the feline brain.

2. Synthesis and Metabolism

Histamine can be synthesized from its precursor, histidine, in the brain *in vivo* (Fig. 3.12) (White 1960; Jonson and White, 1964). There is a reasonable correlation between the distribution of histamine and the distribution of its synthesizing enzyme, histidine decarboxylase, in the

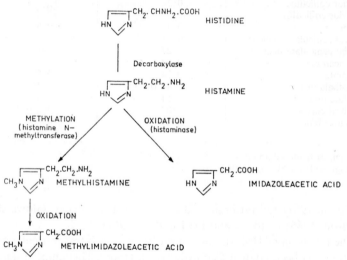

FIG. 3.12. Pathways for the synthesis and degradation of histamine.

brain (White 1959). In regions where this correlation fails, such as the area postrema, which is rich in histamine but poor in histidine decarboxylase activity, histamine may be concentrated from the blood (Green, 1964). The histidine decarboxylase in the brain appears to be the same enzyme that decarboxylates 5-hydroxytryptophan and dopa (Green, 1964) and is inhibited by α-methyldopa (Werle, 1961). The decarboxylating activity in mast cells is apparently due to a different enzyme (Weissbach, Lovenberg and Udenfriend, 1961).

The mammalian brain contains the two enzymes which have been implicated in the metabolism of histamine (Fig. 3.12) (Schayer, 1959).

Histamine-N-methyltransferase is widely distributed in the brain, and in the presence of S-adenosyl-methionine (Brown, Tomchick and Axelrod, 1959) converts histamine into methylhistamine. Formation of methylhistamine and its oxidation product, methylimidazoleacetic acid, from histamine has been demonstrated in several areas of the feline brain (Axelrod, MacLean, Albers and Weissbach, 1961; Wurtman, Axelrod and Barchus, 1964). The methylation of histamine can be regarded as the major route of inactivation of histamine in the feline brain, as significant amounts of labelled imidazoleacetic acid were not detected. The major metabolite of histamine in rat brain, however, appears to be imidazoleacetic acid (Snyder et al., 1966), and only small amounts of H^3-methylhistamine were formed. This is in accordance with the relatively low levels of histamine-N-methyltransferase which occur in the rat brain in comparison with the feline brain (Brown et al., 1959). It is possible that the active methylating enzyme in the feline brain competes with the binding of histamine, for 40 min after ventricular perfusion of the cat brain with C^{14}-histamine, only $0 \cdot 5\%$ of the perfused amine was retained in the brain (White, 1960). Robinson and Green (1964) have also detected the formation of imidazoleacetic acid riboside or ribotide as metabolites of C^{14}-histamine in rat brain.

The disappearance of H^3-histamine from rat brain is retarded by pretreatment with β-phenylisopropylhydrazine, a monoamine oxidase inhibitor, but not by aminoguanidine, an inhibitor of diamine oxidase (Snyder et al., 1966). This finding suggests that H^3-histamine in rat brain is metabolized predominantly by monoamine oxidase. However, β-phenylisopropylhydrazine may also inhibit diamine oxidase (Shore and Cohn, 1960). Histamine methylation is inhibited both in vivo and in vitro by chlorpromazine, 5-hydroxytryptamine and bufotenine (Green, 1964). Methylhistamine is oxidatively deaminated by monoamine oxidase, as a consequence of which, inhibitors of this enzyme cause an increase in the excretion of methylhistamine (Green, 1964). It is likely, therefore, that the psychotropic monoamine oxidase inhibitors would increase the brain levels of methylhistamine.

CONCLUSIONS

1. The recent development of fluorescent histochemical techniques has contributed to a rapid advance in the elucidation of the roles of dopamine,

noradrenaline and 5-hydroxytryptamine in the central nervous system. A schematic outline of the major monoaminergic pathways in the brain and spinal cord is presented in Fig. 3.2.

2. In comparison with the catecholamines and 5-hydroxytryptamine, relatively little is known about histaminergic pathways in the brain.

3. The distribution of these monoamines in the brain is comparable in many respects, for example, they are concentrated in the brain stem and hypothalamus. Studies on the intracellular localization of the monoamines by differential centrifugation reveal that they are associated with the synaptic vesicle fractions.

4. Noradrenaline is synthesized from tyrosine; dihydroxyphenylanine (dopa) and dopamine being intermediaries in the biosynthetic pathway (Fig. 3.3). Conversion of tyrosine to dopa by the enzyme tyrosine hydroxylase appears to be the rate-limiting step in this pathway. The pathways for noradrenaline metabolism are illustrated in Fig. 3.4. Dopamine is metabolized to homovanillic acid (Fig. 3.5).

5. 5-Hydroxytryptamine is synthesized from tryptophan, with 5-hydroxytryptophan as an intermediary (Fig. 3.10) and metabolized to 5-hydroxyindoleacetic acid (Fig. 3.11).

6. Histamine is synthesized from histidine and metabolized to methylimidazoleacetic and imidazoleacetic acids (Fig. 3.12).

7. The decarboxylating enzymes which convert the precursor amino acids, dopa, 5-hydroxytryptophan and histidine, into dopamine, 5-hydroxytryptamine and histamine, appear to be identical. There is evidence that the various monoamines and their precursors may be taken up by neurones which normally do not release them. The possibility therefore arises that administration of a particular precursor, for example dopa, may result in the release of dopamine from 5-hydroxytryptaminergic or histaminergic neurones. Examples of the release of "false transmitters", for example octopamine, from adrenergic nerve terminals are discussed.

8. The enzyme, monoamine oxidase, is involved in the degradation of all these monoamines, and drugs which reduce its activity potentiate their actions.

9. The pharmacology of the adrenergic neurone is discussed in detail. Relatively less information is available concerning 5-hydroxytryptaminergic and histaminergic systems.

CHAPTER 4

NEUROMUSCULAR TRANSMISSION IN VERTEBRATES: THE SKELETAL NEUROMUSCULAR JUNCTION

THIS synapse has afforded unusual opportunities for the study of the electrophysiological, biochemical and ionic factors controlling the release and action of transmitter substances. As the most firmly established example of a chemically transmitting synapse, it has served as a model for the investigation of synapses in the autonomic and central nervous system.

A. ACETYLCHOLINE RELEASE

The release of acetylcholine from motor axon terminals and cholinergic transmission at the neuromuscular junction has been accepted since the classical experiments of Dale and his colleagues (Dale, Feldberg and Vogt, 1936; Brown, Dale and Feldberg, 1936) which demonstrated a release of acetylcholine during motor axon stimulation and showed that acetylcholine would mimic the actions of the synaptically released transmitter. Potentiation of the effects of nerve stimulation by anticholinesterases and block by curare were also demonstrated (Brown *et al.*, 1936; Bacq and Brown, 1937).

More recently there have been investigations designed to give a quantitative measure of the output of acetylcholine by a single impulse at a motor synapse and to relate this to the amount of acetylcholine required for the generation of an endplate potential. Values for the calculated mean release of acetylcholine per impulse from an average nerve ending have varied. Emmelin and MacIntosh (1956), using a frequency of stimulation of 20–25/sec, calculated a release per impulse per synapse of 5×10^{-17} g. At lower frequencies of stimulation Straughan (1960) obtained an output of $3 \cdot 5 \times 10^{-16}$ g/impulse and Krnjević and Mitchell (1961) an output of $1 \cdot 8 \times 10^{-15}$ g/impulse.

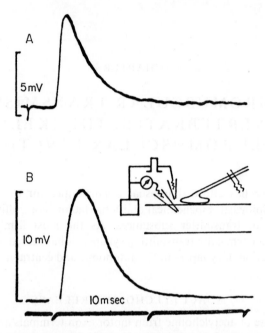

FIG. 4.1. A. Endplate potential evoked by stimulation of phrenic nerve in a rat diaphragm muscle fibre paralysed by 15·0 mM magnesium. B. Acetylcholine potential evoked in another fibre by a 1 msec pulse of current ($3\cdot5 \times 10^{-8}$ A) from an acetylcholine-filled micropipette in close proximity to an endplate (see inset diagram). Both potentials were recorded with an intracellular electrode situated adjacent to the junctional region (Krnjević and Miledi, 1958a).

A direct comparison between the liberation of acetylcholine and the amounts needed to excite a muscle has only recently become feasible. With the development of the iontophoretic method of drug application, it has been possible to apply minute quantities of acetylcholine in close proximity to a neuromuscular synapse, whose responses are registered with an intracellular microelectrode, as illustrated in Fig. 4.1 (Nastuk, 1953, 1959; del Castillo and Katz, 1955a, 1956, 1957a, b, c; Thesleff, 1958; Krnjević and Miledi, 1958a). Under optimal conditions, the acetylcholine emission produced by a very brief (0·1–1·0 msec) current causes a depolarization of the muscle fibre that has a time course almost as fast as the endplate potential produced by a nerve impulse (Krnjević and Miledi, 1958a). It has been calculated that $1 \cdot 8 \times 10^{-15}$ g of acetylcholine will reproduce endplate potentials in the rat diaphragm (Krnjević and Miledi, 1958a). This amount is comparable in order of magnitude with the mean ACh release from a phrenic nerve ending per impulse during activity (Krnjević and Mitchell, 1961).

There is, therefore, a surprisingly good agreement between the quantity of acetylcholine released in muscle and that needed for effective depolarization. Some intriguing possibilities concerning the origins of the acetylcholine released by muscles have arisen from experiments on resting and denervated muscle. One of the most important controls performed by Dale *et al.* (1936) was to show that acetylcholine is not obtained from a denervated muscle. More recently it has been claimed that even after denervation, acetylcholine can be released from muscle by direct stimulation (McIntyre, 1959; Hayes and Riker, 1963). According to the latter authors, normal and denervated rat diaphragms yield identical amounts of acetylcholine on stimulation. However, Mitchell and Silver (1963) and Krnjević and Straughan (1964) have shown that the mean release of acetylcholine in resting, denervated, rat diaphragm was one half of that in normal muscle. Moreover, Krnjević and Straughan (1964) and Bowman and Hemsworth (1965) reported that whilst direct stimulation of the normal right hemidiaphragm increased release fivefold; only a small increase was recorded in the case of the denervated hemidiaphragm. Krnjević and Straughan ascribed the release of acetylcholine in the resting, denervated muscle to Schwann cells and other cell remnants (Birks, Katz and Miledi, 1960).

Several authors have described a small but variable release of acetylcholine from resting muscle (Brooks, 1954; Straughan, 1960; Krnjević and Mitchell, 1961) and this spontaneous release has been analyzed in detail by Mitchell and Silver (1963). The resting output of acetylcholine has been given as $300-400 \times 10^{-12}$ g/min from the rat hemidiaphragm (Straughan, 1960; Mitchell and Silver, 1963). This is considerably larger than the value expected from the resting quantal release of acetylcholine that is responsible for the miniature endplate potentials. Presumably it arises, in part, from structures other than the nerve endings because after denervation it continues at about 50% of normal (Mitchell and Silver, 1963).

SOME ASPECTS OF THE PHARMACOLOGY OF
NEUROMUSCULAR TRANSMISSION

For neuromuscular transmission to take place, the nerve impulse must cause the release of an amount of transmitter sufficient to elicit a pro-pagated action potential in the muscle fibre. Normally the quantity liber-ated is more than adequate, there being a large safety margin for trans-mission. Consequently it is only when neuromuscular transmission has been depressed to such an extent that endplate potentials are only a little above or below fibre threshold, that transmission is particularly sensitive to changes in the amount of acetylcholine released. Under normal circum-stances, facilitation of the release process is devoid of effect and a relatively large inhibition of release is necessary before transmission becomes blocked.

1. *Substances which act Presynaptically*

Many agents have been shown to influence the release of transmitter from motor nerve terminals.

(a) *Calcium and magnesium.* Studies on the relationship between acetyl-choline release and calcium and magnesium have been conducted by assessing the effects of these ions on the quantal content of endplate potentials or the frequency of miniature endplate potentials. Presynaptic-ally the two ions oppose one another; either a high concentration of mag-nesium or a low concentration of calcium can block transmission and raising the calcium concentration antagonizes a block caused by mag-nesium. A reduction in the quantal content of the endplate potential has been shown to account for the transmission failure (Boyd and Martin, 1956; del Castillo and Katz, 1954a; del Castillo and Engbaek, 1954; Liley, 1956). A decrease in calcium or increase in magnesium in the perfusion fluid reduces the frequency of miniature endplate potentials in isolated rat diaphragm preparations (Fig. 4.2) (Hubbard, 1961), although some miniature endplate potentials can still be recorded in the absence of calcium (Hubbard, 1961; Hubbard, Jones and Landau, 1968).

Miniature endplate potentials have been detected even after treatment of rat diaphragm–phrenic nerve preparations with chelating agents, such as ethylenediamine tetraacetate (EDTA) (Hubbard *et al.*, 1968). Such activity has been attributed to residual free calcium ion in the solution.

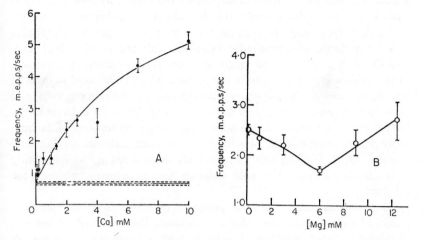

FIG. 4.2. Influence of calcium and magnesium concentrations on miniature endplate potential (m.e.p.p.) frequency in single fibres of rat diaphragm-phrenic nerve preparations. The osmotic pressure of all the solutions was corrected to approximately the same value by the addition of sucrose. The bars indicate ± 1 S.E. of the mean and both ordinate and abscissal scales are linear. A. Influence of [Ca] on m.e.p.p. frequency. The curve was derived from theoretical considerations of the relationship between [Ca] concentration and m.e.p.p. frequency and fitted to the points obtained experimentally. The horizontal line indicates the mean frequency in the presence of 10^{-5} M Ca and the dotted lines above and below this line indicate ± 1 S.E. of this mean value. B. Effect of [Mg] on m.e.p.p. frequency. M.e.p.p. frequency fell as [Mg] was raised from $0 \cdot 1$ to 6 mM and increased again as the [Mg] was raised to 12 mM. The normal levels of [Ca] and [Mg] in bathing solutions for muscle preparations are 2 and 1 mM respectively (Hubbard, Jones and Landau, 1968).

Interestingly enough, the addition of magnesium to calcium-depleted solutions caused an acceleration of miniature endplate potential frequency and the interactions between calcium and magnesium indicated that they competed for the same sites (Hubbard *et al.*, 1968).

Katz and Miledi (1965a, 1967) have applied calcium iontophoretically to frog motor nerve terminals bathed in high magnesium, low calcium media and demonstrated a rapid increase in the number of quantal components of the endplate potential. Calcium, therefore, appears to be an essential factor for the discharging of acetylcholine by nerve terminals. Related studies on the squid giant synapse have shown that electrophoretically applied calcium affects transmitter release only when applied extracellularly, whilst intracellular application is without effect (Miledi and Slater, 1966). A surface action of calcium and magnesium is therefore probable at the vertebrate neuromuscular junction. Hubbard *et al.* (1968) have postulated that calcium and magnesium compete for receptor sites on a carrier molecule X in the membrane surface, which is involved in quantal release, and modify its activity. Barium (Elmqvist and Feldman, 1965) and strontium (Miledi, 1966) appear to be able to substitute for calcium as cofactors in the release of acetylcholine. Higher concentrations of calcium depress transmitter release, possibly by inactivating molecule X (Gage and Quastel, 1966). Sodium ions competitively depress release by competing with calcium for association with molecule X or by reducing its affinity for calcium.

(b) *Botulinum toxin.* The toxin produced by *Clostridium botulinum* is a potent blocker of neuromuscular transmission. The action of the toxin is to inhibit transmitter release drastically, with a progressive reduction in endplate potential size until inhibition becomes complete (Burgen, Dickens and Zatman, 1949). Unlike magnesium, the toxin blocks the spontaneous release of acetylcholine quanta responsible for the generation of miniature endplate potentials (Brooks, 1956; Thesleff, 1960). The effect of the toxin can only partially be reversed by raising the calcium concentration. As there is no evidence that it affects the propagation of nerve impulses or the acetylcholine stores, the action of the toxin is presumably on the depolarization-release coupling system. From electron microscopic studies with ferritin-tagged toxin, it appears that the toxin molecules may mechanically obstruct the sites of quantal efflux of acetylcholine (Zacks, Metzger, Smith and Blumberg, 1962).

(c) *Hemicholiniums.* The drug hemicholinium-3 (HC-3), which was described by Schueler in 1955, has been shown to inhibit the synthesis of acetylcholine and block neuromuscular transmission (Schueler, 1960). Neuromuscular blockade by HC-3 is characteristically slow in onset and develops first at junctions which are stimulated repetitively. A progressive diminution in the size of endplate potentials and miniature endplate potentials occurs when nerves are stimulated in the presence of HC-3 (Elmqvist and Quastel, 1965). The change in quantum size is presumably related to depletion of the presynaptic acetylcholine store as a result of an inhibition of acetylcholine synthesis. Triethylcholine is a drug with pharmacological actions resembling those of HC-3 (Bowman and Rand,

1961; Bowman, Hemsworth and Rand, 1962). It produces a delayed neuro-muscular blockade, the onset and degree of which depends on the rate of nerve stimulation. Like HC-3, it has been shown to block acetylcholine synthesis (Bull and Hemsworth, 1963) and like HC-3, it causes a decline in the amplitude of endplate potentials due to a decreasing quantum content (Elmqvist and Quastel, 1965).

Like most quaternary ammonium compounds, HC-3 and triethylcholine depress the sensitivity of the endplate receptor to acetylcholine (Martin and Orkand, 1961; Thies and Brooks, 1961; Bowman et al., 1962). As Roberts (1962) blocked the response of isolated frog muscle to electrophoretically applied acetylcholine with triethylcholine but did not demonstrate a block of the response to indirect stimulation, it appears that the action of this compound in the frog may be predominantly curarimimetic.

(d) *Acetylcholine and anticholinesterases.* Released from the nerve terminal, acetylcholine classically activates transmission by its post-synaptic action. An additional action of acetylcholine on the nerve terminal was proposed by Masland and Wigton (1940) to account for the repetitive discharges in motor nerve fibres after injections of acetylcholine or prostigmine. They confirmed earlier findings (Langley and Kato, 1915; Feng and Li, 1941) that curare abolishes both these repetitive discharges and the associated muscle twitching in doses much lower than those required for blocking neuromuscular transmission. It was concluded that the nerve terminals are directly excited by acetylcholine and that anti-cholinesterases may excite nerve terminals secondarily, as a result of the accumulation of acetylcholine that occurs when cholinesterase is inhibited. Eccles, Katz and Kuffler (1942) showed that a repetitive discharge from motor endplates often occurs in the absence of any discharge from the nerve terminals and that the nerve discharge sometimes occurs at a time that precludes its initiation by muscle impulses. It was therefore proposed that, in the presence of anticholinesterases, acetylcholine liberated from the nerve terminals can generate impulses at both the motor endplate and the nerve terminals. The nerve impulses would also be likely to generate some of the later discharges from motor endplates. It was also shown that action potentials in the muscle could generate impulses ephaptically in the motor nerve fibres.

The detailed analyses of Werner (1960, 1961) and Barstad (1962) have demonstrated that the generation of impulses at motor nerve terminals can occur in two independent ways. By the use of varied criteria, Werner was able to distinguish the short latency, ephaptic, back response of Lloyd (1942) from the drug conditioned back response. Barstad (1962) demonstrated that the acetylcholine-induced antidromic discharges could still be detected when muscle fibres were so damaged (by cutting) that they could not develop action potentials.

These experiments did not provide conclusive evidence for a presynaptic action of acetylcholine, for it is known (Fatt and Katz, 1951; Takeuchi and Takeuchi, 1960a) that in generating the endplate potential, acetylcholine increases the extracellular potassium ion concentration in the synaptic cleft. Even in cut muscle fibres, this mechanism is still operative (Randić and Straughan, 1964). It has been suggested (Diamond, 1959; Katz, 1962) that, in the presence of anticholinesterases, this increase in extracellular potassium concentration might be large enough to depolarize the nerve terminals and thus generate a discharge.

The lack of unequivocal evidence for a direct action of acetylcholine in motor nerve terminals has not prevented speculation about the possible physiological significance of this action. Thus Riker, Werner, Roberts and Kuperman (1959) have argued that the presence of antidromic nerve discharges reveals the presence of a generator potential set up in the nerve terminals. The generator potential was thought to release acetylcholine from its bound state. This acetylcholine then reacted with further presynaptic receptors (Riker, Roberts, Standaert and Fujimori, 1957) to release still more acetylcholine, which then acted on the postsynaptic membrane (Koelle, 1962).

However Hubbard, Schmidt and Yokota (1965) have shown that acetylcholine applied electrophoretically at the neuromuscular junction does not increase the frequency of miniature endplate potentials or the quantal content of the endplate potential. In the presence of prostigmine, acetylcholine decreased the quantal content of the endplate potential but did not affect miniature endplate potential frequency. It was concluded that acetylcholine did not depolarize at the site of release of transmitter. To account for the reduction in threshold of the nerve terminal to cathodal stimulation, it was suggested that depolarization occurred at sites more proximal than the site of release of transmitter, presumably the nodes of Ranvier. The depolarization at this site would be insufficient to increase acetylcholine release but sufficient to lower the threshold. Endogenous acetylcholine released by nerve impulses would also be capable of action at this site, particularly in the presence of cholinesterase inhibitors, causing fasiculation and antidromic firing. Hubbard (1965) concluded that contrary to Koelle's (1962) hypothesis, acetylcholine does not appear to have any essential role in transmitter release at the neuromuscular junction.

2. Drugs Acting on the Subsynaptic Membrane

(a) *Acetylcholine*. The ionic permeabilities that are responsible for the currents generating the endplate potential have been studied in some detail. As Katz (1962) has pointed out, the reaction between excitatory transmitter and the membrane receptors has no regenerative link; the local conductance change produced by acetylcholine being independent of the level of membrane potential (Fatt and Katz, 1951; Takeuchi and Takeuchi, 1960a, b). The original "short-circuit" hypothesis of Fatt and Katz (1951) and del Castillo and Katz (1954b) proposed that acetylcholine increased the membrane permeability to sodium, potassium and chloride, the only ions present in sufficient abundance to contribute appreciably to the conductance changes. The fraction of the total conductance due to each of these ion species has been assessed by observing the effects that changes in concentration of each have on the equilibrium potential for the endplate current (Takeuchi and Takeuchi, 1960a). As replacement of chloride by the impermeable glutamate ion caused virtually no change in the equilibrium potential for the endplate current, it appears that increased chloride conductance can make little, if any, contribution to the endplate current. On the other hand, changes in the relative concentrations of sodium or of potassium across the membrane alter the equilibrium potential of the endplate current (Fig. 4.3), which indicates that almost all of the increased conductance is shared between these two ion species, that for sodium being rather larger. The displacement of membrane potential produced by applied acetylcholine has the same equilibrium potential as the endplate current (Axelsson and Thesleff, 1959) and is due to the same changes in ionic permeability (Takeuchi, 1963).

It has been shown that ammonium ions, various substituted ammonium ions and hydrazinium can substitute for sodium ions at the neuromuscular junction (Nastuk, 1959; Furukawa and Furukawa, 1959; Koketsu and Nishi, 1959). For example, the various methylammoniums are good substitutes, while larger ions, such as trimethylethylammonium, choline and dimethyldiethanolammonium are poor, which suggests that acetylcholine has quite a limited action in increasing the permeability of the subsynaptic membrane to cations, there being a probable size limitation to ions with a hydrated diameter of twice that of a hydrated potassium ion. The ability of acetylcholine to produce an alteration in membrane conductance is basically restricted to the external surface of the muscle at the endplate region. When the injecting micropipette is inserted intracellularly, injections of acetylcholine fail to produce a depolarization (del Castillo and Katz, 1955a). Miledi (1960b) has shown that the acetylcholine receptor sites are not confined to the actual subsynaptic membrane, but extend in progressively diminishing concentration for up to 300μ away from the endplates on muscle fibres of the rat diaphragm (Fig. 4.4), where the actual

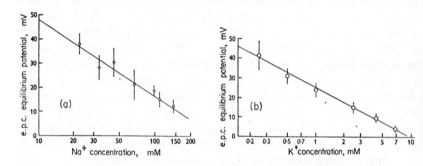

FIG. 4.3. The effects of sodium and potassium on the endplate current (e.p.c.) equilibrium potential of frog sartorius muscles. A. E.p.c. equilibrium potential plotted against sodium concentration in the external solution on a semilogarithmic scale (mean ± standard deviation of mean). B. E.p.c. equilibrium potential plotted against external potassium concentration. (Takeuchi and Takeuchi, 1960).

endplate is less than 30μ in diameter (Cole, 1957). These sparsely distributed receptor sites contribute to the depolarization produced by relatively large injections of acetylcholine at sites remote from the endplate. The sensitivity of the nonjunctional membrane is low in comparison with that at the endplate, reaching a maximum at the muscle–tendon junction, which was found to be one-thousandth as sensitive as the endplate (Katz and Miledi, 1964a). This is of interest, because of the local concentration of acetylcholinesterase which has been reported at myoneural and muscle-tendon junctions by Couteaux (1953), Gerebtzoff (1954) and Schwarzacher (1960, 1961).

After nerve section, chemosensitivity to acetylcholine spreads from the

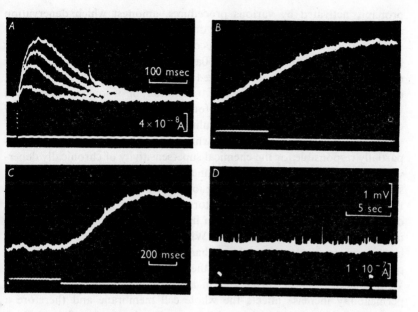

FIG. 4.4. Intracellular potential changes caused by acetylcholine on a rat diaphragm muscle fibre. Upper traces illustrate depolarizations produced by acetylcholine released iontophoretically from a micropipette by current pulses monitored in bottom traces. In A and B acetylcholine was applied at points 75μ (A) and 375μ (B) from a recording electrode placed near the endplate. In C and D the acetylcholine pipette was in the same longitudinal position as in A but displaced 35μ (C) or 100μ (D) transversely from the fibre's edge. Time calibration for B as in C. Voltage calibration same for all records. Monitor trace calibration for B and C as in D (Miledi, 1960b).

motor endplate towards the tendon (Ginetzinsky and Shamarina, 1942; Axelsson and Thesleff, 1959; Miledi, 1960a). It has been suggested that this depends upon a special chemical process at the endplate region, which gradually causes adjacent parts of the fibre surface to become sensitized. This hypothesis has been refuted by experiments in which frog sartorius muscles were divided into innervated and aneural segments (Katz and Miledi, 1964b). Within two weeks of separation from the innervated portion of the muscle, the aneural segments developed a high degree of acetylcholine sensitivity which greatly exceeded the change brought about by ordinary nerve section. The ability to produce acetylcholine-receptive sites appears to be inherent in all regions of the muscle membrane and is probably activated by various procedures, amongst which denervation and myotomy may only be specially drastic examples. The finding that the whole surface of the muscle fibre becomes sensitive to acetylcholine after botulinum poisoning (Thesleff, 1960a) is of considerable interest. Since degenerative changes are not observed in the motor nerve or its terminals, it has been suggested that the lack of transmitter, or of some agent released with the transmitter, is responsible for the changes produced in a muscle cell following denervation or in botulinum poisoning.

The increase of receptor surface which occurs following denervation is partially responsible for the chemical supersensitivity of chronically denervated muscles. As previously mentioned, the action of acetylcholine on a skeletal muscle fibre is to change the ionic permeability of that part of the membrane which is covered by receptors, the resulting depolarization being determined by the relative reduction in the effective resistance across the membrane produced by this shunt. With a small membrane area, even a large increase in its permeability has little effect on the total "input resistance" of the fibre and hence the resulting depolarization is small. With a large receptor surface, as in a chronically denervated fibre, the permeability increase affects the whole cell membrane and therefore a proportionally larger depolarization is produced. Another factor which contributes to denervation supersensitivity is a reduction in the ionic permeability of the resting membrane (Nicholls, 1956; Klaus, Lüllman and Muscholl, 1960). Membrane resistance increases about two-fold and therefore the depolarization produced by a given electric current is enhanced. The absence of acetylcholine uptake by nerve endings may also contribute, in a small measure, to denervation supersensitivity of skeletal muscles.

Electrophoretic application of acetylcholine onto the endplate receptor sites has been employed to study the desensitization of these receptors by prolonged doses of acetylcholine (Thesleff, 1955; Axelsson and Thesleff, 1958). A steady slow rate of ejection produces, in a few seconds, a considerable desensitization that is best demonstrated by the decreasing depolarizations produced by standard testing pulses of acetylcholine. The rapidity with which receptor desensitization develops under the influence of the depolarizing action of acetylcholine has led to the suggestion that the progressive decline in endplate potential amplitude early in a high frequency train of impulses might be attributable to postsynaptic desensitization by the transmitter (Axelsson and Thesleff, 1958). Support for this hypothesis was obtained when it was observed that postsynaptic sensitivity to a pulse of electrophoretically applied acetylcholine was sometimes reduced (Fig. 4.5(i)) during a few tenths of a second following a train of nerve impulses at frequencies above twenty per second (Thesleff, 1959). However, other investigators have not been able to confirm this observation (Fig. 4.5(2)) (Otsuka, Endo and Nonomura, 1962). The most important factor in the development of neuromuscular depression or "Wedensky inhibition" during high frequency stimulation is a gradual decrease of transmitter release per nerve impulse as a result of transmitter depletion (Otsuka *et al.*, 1962).

Many tertiary and quaternary ammonium compounds have been shown to depress postsynaptic sensitivity to synaptically or artificially applied acetylcholine. With most of these, it is probable that the blocking action is a result of an association of the drug with the acetylcholine receptor molecule, thus preventing acetylcholine from reacting with its receptor. The combination between blocking drug and receptor may or may not lead to ionic permeability changes like those which normally result from the combination of acetylcholine with receptor. On the basis of whether or not a drug causes postsynaptic depolarization, it can be classified as either a non-depolarizing or depolarizing receptor-blocking drug.

(b) *Non-depolarizing receptor-blocking agents.* With few exceptions these are completely ionized tertiary or quaternary ammonium salts; bis-quaternaries are generally more active than monoquaternaries. Sterically the molecular structure is bulky and rigid or has hindering groups attached to the onium N atom. It is believed that these agents owe their blocking activity to electrostatic bonding with anionic sites in the acetylcholine receptor molecule.

The best known example of a non-depolarizing receptor-blocking drug is *d*-tubocurarine. Studies with electrophoretically applied d-tubocurarine have confirmed that it does not alter membrane potential or ionic permeability of the endplate membrane (del Castillo and Katz, 1957a, b). Its equivalent effectiveness in blocking both neuromuscular transmission and the depolarizing action of electrophoretically applied acetylcholine can be explained by its competitive occupation of the acetylcholine receptor sites (Jenkinson, 1960). As would be expected, *d*-tubocurarine is ineffective when injected into the muscle fibre at the endplate region. As a competitive blocker, *d*-tubocurarine is antagonized by agents which release acetylcholine, such as tetraethylammonium ion (Koketsu, 1958) and calcium or by anticholinesterase agents.

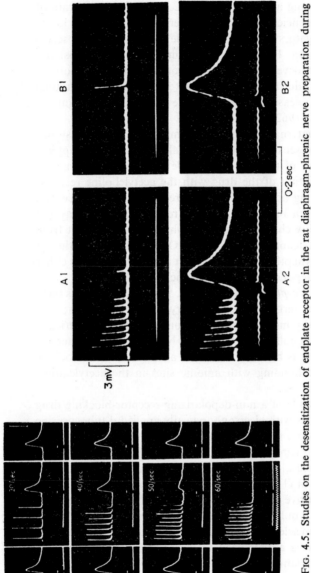

FIG. 4.5. Studies on the desensitization of endplate receptor in the rat diaphragm-phrenic nerve preparation during repetitive nerve stimulation. (1) Endplate desensitization produced by repetitive nerve stimulation at frequencies of 40, 50 and 60/sec. The entire period of stimulation (150 msec) is shown in each record. Responses to test pulses of ACh are shown: 5 sec before nerve stimulation (left-hand records) 50 msec after the end of stimulation (middle records); and 5 sec later (right-hand records). The current pulse responsible for the release of ACh is monitored in the lower tracing of each record. Time marker, 100 c/s; voltage calibration. 10 mV; monitor calibration (voltage scale) = $3 \cdot 3 \times 10^{-7}$ A. To reduce mechanical movements, the preparation was immersed in a salt solution containing $2 \cdot 0$–$2 \cdot 5$ times the normal concentration of NaCl (Thesleff, 1959). (2) Endplate potentials and acetylcholine potentials following a 50/sec conditioning tetanic stimulation. The preparation was treated with d-tubocurarine (5×10^{-7} g/ml) to reduce contractions. In each record, the upper trace shows the membrane potential recorded from endplate region. In the lower trace the strength of the current through the acetylcholine pipette is monitored. A, endplate potential (A1) and acetylcholine potential (A2) $0 \cdot 08$ sec after repetitive stimulation. B, endplate potential (B1) and acetylcholine potential (B2) $1 \cdot 9$

Although these actions of d-tubocurarine are consistent with a competitive blockade of the postsynaptic membrane, Riker and his colleagues (Riker, 1960; Riker and Standaert, 1966) believe that the nerve terminal is also involved. The repetitive antidromic firing, originating in the nerve terminals, due to anticholinesterases, hydroxyaniliniums or tetanic orthodromic stimulation is readily antagonized by d-tubocurarine (Riker, 1960; Werner, 1961; Standaert, 1963, 1964). Standaert (1964) has pointed out that d-tubocurarine was twenty five times more potent in abolishing posttetanic antidromic impulses as in blocking transmission and suggested that a presynaptic action of this substance was of major significance in its neuromuscular blocking action. Katz and Miledi (1965a) were unable to demonstrate an action of d-tubocurarine on the electrical excitability of motor nerve terminals. More complex effects of d-tubocurarine on the motor nerve terminal have been demonstrated by Hubbard et al. (1965). d-Tubocurarine shortened the refractory period and the supernormal period as well as blocking the acetylcholine-induced reduction in threshold of the nerve terminal. Used in the absence of acetylcholine, d-tubocurarine also decreased the threshold for cathodal stimulation of nerve terminals. Hubbard and his colleagues have suggested that the actions of d-tubocurarine, like those of acetylcholine, occur at the nodes of Ranvier rather than at the site of transmitter release and that the abolition of antidromic discharges can be fully explained by the acetylcholine-tubocurarine antagonism at this site.

A great many tertiary and quaternary ammonium compounds, such as dihydro-β-erythroidine, gallamine, benzoquinonium, the hemicholinium and tetraethylammonium appear to have a similar mode of action to d-tubocurarine, but quantitative studies of their interaction with acetylcholine at the endplate receptor are still lacking.

(c) *Depolarizing receptor-blocking drugs.* Drugs with this mode of action are mono- or bis-quaternary compounds, but the molecule is slender and flexible and the cationic head has a minimum of steric hindrance. Typical depolarizing receptor blockers are acetylcholine itself, choline, carbachol, succinylcholine, decamethonium and tetramethyl-ammonium. The combination between these agents and endplate receptors produces an initial depolarization at the endplate region which is followed by a reduction in the sensitivity of the endplate to the transmitter. The mechanism responsible for the initial depolarization by these agents is presumably similar to that of the transmitter and involves a local conductance increase of the endplate membrane to sodium and potassium (Takeuchi and Takeuchi, 1960a). Persistent depolarization of the muscle fibre results in inactivation of the sodium-carrying mechanism responsible for the generation of the action potential. Endplate potentials are both reduced in amplitude by the drug-induced depolarization and unable to elicit action potentials because of the inactivation of the spike generating mechanism and transmission block results. The localized endplate depolarization produced by these agents necessarily causes current to flow through the adjoining muscle fibre membrane, depolarizing it and frequently generating isolated or brief trains of action potentials. Whether action potentials occur is determined by the rapidity and extent of the depolarization and also on the electrical properties of the membrane. The neuromuscular block induced by these substances seems to be initially a result of the persistent and excessive depolarization of the endplate, but subsequently an important role is played by receptor desensitization which may or may not be accompanied by some repolarization (Thesleff, 1955, 1958; Karczmar, Kim and Koketsu, 1961). This desensitization differs from the competitive blockade by the curarimimetics, since it is generally not found to be competitive and responds poorly to attempts to reverse it with high concentrations of acetylcholine or with anticholinesterases (Kim and Karczmar, 1967).

This concept of the action of the depolarizing receptor-blocking agents has to be modified for some muscles. Amphibian slow or "tonic" muscles (Kuffler and Williams, 1953a, b) and mammalian slow muscle fibres such as those in the extraocular muscles of the cat (Hess and Pilar, 1963), which are not electrically excitable, respond to acetylcholine with prolonged sustained contractions, the contraction tension being proportional to the acetylcholine concentration. Relaxation occurs slowly, indicating that desensitization of the receptor is not an important factor.

Attention has also been directed to the presynaptic actions of the depolarizing receptor-blocking agents and to their efficacy as inhibitors of acetylcholinesterase. Succinylcholine and the other fatty acid esters of choline are hydrolyzed by pseudo- but not by acetylcholinesterase (Foldes and Foldes, 1965). Succinylcholine and decamethonium are weak inhibitors of acetylcholinesterase (Long, 1963) and a potentiation of endogenously released acetylcholine may contribute to their effects.

Standaert and Adams (1965) found that succinylcholine will evoke repetitive firing at nerve terminals in doses below those required to depress the evoked twitch. They concluded that the block of transmission was due to impairment of the nerve terminal by succinylcholine following its initial facilitatory action. Blaber (1967), however, did not observe an increase in the frequency of miniature endplate potentials with succinylcholine, which suggests that, like acetylcholine (Hubbard et al., 1965), it does not depolarize at the site of transmitter release but may do so at the adjacent nodes of Ranvier. A postsynaptic mechanism of succinylcholine blockade of neuromuscular transmission appears to explain the available data most satisfactorily, although the drug undoubtedly has some actions on the presynaptic terminals.

(d) *Anticholinesterases.* Diffusion and the enzyme, acetylcholinesterase, are jointly responsible for the rapid removal of transmitter from the endplate receptors. Histochemical studies have established that the enzyme, which hydrolyzes acetylcholine into acetic acid and choline, is concentrated on the subsynaptic membrane of the neuromuscular junction, especially in the region of the junctional folds (Couteaux, 1953, 1958; Barnett, 1962). Thus the enzymic receptor sites for acetylcholine hydrolysis are located in close apposition to the receptor sites responsible for its depolarizing action, and there is reason to believe that the chemical forces binding acetylcholine to the enzyme are very similar to those between acetylcholine and its receptor. It is generally accepted that two groups at the active site of the enzyme are essential for bringing about hydrolysis of substrate: the esteratic site, where the ester bond is activated; and the anionic site, consisting of one or more negative groups which interact by ionic bonding with the cationic head of the acetylcholine molecule.

Numerous agents from many classes of pharmacologically active drugs have been reported to inhibit acetylcholinesterase, although this is usually only a weak side action which may not be of any significance. Many of the drugs which inhibit acetylcholinesterase, including the organophosphorus compounds also react to some extent with the acetylcholine receptor. As a result, most inhibitors, in sufficient concentration, also have a"curarizing" action and block neuromuscular transmission. The type of receptor blockade evidently varies with the structure of the inhibitor and can be either predominantly depolarizing or non-depolarizing. The accumulation and persistance of acetylcholine at the endplate may also contribute to the blocking action of the anticholinesterases.

3. *Catecholamines*

Adrenaline, and some of the other sympathomimetic amines have been shown to produce two opposing effects on neuromuscular transmission in partially curarized mammalian skeletal muscles; the ability to demonstrate either depending on the experimental conditions. An anti-curare effect of adrenaline has been demonstrated by various investigators (Wilson and Wright, 1937; Bowman, Goldberg and Raper, 1962), whereas under different conditions it has been shown to enhance the blocking action of *d*-tubocurarine (Paton and Zaimis, 1950; Naess and Sirnes, 1953). A dual action of adrenaline has also been demonstrated when it is administered in conjunction with anticholinesterases or depolarizing drugs. Adrenaline enhances the twitch potentiation and repetitive firing produced by a single injection of an anticholinesterase drug (Bulbring and Burn, 1942; Blaber and Bowman, 1963) or a small dose of a depolarizing drug (Paton and Zaimis, 1950). If the anti-cholinesterase drug is infused continuously, the potentiated contractions are first augmented and then depressed by adrenaline (Naess and Sirnes, 1954) and if a dose of the depolarizing drug sufficient to produce neuromuscular block is injected simultaneously with or after adrenaline, its blocking action is reduced (Paton and Zaimis, 1950).

Bowman and Raper (1966) have compared the actions of adrenaline and isoprenaline on neuromuscular transmission and demonstrated two distinct types of effect. The facilitatory action of adrenaline on transmission is exemplified by its anti-curare action (Fig. 4.6a and b) and ability to potentiate the stimulant actions of decamethonium and neostigmine. It is not reproduced by isoprenaline, and is antagonized by *a*-receptor blocking drugs. An inhibitory action of adrenaline is reflected by its ability to augment *d*-tubocurarine paralysis and to depress contractions produced by acetylcholine. These inhibitory effects of adrenaline, as well as its actions in hyperpolarizing the muscle membrane, were slower in onset and longer lasting than the initial facilitatory actions. They were reproduced by isoprenaline and blocked by *β*-receptor blocking drugs.

Bowman and Raper (1966) concluded that the facilitatory actions of adrenaline and noradrenaline are due to the effects of these substances on the motor nerve terminals. Adrenaline has been shown to increase the amplitude of endplate potentials produced by motor nerve stimulation (Hutter and Loewenstein, 1955; Krnjević and Miledi, 1958b) but not to

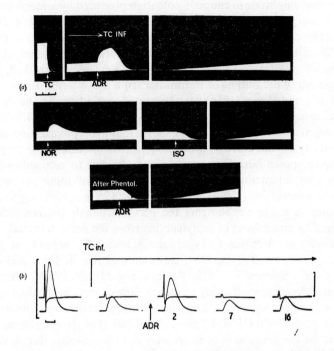

FIG. 4.6. (a) Maximal twitches of a feline tibialis anterior muscle elicited indirectly once every second. At TC a single IV injection of tubocurarine (0·3 mg/kg) was given. During recovery from this dose an intravenous infusion of tubocurarine was started and adjusted to give a constant degree of partial block. The infusion (0·58 mg/kg per hr) was then maintained constant for the remainder of the experiment. At ADR, NOR and ISO, 10 μg/kg of adrenaline, noradrenaline and isoprenaline were injected intravenously. The second response to adrenaline was recorded after the I/V injection of phentolamine (2 mg/kg). The gaps in the responses to adrenaline and isoprenaline each correspond to 10 min. Time calibration in minutes. (b) as for (a) but twitches and gross muscle action potentials were recorded on an oscilloscope. In this experiment the dose of adrenaline (ADR) was again 10 μg/kg I/V. Responses are shown at 2, 7 and 16 min after injection of adrenaline. Note that the changes in twitch tension are accompanied by corresponding changes in the amplitude of the gross action potentials. Abbreviations: tension on the left, 1 kg; time below, 30 msec; action potentials on the right, 20 mV (Bowman and Raper, 1966).

increase the amplitude of endplate potentials produced by iontophoretically applied acetylcholine (Krnjević and Miledi, 1958b) indicating that the facilitatory effect is located prejunctionally. Adrenaline relieves the presynaptic failure of transmission which occurs during repeated nerve stimulation (Hutter and Loewenstein, 1955; Krnjević and Miledi, 1958b) by augmenting the output of transmitter from nerve terminals.

Bowman and Raper (1966) have suggested that adrenaline has a hyperpolarizing action on motor nerve endings, as Krnjević and Miledi (1959) and Hubbard and Willis (1962) had shown that hyperpolarization of nerve terminals by anodal currents produces a similar increase in the magnitude of endplate potentials. This conclusion is difficult to reconcile with the finding that adrenaline increases the frequency of miniature endplate potential generation (Krnjević and Miledi, 1958), which suggests that adrenaline is either depolarizing the nerve terminals or facilitating the mobilization and release of acetylcholine from the nerve terminal.

An ability of adrenaline to hyperpolarize muscle fibres has been claimed (Brown, Goffart and Dias, 1950; Bowman and Raper, 1965) and denied (Hutter and Loewenstein, 1955; Krnjević and Miledi, 1958b), although a decreased electrical excitability of muscle fibres during adrenaline application, in the absence of a change in resting potential, was observed by Krnjević and Miledi (1958b). Such a stabilization of the membrane would account for the depression of neuromuscular transmission during circumstances in which the normal safety margin in transmission was already decreased, as in a curarized muscle. Stabilization of the membrane, with or without an accompanying hyperpolarization, undoubtedly accounts for the inhibitory actions of the catecholamines on muscle excitability. These effects are clearly demonstrable when the β-receptor stimulant, isoprenaline, is employed, or after the administration of an α-receptor blocker (Fig. 4.6a) (Bowman and Raper, 1966). The post-junctional hyperpolarizing action of adrenaline may be a result of changes in muscle carbohydrate metabolism (Bowman and Raper, 1964).

4. 5-*Hydroxytryptamine*

5-Hydroxytryptamine has been reported to antagonize the neuromuscular block induced by *d*-tubocurarine in cats and rabbits, but not that due to decamethonium (Philippot and Dallemagne, 1956; Sala and Perris,

1958). It also increased the contractions of fatigued frog gastrocnemius muscle (Gromakovskaya, 1962).

In another series of experiments, 5-hydroxytryptamine was observed to depress neuromuscular transmission in rats and frogs and potentiate the neuromuscular block induced by d-tubocurarine. The effects of 5-hydroxytryptamine were suppressed by both eserine and methysergide (Gawecka and Kostowski, 1966).

The effect of 5-hydroxytryptamine on frog neuromuscular transmission has recently been studied with intracellular recording techniques (Colomo, Rahamimoff and Stefani, 1968). The amplitude of endplate potentials and of potentials elicited by iontophoretic application of acetylcholine were reversibly reduced by 5-hydroxytryptamine either added to the bathing solution or iontophoretically applied close to the endplate. The results indicate that 5-hydroxytryptamine decreases the amplitude of postsynaptic potentials evoked by synaptically released or iontophoretically applied acetylcholine. However, the underlying mechanism of action of 5-hydroxytryptamine has still to be elucidated.

5. *Histamine*

Histamine potentiates the response to acetylcholine of the tibialis muscle of the cat and has some stimulant actions on the denervated muscle. It has been reported to have an antagonistic action on the neuromuscular blockade produced by depolarizing agents, such as suxamethonium and a potentiating action on the neuromuscular block produced by non-depolarizing agents such as d-tubocurarine (Schenk and Anderson, 1958; Bovet-Nitti *et al.*, 1964).

6. *Prostaglandins*

Extracts of human seminal plasma were originally described as having a stimulant effect on frog rectus abdominis muscle by Goldblatt (1935). Sasamori (1965) was unable to demonstrate either a stimulant or relaxant effect of PGE_1 on skeletal muscle preparations.

More recently PGE_1 has been shown to potentiate the responses of frog rectus abdominis preparations to acetylcholine, exhibiting an anti-tubocurarine action, and to decrease the threshold of this preparation to electrical stimulation (Khairallah, Page and Türker, 1967). The same authors found, however, that PGE_1 depressed the contractile response of cat gastrocnemius muscle to sciatic nerve stimulation.

CONCLUSIONS

1. Acetylcholine has been generally accepted as the transmitter at nerve-skeletal muscle synapses. Comparisons between the quantity of acetylcholine released at nerve terminals on skeletal muscles and the amount needed to excite skeletal muscle, reveal a close correlation. The $1 \cdot 8 \times 10^{-15}$ g of acetylcholine released from a nerve terminal by a single impulse is sufficient to reproduce an endplate potential.

2. Acetylcholine release continues from denervated muscles, although at a reduced rate, indicating that it arises in part from structures other than the nerve endings.

3. Many agents have been shown to influence the release of acetylcholine from motor nerve terminals. These include calcium, magnesium and sodium, *botulinum* toxin, hemicholinium-3 and possibly neuromuscular blockers such as *d*-tubocurarine and succinylcholine. Acetylcholine depolarizes nerve terminals, but it has been suggested that it acts at the nodes of Ranvier, rather than at the sites of transmitter release.

4. Acetylcholine increases the permeability of the postsynaptic muscle membrane to sodium and potassium ions, generating the currents which give rise to the endplate potential. Increases in chloride conductance contribute little, if at all, to the endplate current. Acetylcholine receptor sites are not confined to the actual subsynaptic membrane, but extend in a progressively diminishing concentration for up to 300μ away from the junctional region. After nerve section, or during botulinum poisoning, chemosensitivity to acetylcholine becomes a property of the entire muscle membrane.

5. This increase in receptor surface is, in part, responsible for the chemical supersensitivity of denervated muscle. Another factor in this phenomenon is the increased membrane resistance of denervated muscle.

6. The actions of anticholinesterases and depolarizing and non-depolarizing receptor blocking agents on the neuromuscular junction are discussed.

7. Catecholamines have at least two actions on neuromuscular transmission—a facilitatory action, which appears to be due to an increased release of acetylcholine from the presynaptic terminals, and an inhibitory

action, due to stabilization of the muscle membrane. The latter may or may not be accompanied by a hyperpolarization. The facilitatory action is blocked by α-adrenergic antagonists and the inhibitory action by β-antagonists.

8. 5-Hydroxytryptamine, histamine and prostaglandins influence neuromuscular transmission. Their actions have yet to be elucidated.

CHAPTER 5

NEUROMUSCULAR TRANSMISSION IN VERTEBRATES: SMOOTH MUSCLE

FOR a number of reasons experiments with smooth muscle cells have always been difficult and the results frequently ambiguous. In general, smooth muscle occurs as part of a complex aggregation of tissues including nerve cells and their axons and is frequently associated with secretory epithelium. Possibly because of their large surface area relative to volume, smooth muscle cells are very sensitive to small fluctuations in their immediate, local environment, which is therefore more difficult to control experimentally. Furthermore the pharmacological properties of smooth muscle, even within the same organ, may vary greatly with the sex, age and species of the animal from which it was taken.

Considerable progress in the interpretation of drug effects on smooth muscle has been made in the past decade as a result of the rapid development of electrophysiological and morphological techniques for the study of smooth muscle cells. In particular, the use of capillary microelectrodes for recording changes in the membrane potentials of muscle cells during nerve stimulation or drug application and the development of fluorescence histochemistry to localize monoamines have contributed extensively to an understanding of the synaptic transmission process in many smooth muscles.

In spite of the diversity of their physiological properties, Bozler (1948) attempted to subdivide vertebrate smooth muscles into two categories according to their degree of dependence on an extrinsic nerve supply and their ability to respond in an all-or-none manner to various stimuli. Muscles of the first category (multiunit) include the nictitating membrane and iris, ciliary muscles, pilomotor muscles and also some blood vessels. Under normal conditions they contract only in response to excitation of their extrinsic motor nerves, often responding to single volleys. Muscles of the second category (single-unit) include most visceral smooth muscles, such as those in the gastrointestinal tract, ureter and uterus. These muscles frequently show continuous rhythmical activity, and although this may be modified by extrinsic nerves, it does not appear to depend on them and rhythmic activity continues after their removal.

A. ACETYLCHOLINE AND SMOOTH MUSCLES

Acetylcholine excites most single unit smooth muscle including longitudinal intestinal muscle and that of the ureter, uterus, vas deferens and bladder. It also causes contraction of multi-unit smooth muscle such as that in the iris and nictitating membrane. The enhancement of excitability is usually manifested by a sustained contraction or increased spontaneous contractions and is accompanied by depolarization of the smooth muscle membrane. Inhibitory effects of acetylcholine occur on cardiovascular and retractor penis muscle fibres.

1. *Gastro-intestinal Smooth Muscle*

Acetylcholine depolarization is associated with an increase in action potential frequency in spontaneously active muscles, such as the taenia coli. Low doses of acetylcholine increase the rate of depolarization of the prepotentials, from which the action potentials arise (Bulbring and Kuriyama, 1963). In some cells the prepotentials increase in amplitude. The amplitude and rate of rise of the action potentials are reduced and the repolarization phase is prolonged, partly as a result of the depolarization of the cell membrane and partly because of the increase in membrane permeability to potassium.

The cholinergic nature of the parasympathetic innervation of intestinal longitudinal smooth muscle has been established in many experiments. Anticholinesterases potentiate and atropine abolishes the contractions of longitudinal smooth muscle evoked by transmural stimulation (Harry, 1962) and *botulinum* toxin has been shown to paralyze excitatory cholinergic nerves in the intestine of rabbits and kittens (Ambache, 1951; Harry, 1962). Intracellular recording has revealed that the excitatory junctional potentials evoked in guinea-pig taenia coli by transmural stimulation are potentiated by neostigmine and abolished by atropine (Burnstock, Campbell, Bennett and Holman, 1964).

In contrast to the longitudinal intestinal muscle which is highly sensitive to acetylcholine, intestinal circular muscle is rather insensitive to acetyl-choline (Sperelakis and Prosser, 1959; Harry, 1963). Claims that the con-tractions of circular muscle in the guinea-pig ileum evoked by transmural stimulation are abolished by *botulinum* toxin and atropine (Harry, 1962) have recently been challenged (Kottegoda, 1968).

Acetylcholine release by the gut has been extensively investigated since Dikshit (1938) and Goffart (1939; Bacq and Goffart, 1939) measured its release and postulated that its source was the myenteric plexuses. Sugges-tions that acetylcholine release might also occur, in part, from glandular structures in the gut wall (Feldberg and Lin, 1950; Chujyo, 1952) have not been substantiated (Paton, 1957; Harry, 1962; Johnson, 1963). It has recently been demonstrated convincingly that denervated strips of longi-tudinal muscle from the guinea-pig ileum neither contain detectable amounts of acetylcholine nor release it spontaneously or in response to stimulation (Paton and Zar, 1968). The nerve plexus (Auerbach's plexus) attached to the longitudinal muscle accounts for only about one third of the acetylcholine content of the whole gut and for around one fifth of the spontaneous resting release. Paton and Zar (1968) postulate that the remainder of the acetylcholine is also associated with nervous tissues in the other (Meisner's) plexus. Their evidence is that the pattern of acetylcholine release with variations in the frequency of stimulation, and during the application of cocaine and morphine is very comparable for the whole gut and an innervated strip of longitudinal muscle. Increases in intraluminal pressure in the guinea-pig ileum cause an increase in the rate of release of acetylcholine, the amount liberated being proportional to the magnitude of the applied pressure (Kažić and Varagić, 1968). Acetylcholine output is increased, irrespective of whether peristalsis occurs or not, which suggests that the increased intraluminal pressure and not the resultant peristaltic activity is essential for producing the release. These experiments suggest that increased intraluminal pressure stimulates peristalsis by activating cholinergic neurones involved in the peristaltic reflex arc.

2. *Uro-genital Tract*

Acetylcholine depolarizes and evokes contractions of the cat bladder, uterus and vas deferens (Bacq and Monnier, 1935), rat ureter (Prosser, Smith and Melton, 1955) and rat uterus (Marshall, 1959).

In the rat ureter, where the normal spike potential has a plateau form,

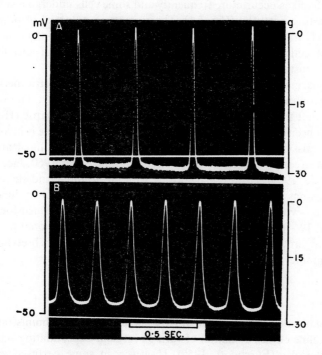

FIG. 5.1. Effects of ACh on estrogen-dominated rat uterine muscle fibre. A. Control record. B. Record 2 min after addition of ACh (10^{-5} g/ml). Note, fall in membrane potential, increase in firing rate of action potentials, their increased duration and decreased overshoot. Note also the slowing of repolarization rate. Muscle tension; upper trace in A, bottom trace in B (Marshall, 1959).

acetylcholine slightly prolongs the duration of the plateau, induces repetitive firing and initiates spontaneous contractile activity. Local application of acetylcholine to any region of the rat ureter can cause this region to become a pacemaker, whereas impulses normally originate at the renal end (Prosser *et al.*, 1955). The rhythmicity induced by acetylcholine often occurs at a higher frequency than normal spontaneous rhythms and is even faster than the ureter can be driven electrically. The stimulating action of acetylcholine is markedly enhanced by eserine.

Low doses of acetylcholine alter the pattern of spontaneous activity in the isolated rat uterus (Marshall, 1959; Csapo and Kuriyama, 1963).

Trains of spikes occur more frequently and some cells undergo a sustained fall in resting potential (Fig. 5.1). The membrane potential of other cells shows only transient depolarizations, which are frequently associated with bursts of action potentials. With higher concentrations of acetylcholine there is a sustained discharge of action potentials.

The pharmacology of the isolated vas deferens-hypogastric nerve preparation of the guinea pig has been discussed extensively. The original concept that this junction was typical of an adrenergic synapse (Huković, 1961) has been challenged by the suggestion that acetylcholine is involved in the transmission process according to the theory of Burn and Rand, discussed in an earlier chapter of this book (Chang and Rand, 1960; Jacobowitz and Koelle, 1965). However, recording with intracellular and sucrose gap electrodes has shown that atropine has no effect on excitatory junctional potentials evoked by hypogastric nerve stimulation (Burnstock and Holman, 1964) and Kuriyama (1963) found that the junctional potentials in this preparation were abolished by the adrenergic blockers bretylium and phentolamine.

3. *Cardio-vascular Muscles*

Stimulation of the parasympathetic nerve supply or administration of acetylcholine causes a dilation of various vascular beds, dilating small and large arterioles (Furchgott, 1955). However, in some perfused vascular systems, such as those associated with the lungs and abdominal viscera, acetylcholine often causes an increase in resistance.

Local application of acetylcholine to isolated arteries and veins has yielded variable results. Acetylcholine-induced contractions have been recorded from the posterior vena cava and anterior mesenteric veins of the rabbit (Sutter, 1965) and sheep mesenteric vein (Holman and McLean, 1967). As the contractions evoked by acetylcholine were blocked by α-receptor antagonists and guanethidine in doses which also abolished the responses to nerve stimulation, it is possible that acetylcholine was releasing noradrenaline from axon terminals of the sympathetic ground plexus. After hexamethonium, acetylcholine had an inhibitory action on the sheep mesenteric veins (Holman and McLean, 1967).

Acetylcholine had a diphasic action on muscle of the rat portal vein (Funaki and Bohr, 1964), causing a hyperpolarization, which was associated with an increased level of mechanical and electrical activity.

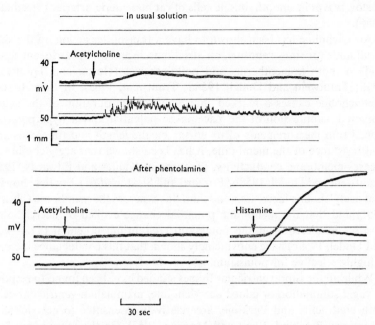

FIG. 5.2. (Top) electrical (sucrose gap) and mechanical response of sheep carotid artery to acetylcholine, 25 μg/ml. (Bottom) response of same artery to acetylcholine (left) and histamine (right), 25 μg/ml, after exposure to phentolamine 100 μg/ml for 20 min. In all records upper trace is mechanical, lower electrical.
* Mechanical calibration refers to all mechanical traces and gives actual shortening of arterial segment; contraction upwards (Keatinge, 1966).

Acetylcholine induced relaxation was observed with the central ear artery of rabbits when the tone of the artery had been raised by sympathetic stimulation (de la Lande and Rand, 1965), but it constricts the isolated rabbit pulmonary artery (Bevan and Su, 1964). Acetylcholine (25 μg/ml) elicited an irregular electrical discharge in sucrose gap records from isolated carotid arteries; which was associated with a contraction (Keatinge, 1966). This effect was blocked by hexamethonium and the α-adrenergic antagonist phentolamine (Fig. 5.2), providing evidence that acetylcholine causes activation by releasing noradrenaline. By contrast, the excitant effects of histamine were not antagonised by phentolamine (Fig. 5.2). High concentrations of acetylcholine abolished spike activity and reduced the amplitude of slow waves in smooth muscle cells of rat mesenteric arteries (Steedman, 1966).

Acetylcholine has been shown to have a transmitter action on the sino-atrial node (or sinus venosus), on atrial muscle and on the atrioventricular node of both homeotherms and poikilotherms (Hutter and Trautwein, 1956; Trautwein and Dudel, 1958a; Trautwein, 1963). In these tissues, acetylcholine causes a marked shortening of the duration of the action potential, suppression of the pacemaker potential and a hyperpolarization. From measurements of its effects on the length and time constants and resistance of the membrane, it has been shown that acetylcholine increases membrane conductivity. (Trautwein, Kuffler and Edwards, 1956; Trautwein and Dudel, 1958b; Fozzard and Sleator, 1967). Studies showing that acetylcholine increases potassium fluxes across the membrane (Hutter, 1961) and that the membrane potential change evoked by acetylcholine reverses in direction at the potassium equilibrium potential (Trautwein and Dudel, 1958b) have convincingly shown that this conductance increase is highly selective for potassium.

While all the supraventricular tissues studied have been found to respond to vagal stimulation or added acetylcholine, mammalian ventricular cells, both contractile and Purkinje, are relatively insensitive to acetylcholine (Schreiner, Berglund, Borst and Monroe, 1957). On the other hand, frog ventricular muscle is quite sensitive to acetylcholine, which appears to induce an increase in potassium permeability, with a resultant hyperpolarization and shortening of the action potential. The maximum depolarization rate during excitation was also increased, which indicates that acetylcholine may also have an effect on the sodium-carrier mechanism (Ware and Graham 1967).

4. Dog-retractor Penis Muscle

Acetylcholine hyperpolarizes single smooth muscle cells of this preparation and therefore reproduces the effects of stimulation of the parasympathetic nerves (Orlov, 1961, 1963). Repetitive stimulation of the parasympathetic nervous supply was necessary to evoke hyperpolarizations, and these were abolished by atropine or d-tubocurarine. Eserine potentiated the response so that lower frequencies of stimulation were adequate to produce a hyperpolarization.

B. CATECHOLAMINES AND TRANSMISSION IN SMOOTH MUSCLE

The actions of adrenaline and noradrenaline vary considerably from preparation to preparation and species to species. These actions may be reversed under a variety of different conditions. For example, in fetal guinea-pigs the ileum is contracted by adrenaline whereas in adults it is relaxed (Munro, 1933). Adrenaline relaxes a rat uterus, contracts that of a rabbit or human, while in cats adrenaline relaxes the oestrogen-dominated non-pregnant uterus but contracts the pregnant uterus (Burnstock, Holman and Prosser, 1963).

1. *Excitatory Effects*

Excitatory effects of adrenaline and noradrenaline on various smooth muscles have been recorded and some of these will be described in this section. No evidence is available so far which suggests that the ionic basis of these excitatory actions of the catecholamines on smooth muscle differ in any way from that of acetylcholine at the neuromuscular junction.

(a) *Gastro-intestinal tract.* Although its dominant action on gastro-intestinal smooth muscle is inhibition, Burnstock (1960) has shown that in the muscularis mucosa of the pig oesophagus, adrenaline causes depolarization and the initiation of action potentials, or an increase in their frequency. In the dog stomach adrenaline has a diphasic action, an initial relaxation with an associated hyperpolarization being followed by a contraction associated with depolarization (Ichikawa and Bozler, 1955).

(b) *Uro-genital tract.* The excitant action of adrenaline on cat uterus, bladder and vas deferens was described by Bacq and Monnier (1935).

Electrophysiological studies on the vas deferens have contributed greatly to our understanding of autonomic control of smooth muscle and will therefore be discussed in some detail. A spontaneous discharge of small excitatory junctional potentials has been recorded from smooth muscle cells in the vas deferens of guinea-pig, rat and mouse. The amplitudes of these potentials vary over a wide range (Fig. 5.3) occasionally reaching 22mV. The potentials appear to be comparable with miniature endplate potentials recorded at the skeletal neuromuscular junction and are therefore thought to be a result of quantal release of transmitter (Burnstock and Holman, 1966). The large amplitude of some of these spontaneous excitatory junctional potentials may indicate that the "quanta" of noradrenaline

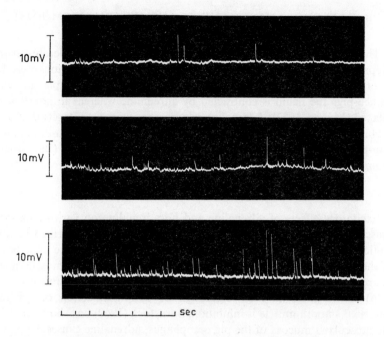

FIG. 5.3. Intracellular records from guinea pig (upper record), rat (middle record) and mouse (lower record) vas deferens, showing spontaneous excitatory junctional potentials in the absence of nerve stimulation (Burnstock and Holman, 1966).

released from sympathetic nerve terminals are larger or more effective in depolarizing the smooth muscle membrane than the packets of acetyl-choline at cholinergic junctions.

In the guinea-pig, stimulation of the hypogastric nerve or intramural nerve fibres evokes excitatory junctional potentials in muscle cells of the vas deferens (Fig. 5.4). Excitatory junctional potentials of 25–35 mV amplitude are necessary to generate an action potential and several successive nerve impulses are required for a maximum contraction of the vas deferens. The junctional potentials generated in any one cell increase in amplitude in a step-wise manner as the strength of stimulation is increased, suggesting that individual muscle fibres are innervated by several axons (Burnstock and Holman, 1961; Kuriyama, 1963).

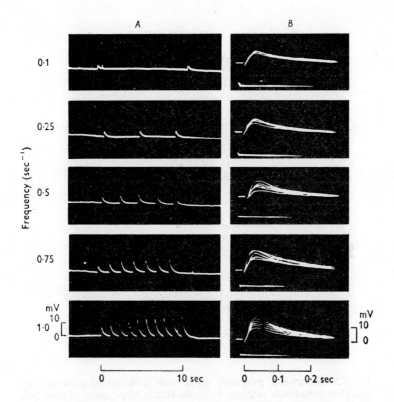

FIG. 5.4. Junctional potentials recorded from smooth muscle cells of the guinea-pig vas deferens and evoked by repetitive field stimulation of the muscle, at frequencies as indicated from 0·1 to 1·0/sec. Pulses 0·05 msec, 10V. A. Trains of successive stimulation for 10 sec. B. Five superimposed junction potentials at various frequencies (Kuriyama, 1963).

The rat vas deferens will give a maximal contraction in response to a single supramaximal pulse and excitatory junctional potentials are more constant in amplitude. Consequently it is difficult to obtain a graded response in this species. Morphological studies have shown that the density of innervation of muscle cells is greater in the rat than in the guinea-pig vas deferens (Burnstock and Holman, 1966).

The actions of a number of drugs on transmission of excitation during stimulation of the hypogastric nerve or its intramural extensions have been

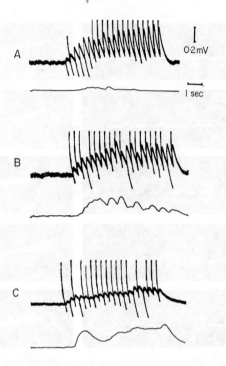

FIG. 5.5. Responses of guinea-pig vas deferens in the sucrose gap apparatus. Electrical stimulation at 3/sec, 0·5 msec pulses. Upper trace of each pair, membrane potential, shows depolarization upwards; lower trade, tension, shows increase upwards. A. Control. B. 5 min after treatment with phenoxybenzamine (1 × 10⁻⁵ gm/ml). C. After 60 min exposure to phenoxybenzamine (Bentley and Smith, 1967).

intensively studied in the guinea-pig vas deferens. High concentrations of α-receptor adrenergic blocking agents such as phentolamine, ergotamine, phenoxybenzamine and yohimbine are needed to block the excitatory junctional potentials in response to nerve stimulation recorded with microelectrodes or with the sucrose gap (Kuriyama, 1963; Burnstock and Holman, 1964; Bentley and Smith, 1967). The rate of discharge of spontaneous excitatory junctional potentials is reduced by both α- and β-adrenergic antagonists (Burnstock and Holman, 1966). In spite of this reduction in junctional potential amplitude, action potentials and contractions in response to transmural stimulation are more marked in vas deferens preparations treated with α-blockers (Fig. 5.5) and the muscles often become spontaneously active (Bentley and Smith, 1967). The reasons for this augmentation of the electrically induced response are not yet understood, but may be a result of alterations in the excitability of the muscle cells by α-blockers.

Bretylium reduces the amplitude of excitatory junctional potentials and initially also lowers the frequency of occurrence but not the amplitude of

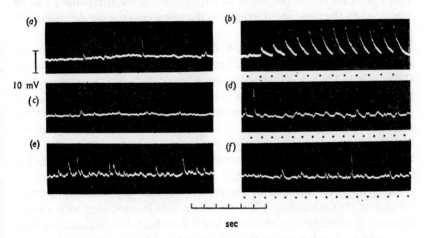

FIG. 5.6. The effect of bretylium (10^{-5} g/ml.) on the membrane potential of the vas deferens (intracellular recording). The tracings on the left show spontaneous potentials, and those on the right the response to stimulation of the hypogastric nerve as indicated by the dots. Tracings (a) and (b) are controls; tracings (c) and (d) were taken after 12 min; and records (e) and (f) after 30 min exposure to the drug (Burnstock and Holman, 1964).

spontaneous junctional potentials, though after further exposure, the frequency of spontaneous junctional potentials increases (Fig. 5.6) (Burnstock and Holman, 1964). This finding supports the concept that bretylium blocks transmission at a prejunctional site, although it appears that the spontaneous release of transmitter occurs by an independent process. Guanethidine, like bretylium, blocks excitatory junctional potentials evoked by nerve stimulation but not the spontaneously occurring junctional potentials (Burnstock and Holman, 1964).

Excitatory junctional potentials in the vas deferens of reserpinized guinea-pigs are smaller than those in normal animals and facilitation slower, so that many stimulating pulses are required before spike initiation and contraction occurs (Burnstock and Holman, 1962). Both the frequency and amplitude of spontaneous excitatory junctional potentials are reduced.

Various ganglion blockers, including hexamethonium, do not affect the response of the vas deferens to transmural stimulation although the responses to hypogastric nerve stimulation are reduced (Kuriyama, 1963). This reduction in the responses to hypogastric nerve stimulation can be explained by the presence of ganglia in the nerve near the vas deferens itself (Ferry, 1967).

The transmission of excitation from sympathetic nerves to smooth muscle cells in the retractor penis muscle of the dog has been studied by Orlov (1961, 1962, 1963). Facilitation of excitatory junctional potentials by repetitive stimulation, eventually reaching threshold for action potential generation was observed. Adrenaline potentiated neuromuscular transmission. Spontaneous excitatory junctional potentials were also observed, their frequency and amplitude being reduced by reserpinization.

(c) *Cardiovascular muscle*. Adrenaline affects the shape of the guinea-pig atrial action potential, making the plateau more prominent without increasing the total duration of the action potential very markedly (Sleator, Furchgott, de Gubareff and Krespi, 1964). This is associated with a small decrease in membrane conductivity and a depolarization, which have been attributed to a reduction in the permeability of the muscle membrane to potassium both during the resting and active states (Fozzard and Sleator, 1967). Trautwein and Schmidt (1960) examined the effect of adrenaline on sodium permeability changes in atrial and Purkinje fibres of the dog. No influence was detected, although effects consistent with activation of the membrane sodium/potassium pump were found.

An increase in the mechanical activity of various vascular muscles has been observed during local application of catecholamines. These include turtle aorta and vena cava (Roddie, 1962), sheep common carotid artery (Keatinge, 1964), rabbit pulmonary artery (Che Su, Bevan and Ursillo, 1964), rat mesenteric arteries (McGregor, 1965; Steedman, 1966), rabbit central ear artery (de la Lande and Rand, 1965; Bentley and Smith, 1967), rat portal vein (Funaki and Bohr, 1964), sheep mesenteric vein (Holman and McLean, 1967), rabbit portal vein (Hughes and Vane, 1967) and rabbit external jugular, mesenteric and posterior caval veins (Sutter, 1965). When electrical activity was recorded, an increase was usually associated with the contraction.

The excitatory effect of the catecholamines on arterial smooth muscle was studied by Keatinge (1964), using a modification of the sucrose gap technique. Adrenaline, noradrenaline and histamine caused an abrupt depolarization of about 10 mV from a resting potential of 60 to 70 mV. The depolarization usually took the form of a spike followed by a sustained

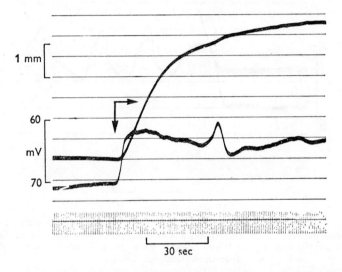

FIG. 5.7. Electrical (sucrose gap) and mechanical responses of sheep carotid artery to noradrenaline (2·5 mg/100 ml), added at arrow. Temperature 35°C. Upper trace—tension; lower trace—membrane potential alterations (Keatinge, 1964).

depolarization and was associated with a smooth contraction (Fig. 5.7). Repeated spikes, each followed by contraction, were occasionally produced by normal arteries and were the usual response of arteries whose oxidative metabolism had been inhibited by cyanide, fluoroacetate or anoxia (Fig. 5.8).

The electrical activity of turtle arteries has been recorded with intracellular electrodes (Roddie, 1962). In this preparation, spontaneous action potentials consist of spikes followed by plateaus of 10–12 sec duration, accompanied by contractions which last for up to 200 sec. Electrical

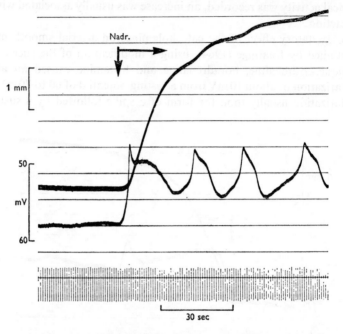

FIG. 5.8. Electrical and mechanical responses of sheep carotid artery to noradrenaline (2·5 mg/100 ml) added at arrow in presence of sodium cyanide (10 mg/100 ml). Upper trace—tension; lower trace membrane potential alterations (Keatinge, 1964).

activity recorded from turtle veins was more variable, and ranged from trains of simple spikes with negative after potentials to "plateau-type" action potentials. In both veins and arteries, adrenaline caused an increase in frequency of the action potentials, and a summation of contractions.

The responses of rat mesenteric arteries to sympathetic nerve stimulation were duplicated by noradrenaline, blocked by bretylium and guanethidine, and markedly reduced or abolished by reserpine and phenoxybenzamine (McGregor, 1965). Microelectrodes have also been used to record the intracellular potentials in rat mesenteric arteries (Steedman, 1966). Intracellular potentials varied continuously as a result of rhythmical slow waves. Electrical stimulation of the splanchnic nerves or local applications of adrenaline or noradrenaline increased the amplitude of these slow waves and the frequency of action potentials which occurred during the maximum period of depolarization of the slow waves.

The contractile response of the rabbit central ear artery to transmural stimulation and noradrenaline was abolished by the α-adrenergic blockers, phentolamine and phenoxybenzamine (Bentley and Smith, 1967). *Alpha*-receptor blocking drugs also abolished the excitant effects of noradrenaline

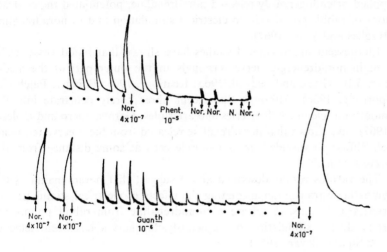

FIG. 5.9. Mechanical responses of sheep superior mesenteric vein. Upper record: effect of phentolamine (10^{-5} g/ml) on responses of vein to transmural stimulation (●) and added noradrenaline (Nor). Note "wash-out" artifacts when noradrenaline was given after phentolamine. Lower record: effect of guanethidine (10^{-6} gm/ml) on responses to periarterial nerve stimulation (●) and added noradrenaline (Nor). Note the large potentiation of the response to noradrenaline in the presence of guanethidine. Vertical calibration: $1 \cdot 0$g for upper record, $0 \cdot 5$g for lower record. Interval between nerve stimuli, 2 min (Holman and McLean, 1967).

and both periarterial and intramural nerve stimulation on rabbit portal and sheep mesenteric veins (Fig. 5.9) (Hughes and Vane, 1967; Holman and McLean, 1967).

Venous responses to nerve stimulation were also abolished by bretylium and guanethidine (Fig. 5.9). Isoprenaline caused a marked reduction in the responses of these preparations to transmural stimulation, indicating that inhibitory β-adrenotrophic receptors are also present on some vascular smooth muscle. β-receptor blockers, such as propanolol, pronethalol and INPEA abolished the relaxation induced by isoprenaline (Hughes and Vane, 1967). Evidence for excitatory β-receptors on the posterior caval vein and ear artery of the rabbit has also been presented (Sutter, 1965; Gay, Rand and Wilson, 1967).

Cocaine, which blocks the uptake by sympathetic nerve terminals of applied or endogenously released noradrenaline, potentiated the contractions of rabbit portal vein to electrical stimulation and to noradrenaline (Hughes and Vane, 1967).

Fluorescent microscopical studies have shown that blood vessel walls contain noradrenergic nerve terminals in the outer part of the media (Fig. 5.10) (Fuxe and Sedvall, 1965; Keatinge, 1966; Ehinger, Falck and Sporrong, 1966). Although fluorescent fibres barely penetrate into the smooth muscle of small arteries and arterioles, Gerova, Gero and Dolezel (1967) have shown that noradrenaline released from these nerve terminals will diffuse to vascular smooth muscle cells at some distance from the nerve terminals.

The various results described above suggest that noradrenaline is the sympathetic transmitter mediating the effects of electrical stimulation in arteries and veins. A release of noradrenaline from rabbit pulmonary artery during stimulation of vasoconstrictor nerves has been detected (Che Su and Bevan, 1967).

2. *Inhibitory Actions of Adrenaline*

In those preparations where adrenaline and noradrenaline cause a relaxation, this effect is associated with hyperpolarization of the smooth muscle membrane and a reduction or cessation of spike activity. Examples of these are the guinea-pig taenia coli (Bulbring, 1954, 1957), the oestrogen and progesterone-dominated rat uterus (Marshall, 1959), circular (Sperelakis and Prosser, 1959) and longitudinal intestinal muscle (Bortoff, 1961) of the cat.

With low concentrations of adrenaline, the membrane potential of the guinea-pig taenia coli tends to fluctuate and spike potentials occasionally appear. These spikes are characterised by their large size, short duration, fast decay and prominent afterhyperpolarization (Bulbring 1957; Burnstock, 1958). During adrenaline-induced relaxation the longitudinal intestinal muscle and taenia coli become inexcitable and conduction of an

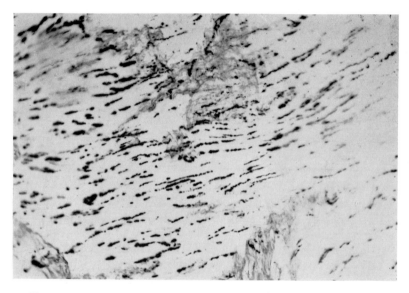

FIG. 5.10. Fluorescent noradrenergic fibres in a freeze-dried sheep carotid artery treated with hot formaldehyde vapour. Tangential section through the outer part of the media (Keatinge, 1966).

action potential is not possible (Bozler, 1940; Bulbring, 1954; Burnstock, 1958). The relaxing action of adrenaline on the taenia coli is accompanied by a hyperpolarization. In the presence of high concentrations of potassium, its action reverses to a depolarization and contraction. This reversal takes place after a period of about 40 sec, during which time there is a normal relaxation (Burnstock, 1958).

Both α- and β-adrenergic antagonists in combination are required to block the relaxant effect of adrenaline on isolated guinea-pig taenia coli (Diamond and Brody, 1966), confirming an earlier finding for canine ileum (Ahlquist and Levy, 1959). Bulbring and Tomita (1968) have used the double sucrose gap technique (Berger, 1963) to investigate the action of catecholamines on the membrane resistance of taenia coli. Noradrenaline caused a block of spike discharge, a hyperpolarization and a reduction in the electrotonic potentials, evoked by brief anodal polarizing currents (indicating a decrease in membrane resistance), developed by the muscle (Fig. 5.11(a)). In the presence of the α-blocker, phentolamine, the hyperpolarization and the reduction of the electrotonic potential by adrenaline were abolished but suppression of spontaneous spikes was still observed (Fig. 5.11(b)). Addition of the β-blocker, propranolol, blocked this remaining effect of noradrenaline (Fig. 5.11(c)).

The reduction of membrane resistance by noradrenaline (α-action) was potentiated by high potassium or by replacement of chloride ion by nitrate ion in the perfusion fluid. It was reduced by low potassium and replacement of chloride with ethanesulphonate or benzenesulphonate. Since raising the external calcium ion concentration had a similar effect to the catecholamines, Bulbring and Tomita have suggested that the α-action may be due to increased calcium-binding by the membrane, resulting in an increased potassium and chloride conductance. It had previously been shown that adrenaline and noradrenaline increase the ^{42}K-efflux in depolarized muscle (Bulbring, Goodford and Setekliev, 1966; Jenkinson and Morton, 1967a).

The β-action of noradrenaline and adrenaline appeared to be due to suppression of the generator potential, as spikes were easily evoked by depolarizing currents of threshold intensity, even when the spontaneous spikes were suppressed. As the action potential in taenia coli is probably a calcium spike (Nonomura, Hotta and Ohashi, 1966), there may be a coupled calcium/potassium pump. Removal of calcium from the cell membrane would decrease the potassium conductance and subsequent depolarization of the membrane would give rise to a generator potential. Catecholamines may oppose the removal of calcium, resulting in a suppression of the generator potential (Bulbring and Tomita, 1968).

The presence of both α- and β-adrenergic inhibitory receptors in taenia coli has also been demonstrated by Jenkinson and Morton (1967b). Evidence was presented to show that α-receptors only were involved in increasing the influx and efflux of potassium. Isoprenaline was about

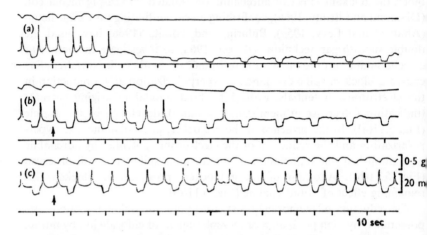

Fig. 5.11. The effect of noradrenaline on membrane resistance and spike generation in guinea-pig taenia coli muscle. Double sucrose gap. Upper trace of each pair of records—tension; lower trace—electrical record. Electronic potentials evoked by hyperpolarizing current pulses of 4 sec duration every 20 sec. Noradrenaline (2×10^{-7} g/ml) added at arrows, (a) before (b) in the presence of an α-blocker, phentolamine (10^{-5} g/ml) and (c) in the presence of phentolamine and a β-blocker, propranolol (10^{-5} g/ml). See text for further explanation (Bülbring and Tomita, 1968).

30 times more active than noradrenaline in inhibiting calcium contractures of the depolarized taenia, suggesting that β-receptors were concerned in this action. This was confirmed by showing that this action of noradrenaline in blocking calcium contractures was antagonized by the β-blocker, pronethalol but not by phentolamine, an α-blocker. Jenkinson and Morton (1967b) postulate that the β-effect may be a result of a lowered calcium permeability of the membrane and a consequent reduction in ionized calcium within the cell. It has already been established that the develop-

ment of tension by both cardiac and skeletal muscles is determined by the concentration of calcium ions within the cells. An alternate possibility is that activation of β-receptors increases the effectiveness of the energy-dependent processes by which cells normally maintain the concentration of ionized calcium at low levels.

A further possibility is that activation of β-receptors interferes with the metabolic processes which supply energy to the contractile apparatus. Brody and Diamond (1966) examined the influence of adrenergic drugs on phosphorylase activity in the guinea-pig taenia. Adrenaline caused both relaxation and the activation of phosphorylase. In the presence of a β-blocker, adrenaline still caused relaxation without influencing the level of active phosphorylase.

Bulbring and her colleagues (Bueding *et al.*, 1967) have recently summarized their evidence for an action of adrenaline on cell metabolism. Adrenaline increased the content of energy-rich phosphate compounds in the taenia coli coincidentally with its inhibitory action on this muscle. The possibility that the increase occurred as a result of decreased metabolic activity in the inhibited, relaxed, muscles was also eliminated. The relationship between the metabolic effects of adrenaline and its physiological action as a relaxant of smooth muscle cells in the taenia coli has, however, yet to be established.

C. ACTIONS OF 5-HYDROXYTRYPTAMINE ON SMOOTH MUSCLE

An extensive review of 5-hydroxytryptamine on smooth muscles has recently been prepared by Erspamer (1966) and the effects of this substance on various groups of smooth muscles will be described in considerably less detail in this section.

1. *Gasto-intestinal Tract*

5-Hydroxytryptamine has a spasmogenic action on intestinal muscles of several mammalian species, including man (Erspamer, 1966).

As most of the experimentation on the role of 5-hydroxytryptamine in the physiological control of intestinal peristalsis has involved the guinea-pig intestine, the responses of this structure will be described in some detail. Longitudinal muscle of the isolated small intestine of the guinea-pig is contracted by 5-hydroxytryptamine in dilutions down to $10^{-8} - 10^{-9}$ g/ml. Tachyphylaxis develops rapidly, and the smooth muscle becomes refractory to further applications (Gaddum, 1953; Gaddum and Picarelli, 1957). Guinea-pig ileum exposed to large doses of 5-hydroxytryptamine not only becomes desensitized to it, but the response to histamine, nicotine and to a lesser extent, acetylcholine is also depressed (Szerb, 1958). There is general agreement that the spasmogenic action of 5-hydroxytryptamine is diminished by atropine, although opinions differ as to the extent of the antagonism (Gaddum, 1953; Rapport and Koelle, 1953; Rocha e Silva, Valle and Picarelli, 1953). A partial explanation of this discrepancy is suggested by Robertson (1953) who found that $0 \cdot 01 - 0 \cdot 1$ μg/ml of atropine blocked the action of 2 μg of 5-hydroxytryptamine, but not the response to 20 μg.

The mode of action of 5-hydroxytryptamine on longitudinal intestinal muscle remains a subject of controversy, in spite of many experimental attacks. According to Rocha e Silva et al. (1953), 5-hydroxytryptamine acts on the postganglionic cholinergic fibres of the intramural plexus. Levy and Michel-Ber (1956) have suggested that it stimulates both postganglionic cholinergic and postganglionic adrenergic fibres. Gaddum and Picarelli (1957) have claimed that there are two kinds of tryptamine receptor in the guinea-pig ileum, namely M receptors which can be blocked with morphine and D receptors which can be blocked with dibenzyline. Atropine, cocaine and methadone inhibit effects due to the M receptors, even after dibenzyline but have no additional effects after morphine. Lysergic acid diethylamide, dihydroergotamine and 5-benzyloxygramine inhibit effects due to the D receptors, even after morphine but have no effect after dibenzyline. M receptors are probably in the nerve plexuses and D receptors in the muscle cells. The smooth muscle receptors are considered to be of secondary importance, as stimulation of specific receptors on the intramural parasympathetic ganglion cells appears to have the predominant effect (Day and Vane, 1963; Brownlee and Johnson, 1963). The demonstration of a 5-hydroxytryptamine-induced release of acetylcholine from the guinea-pig ileum is consistent with the concept that it stimulates intramural parasympathetic nerves (Brownlee and Johnson, 1965).

5-hydroxytryptamine also contracts circular muscle of the guinea-pig isolated ileum, but only after inhibition of cholinesterase (Harry, 1963). Contractions of this preparation by 5-hydroxytryptamine and nicotine were abolished by *botulinum* toxin, hemicholinium and atropine or hyoscine. Harry (1963) concluded that 5-hydroxytryptamine was stimulating

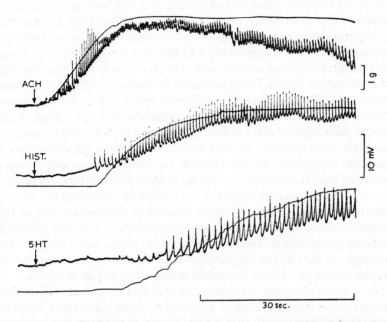

FIG. 5.12. Mechanical (lower) and electrical (upper, sucrose gap) records from a guinea-pig taenia coli in the presence of acetylcholine (10^{-6} g/ml), histamine (10^{-7} g/ml) and 5-hydroxytryptamine (5×10^{-8} g/ml) (Bülbring and Burnstock, 1960).

specific receptor sites in the intramural nerve plexuses of the muscle. Tachyphylaxis to 5-hydroxytryptamine, which is characteristic of the longitudinal muscle of the guinea-pig ileum, was only observed to a small extent in the circular muscle preparation.

Bulbring and Burnstock (1960) have studied the membrane potential changes induced by brief applications of 5-hydroxytryptamine to intestinal smooth muscle taken from the taenia coli of the guinea-pig. 5-Hydroxytryptamine, like histamine and acetylcholine, causes a depolarization which is followed, after removal of the drug, by a hyperpolarization and a sequence of damped oscillations of the membrane potential. The rate of depolarization was slowest with 5-hydroxytryptamine and fastest with acetylcholine (Fig. 5.12). Increasing concentrations of 5-hydroxytryptamine caused a progressively slower rate of depolarization.

A major site of production and storage of 5-hydroxytryptamine in the mammal is the enterochromaffin cell of the gastro-intestinal mucosa, and as 5-hydroxytryptamine has a powerful stimulating action on intestinal motility, it has been suggested the 5-hydroxytryptamine may be involved in the control of motor activity in the gut (Haverback and Wirtschaftler, 1962; Erspamer, 1966). The experiments of Bulbring and Lin (1968) and Lembeck (1958) have figured prominently in the substantiation of this hypothesis. Introduction of 5-hydroxytryptamine into the lumen of the isolated guinea-pig intestine in concentrations of 10^{-9}-10^{-5} g/ml stimulates peristalsis. The threshold of intra-abdominal pressure required to elicit peristalsis is lowered, the contractions are more frequent and a larger volume of fluid is propelled. According to these investigators, 5-hydroxytryptamine stimulates intestinal motility mainly by sensitizing the sensory receptors in intestinal mucosa which respond to pressure and trigger the peristaltic reflex. In addition, 5-hydroxytryptamine might also stimulate chemoreceptors whose fibres converge, with fibres from the pressure receptors, on the same motor ganglion cells. Stimulation of both types of receptor would be additive and would more readily trigger the reflex.

Paton and Vane (1963) have demonstrated that procedures which alter the tone of the stomach, whether produced by nerve stimulation, drugs or mechanical distension, will alter the rate of release of 5-hydroxytryptamine and histamine. However, it has yet to be demonstrated decisively that distension or hypermotility of the intestine, kept within physiological limits, actually produce a local discharge of 5-hydroxytryptamine from the enterochromaffin cells of the intact animal.

2. Uro-genital System

The isolated dioestrus uterus of the rat is barely sensitive to 5-hydroxytryptamine and shows marked tachyphylaxis. The oestrus uterus, on the other hand, is highly sensitive and shows little indication of tachyphylaxis (Gaddum and Hameed, 1954; Erspamer, 1966). Owing to its high sensitivity and specificity to 5-hydroxytryptamine, and the lack of tachyphylaxis, the oestrus uterus of the rat has become a frequently used preparation for the assay of this substance.

The urinary bladders of the rat, guinea-pig and rabbit are insensitive to 5-hydroxytryptamine (Erspamer, 1966). The isolated dog urinary bladder responds to the 5-hydroxytryptamine in doses of above 10^{-5} g/ml. The bladder contraction caused by 5-hydroxytryptamine is highly resistant to atropine and hexamethonium, but is blocked by dibenamine, chlorpromazine, and lysergic acid diethylamide (Gyermek, 1962; Erspamer, 1966), suggesting that it may act by stimulating the adrenergic nerve plexus.

3. Cardio-vascular System

The effects of 5-hydroxytryptamine on the isolated perfused rabbit heart have been studied by Jacob and Poite-Bevierre (1960). Three successive phases of response were observed which included a negative inotropic and chronotropic effect, antagonized by atropine and therefore probably due to a release of acetylcholine and a positive inotropic and chronotropic effect considered to be mediated by catecholamines, which was abolished when the preparation was reserpinised. The third effect, seen with larger doses of 5-hydroxytryptamine, was an atropine-resistant, negative inotropic action which was often accompanied by an increase in tone. A similar sequence of effects has been observed in the isolated rabbit atria with a short lived inhibition followed by facilitation and then a more marked depression. Atropine and hexamethonium abolish the initial inhibitory effect, but not the subsequent one (McCawley, Leveque and Dick, 1952; Sinha and West, 1953) and reserpine the stimulant action (Trendelenburg, 1960).

A positive inotropic effect of 5-hydroxytryptamine on cat papillary muscle has been observed, which was often preceded by a short depressant phase (Leusen and Lacroix, 1959). 5-Hydroxytryptamine had very little effect on ventricular strips from frog and turtle hearts (Hanson and Magill, 1962).

The effects of 5-hydroxytryptamine on blood vessels *in situ* have been reviewed in some detail by Erspamer (1966). The results have frequently been ambiguous and confusing, and whereas 5-hydroxytryptamine was originally considered to act as a vasoconstrictor and hypertensive agent (Page, 1954; Furchgott, 1955), some authors (Gordon, Haddy and Lipton, 1958, 1959; McCubben, Kaneko and Page, 1962) have now attributed vasodilator actions to this substance. Gordon and co-workers have studied the effects of adrenaline and 5-hydroxytryptamine on vascular resistance and concluded that these agents acted synergistically to constrict large arterial segments and antagonistically in small arterioles where 5-hydroxytryptamine was considered to oppose the vasoconstrictor actions of noradrenaline and adrenaline. Synergism between 5-hydroxytryptamine and noradrenaline vasoconstriction has also been observed in the central ear artery of the rabbit by de la Lande and his colleagues (de la Lande and Rand, 1965; de la Lande, Cannell and Waterson, 1966).

Isolated rings or spiral strips of aorta or carotid artery have frequently been used to study the actions of 5-hydroxytryptamine and its antagonists (e.g. Shaw and Woolley, 1953, 1954). The contractile response of strips of sheep aorta to 5-hydroxytryptamine is inhibited by yohimbine, ergotoxine and various antimetabolites (Shaw and Woolley, 1953, 1954). The vasoconstrictor action of 5-hydroxytryptamine on the central artery of the rabbit ear, described above, which is weak in comparison with that of noradrenaline, is greatly enhanced by noradrenaline. 5-Hydroxytryptamine sensitizes the preparation to noradrenaline, adrenaline, histamine, angiotensin and sympathetic nerve stimulation. Although the portal, external, jugular and posterior caval veins of the rabbit are all relatively insensitive to 5-hydroxytryptamine, the anterior mesenteric vein of this animal contracted in the presence of drug concentrations as low as 10^{-8} g/ml (Sutter, 1965; Hughes and Vane, 1967).

D. HISTAMINE

Histamine evokes a contraction of most smooth muscles, although its effect varies somewhat from tissue to tissue, and in different species. The uterus and bronchioles of certain species are particularly sensitive to histamine (Parrot and Thouvenot, 1966). It has little action on some smooth muscles, such as those of the iris and bladder, and exceptionally it causes relaxation, as in the rat uterus. Arterioles and the muscles of the gastrointestinal tract are moderately sensitive to histamine (Parrot and Thouvenot, 1966).

The evidence suggests that histamine can contract smooth muscle quite independently of an action on nervous elements associated with the muscle. However, a component of the response to histamine has been attributed to excitation of the ganglionic plexuses of the gastrointestinal tract (Ambache, 1946; Paton and Vane, 1963). Histamine causes depolarization of the guinea-pig taenia coli and an increase in spike frequency (Fig. 5.12) qualitatively similar to that produced by acetylcholine (Bulbring, 1957), the only apparent differences between their actions being that the rate of depolarization with histamine is slower and the degree of tachyphylaxis greater (Bulbring and Burnstock, 1960). The rate of loss of K^{42} from intestine is increased in the presence of histamine (Born and Bulbring, 1956).

Histamine continues to cause a contraction of smooth muscles that have been treated with the metabolic inhibitor dinitrophenol (Bulbring and Lullman, 1957) or depolarized by excess potassium in the perfusion fluid (Evans, Schild and Thesleff, 1958). As both procedures render muscles electrically inexcitable, it has been suggested that histamine may have a direct action on the contractile elements (Parrot and Thouvenot, 1966). It appears therefore that histamine excites smooth muscle both by a depolarizing action and by a direct effect on the contractile mechanism. The latter action may involve alterations in metabolic activity.

The specificity of the histamine receptor has been established with histamine antagonists, such as mepyramine, which at concentrations adequate to abolish the action of histamine, do not modify the contractions evoked by acetylcholine or 5-hydroxytryptamine. Atropine abolishes acetylcholine-induced contractions of smooth muscle without significantly altering the responses to histamine (Schild, 1947). The possible structure for histamine receptors has been discussed in some detail by Rocha e Silva (1966).

E. PROSTAGLANDINS

The effects of these on a few selected tissues will be discussed.

1. *Uterus*

Interest in the effects of prostaglandins on smooth muscle has largely been confined in the past to its effect on uterine preparations, as this appeared to be the most likely site for a physiological action of seminal prostaglandin after its deposition in the vagina. Von Euler (1936) demonstrated a prostaglandin-induced increase in the frequency and strength of the contractions of various uterine preparations. Further studies have shown that the usual response of the guinea-pig uterus to both PGE_1 or E_2 and to F_1 or F_2 is a contraction or increase in the rate and frequency of spontaneous contractions (Pickles, 1967). After the application of PGE_1 there often follows a prolonged phase during which the responses to other spasmogens are also increased. Pickles has been able to distinguish between the early "potentiation" phase during which contractions occur and this later "enhancement" response by the insensitivity of the latter to changes in ionic environment and the absence of electrical signs of persistent excitation during the "enhancement" phase. The guinea-pig myometrium sometimes shows traces of the inhibitory type of response which is seen with the human myometrium. The variety of responses of guinea-pig myometrium to prostaglandins suggests that at least three fundamentally different cellular processes may be initiated by these substances.

The uteri of the rat and of the rabbit are less sensitive to a stimulant action of the prostaglandins. Rat uterus does not show an "enhancement" response after PGE_1 (Sullivan, 1966). Inhibition or relaxation appears to be the normal response of non-pregnant human myometrium to seminal prostaglandin and to pure PGE_1, E_2 or E_3 (Eliasson, 1966; Pickles, 1967). An initial stimulant action has been observed either preceding the relaxation or when the concentration of prostaglandin E was below threshold for an inhibitory effect. The usual response of the pregnant human myometrium to prostaglandin E_1 is one of contraction (Bygdeman, Kwon and Wiquist, 1967).

2. *Gastro-intestinal Smooth Muscle*

Isolated segments of intestinal muscle of many species contract in response to low concentrations of prostaglandin. Prostaglandins of both E and F series have been shown to stimulate the intestinal smooth muscle of the guinea-pig ileum and rat jejunum (Eliasson, 1959), of the fowl jejunum and rectal caecum (Bergström, Eliasson, Euler and Sjövall, 1959), of the hamster and rat colon (Ambache, 1957a, b), of the rat duodenum (Horton, 1963) and of the rat stomach (Coceani and Wolfe, 1966). In all instances, the contractions of the longitudinal muscle layer only were recorded, and an effect of prostaglandin on circular muscle has yet to be demonstrated.

On the guinea-pig ileum and rabbit jejunum, the stimulant action of PGE_1 giving a response that is about 50% maximum can be abolished by atropine ($0 \cdot 1$ μg/ml), but increasing the concentration of E_1 again causes a further contraction (Pickles, 1967). These results imply the presence of two sites of action of PGE_1 on intestinal smooth muscle, A "neurotropic" action on the cholinergic nerve cells in the intrinsic plexuses and a "musculotropic" action on smooth muscle cells. The action of PGE_1 on isolated rat fundus muscle was not affected by atropine or hexamethonium

(Coceani and Wolfe, 1966), suggesting that its effects on this tissue were entirely musculotropic.

3. *Respiratory Smooth Muscle*

Main (1964) found that PGE_1 relaxed certain respiratory smooth-muscle preparations. Sweatman and Collier (1968) have shown that PGE_1 and E_2 relax, and PGF_2 stimulates human bronchial smooth muscles.

4. *Vascular Smooth Muscle*

Prostaglandins are potent vasodepressors when administered *in vivo*, decreasing blood pressure and vascular resistance. Considerable interest in renal prostaglandins has arisen because of their possible role in preventing pathological rises in blood pressure.

Prostaglandin E_2 has now been identified as the principal vasodepressor lipid of rabbit renal medulla (Daniels, Hinman, Leach and Muirhead, 1967) and PGA_2 may also be present in the renal medulla (Lee, Covino, Takman and Smith, 1965).

Paradoxically prostaglandins E_1, E_2, A_1 and F_1 cause contraction of isolated aortic strips and coronary smooth muscle. However, the smooth muscle of small arteries from other sites showed a biphasic dose–response relationship with these compounds. Helical strips from small renal, muscular and mesenteric arteries, which had been partially contracted by catecholamines, potassium or plasma contracting factor, were relaxed by prostaglandins in low concentrations and contracted further by prostaglandins in higher concentrations (Strong and Bohr, 1967). This relaxation of smooth muscle from small arteries may account for the vasodepressor actions of prostaglandins.

Prostaglandins have been reported to have both relaxant (Strong and Bohr, 1967) and vasoconstrictor actions on veins (Ducharme and Weeks, 1967).

5. *Smooth Muscle of the Iris*

The irins are prostaglandins and prostaglandin-like substances extractable from the irides of various species. One irin extracted from sheep iris, has been shown to be identical with PGF_2 (Anggärd and Samulesson,

1964a). Rabbit and cat irins also contain PGF_2 and PGE_2 (Ambache, Brummer, Rose and Whiting, 1966). The iris responds to irins by constriction of the pupil (miosis) and there is evidence that these substances are released in the iris by mechanical stimulation (Ambache, Kavanagh and Whiting, 1965).

CONCLUSIONS

1. This chapter describes the actions of acetylcholine, catecholamines, 5-hydroxytryptamine, histamine, and prostaglandins on various smooth muscle preparations.

2. Acetylcholine excites most smooth muscles, depolarizing the muscle membrane and eliciting contractions. It has inhibitory effects on cardiovascular and retractor penis muscles.

3. Evidence for cholinergic transmission in the gastro-intestinal tract, urogenital and cardiovascular systems is discussed.

4. The actions of adrenaline and noradrenaline on smooth muscles are complex and may frequently be a result of two or more actions. Noradrenaline has been identified as the neurotransmitter released by sympathetic nerve terminals, but at many junctions, (for instance those in the vas deferens), the pharmacological findings are currently not altogether reconcilable with this hypothesis. Excitatory responses to adrenaline and noradrenaline are most evident in the urogenital and cardiovascular systems whereas inhibitory effects predominate in the gastro-intestinal tract.

5. 5-Hydroxytryptamine has a spasmogenic action on intestinal muscles, and as it is present in the mucosal layers of the intestine in large amounts, it has been proposed that this amine is involved in the control of intestinal mobility. The effects of 5-hydroxytryptamine on other smooth muscle systems are variable.

6. Histamine evokes a contraction of most smooth muscle cells studies, although the types of effect vary from tissue to tissue and in different species.

7. The actions of prostaglandins on various smooth muscle preparations are described. These vary with the tissue and particular prostaglandins tested.

CHAPTER 6

THE PHARMACOLOGY
OF AUTONOMIC GANGLIA

STUDIES on autonomic ganglia have played an important role in the elucidation of the actions of drugs on nervous tissues, and indeed much of the evidence for chemical transmission has been derived from these structures. With the exception of small differences in such details as the magnitude of the resting membrane potential or latency of depolarization, the generation of impulses in sympathetic ganglia conforms to the pattern of events described at other excitatory junctions. Intracellular recording has shown that preganglionic stimulation produces a typical, slowly increasing and decrementing excitatory postsynaptic potential, which gives rise to an action potential (Fig. 6.1) in isolated sympathetic ganglia of the rabbit (Eccles, R. M., 1955, 1963) and frog (Nishi and Koketsu, 1960; Blackman, Ginsborg and Ray, 1963). If action potential generation is abolished by exposure to an appropriate concentration of a ganglionic blocking compound, such as curare or dihydro-β-erythroidine, preganglionic volleys can be shown to evoke a complex sequence of waves in sympathetic ganglia of turtles and rabbits (Laporte and Lorente de Nó, 1950; Eccles, 1952). When recorded extracellularly between an electrode on the ganglion surface and another on the distal end of the isolated postganglionic trunk, the sequence is composed of an initial negative wave (N) of about 100 msec duration, followed by a slight positive wave (P) that is terminated by a late negative wave (LN) of more than 2 sec in duration (Fig. 6.2). Tetanic stimulation enhances the P and LN potentials.

A long lasting hyperpolarization, which corresponds to the P potential, has been recorded intracellularly from neurones in sympathetic ganglia of rabbits, frogs and bullfrogs (Tosaka and Libet, 1965; Libet and Toska, 1966; Nishi and Koketsu, 1966). The P potential can, therefore, be considered to be an inhibitory postsynaptic potential by virtue of its transsynaptic occurrence, its polarity and its ability to inhibit ganglionic transmission (Koketsu and Nishi, 1967). The LN wave has been shown by

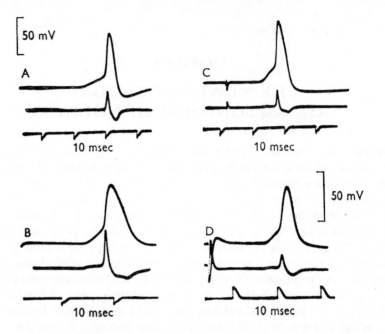

FIG. 6.1. Ganglionic action potentials recorded with microelectrodes from superior cervical ganglion of the rabbit during stimulation of the cervical sympathetic trunk. The records were obtained with four different cells. The middle tracing of each record is an electrotonically differentiated waveform of the evoked potential; the lower tracing a time marker. A synaptic step preceeds the action potential in each record (Eccles, 1963).

intracellular recording to represent a depolarizing postsynaptic response and can be considered as a slow excitatory postsynaptic potential (Tosaka and Libet, 1965; Libet and Tosaka, 1966).

The results of the pharmacological investigations described below are summarized in Table 6.

A. ACETYCHOLINE

The first important account of the actions of a drug on autonomic ganglia was given in a series of papers by Langley (Langley, 1891, 1893) in which the stimulating and blocking actions of nicotine on sympathetic ganglia were described. The nicotine-like activities of choline and several

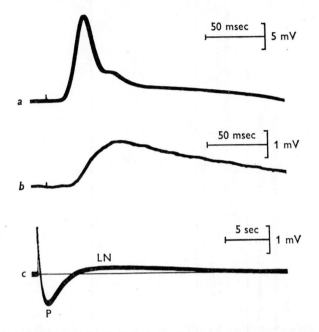

FIG. 6.2. Compound ganglionic action potential set up by single preganglionic volley, recorded by sucrose gap method from rabbit superior cervical ganglion. a, before, b and c, after exposure of the ganglion to hexamenthonium (0·55 mM) for 68 min. In b, the action potential is replaced by an N wave or synaptic potential; in c, the slow P and LN waves are shown (Kosterlitz, Lees and Wallis, 1968).

esters of choline, particularly acetylcholine, were described in detail by Dale in 1914. In this paper, Dale made the distinction between the "nicotinic" and "muscarinic" activities of acetylcholine; the former an excitatory and blocking action in autonomic ganglia and the latter an excitatory action on peripheral parasympathetic postganglionic junctions. The nicotine-like activity of another quaternary ammonium compound, tetramethyl-ammonium, was recognized by Burn and Dale (1915) when, like acetyl-choline, it was found to produce a pressor response in atropinized animals. In addition, they noted that the response to tetramethylammonium could be blocked by tetraethylammonium ion, a structurally similar compound which lacked pressor activity.

TABLE 6.

PHARMACOLOGICAL INVESTIGATIONS ON THE POSTGANGLIONIC RESPONSES OF SYMPATHETIC GANGLIA

— — marked depression; — depression; + potentiation; 0 no effect (further description in text)

Drug	Synaptic transmission and N wave	P wave or potential	LN wave or potential	Intra-arterially injected acetylcholine		Prolonged discharges caused by anticholinesterases
				early discharge	late response	
"Nicotinic" acetylcholine antagonists, e.g. d- tubocurarine and hexamethonium	— —	+	+ or 0	— —	0	+
"Muscarinic" acetylcholine antagonists, e.g. atropine	0	— —	— —	0	— —	— —
Noradrenaline	—	—	—	0	—	— and then +
Adrenaline	—			0		— and/or +
Isoprenaline	+			0		
Dibenamine	0					
5-hydroxytryptamine	+ or —				+++	
Histamine	—					

The identification of acetylcholine as a chemical transmitter in sympathetic ganglia was a result of a series of important experiments. Chang and Gaddum (1933) had isolated an acetylcholine-like substance from sympathetic ganglia and subsequently Feldberg and Gaddum (1934) were able to show that preganglionic stimulation evoked the release of an acetylcholine-like substance from perfused superior cervical ganglia. In further experiments it was established that this acetylcholine-like substance evoked a ganglionic response when added to the fluid perfusing the ganglion (Feldberg and Vartiainen, 1934) and that stimulation of the postganglionic nerve did not evoke a release of the material. Injection of acetylcholine into the perfusion fluid caused ganglionic stimulation, which was antagonized by curare. Curare also antagonized the responses to preganglionic nerve stimulation. Anticholinesterases potentiated the effects of preganglionic stimulation and those of injected acetylcholine (Feldberg and Gaddum, 1934; Feldberg and Vartiainen, 1934; Eccles, 1935). The levels of acetylcholine (Brown and Feldberg, 1936) and cholinesterase (Brücke, 1937) in the ganglion were found to decrease when the preganglionic nerve to the superior cervical ganglion was sectioned. Collectively, these results satisfied most of the criteria for transmitter identification and established that acetylcholine was a transmitter in sympathetic ganglia.

The possibility has been raised that choline esters other than acetylcholine are present in sympathetic ganglia (Kewitz, 1955). Attempts to establish whether only acetylcholine is present, have yielded equivocal results. In one study, no evidence was obtained, using physical and chemical techniques, of the presence of any ester of choline other than acetylcholine in sympathetic ganglia (Friesen, Kemp and Woodbury, 1965). In a second study, in which similar techniques were employed, it was reported that most of the acetylcholine-like activity extractable from ganglia is in the form of coenzyme A esters of betaine (Hosein and Proulx, 1965). This report also described the presence of propionyl- and butyryl-choline in ganglia. Until these differences are resolved, the possibility that other choline esters and substances with acetylcholine-like activity are present in ganglia cannot be eliminated.

1. *Acetylcholine Release from Ganglia*

The relationship between the storage and release of acetylcholine from sympathetic ganglia has been the subject of repeated investigations (Brown and Feldberg, 1936; Kahlson and MacIntosh, 1939; Perry, 1953; Birks and MacIntosh, 1961) and has contributed to our understanding of the metabolism of acetylcholine in nerve terminals, discussed in Chapter 2. The rate of release from an eserinized, resting, ganglion is very small, amounting to about $1 \cdot 5 - 5 \times 10^{-10}$ g/min (Birks and MacIntosh, 1961). Repetitive stimulation of the preganglionic trunk, at frequencies of 10–20/sec, initially increases the rate of release to $31–34 \times 10^{-9}$ g/min, although during a 15 min period of continuous stimulation this subsequently declines to a rate of approximately 4×10^{-9} g/min.

Elevation of the calcium ion content of the perfusion fluid causes an increase in the rate of release of acetylcholine from stimulated ganglia (Harvey and MacIntosh, 1940; Hutter and Kostial, 1954; McKinstry and Koelle, 1967) and a reduction in the external calcium concentration depresses transmitter release. Barium can act as a substitute for calcium (Douglas, Lywood and Straub, 1961) and magnesium is an antagonist, just as at the neuromuscular junction. Using isolated rabbit ganglia depolarized by potassium chloride, Lipicky, Hertz and Shanes (1963) found that a slightly less than one-to-one molar exchange occurred between the influx of radiocalcium and the release of acetylcholine.

The release of acetylcholine from sympathetic ganglia is severely depressed when the levels of sodium in the perfusion fluid are reduced (Birks, 1963). A depletion of potassium ions in the perfusing fluid, which would be expected to cause an accumulation of intracellular sodium, causes an enhancement of the release of acetylcholine. Birks has, therefore, suggested that an inward movement of sodium ions into the nerve ending may be an important part of the mechanism coupling neuronal activity to the synthesis and release of transmitter.

Tetraethylammonium and certain other quaternary ammonium ions enhance the amount of acetylcholine released from sympathetic ganglia by nerve stimulation (Douglas and Lywood, 1961). This is probably a result of a prolongation of the preganglionic nerve action potential (Kusano, Livengood and Werman, 1967). Carbamylcholine (carbachol) causes a release of acetylcholine from the superior cervical ganglion of the cat (McKinstry, Koenig, Koelle and Koelle, 1963). It has been suggested that this release is the result of an actual penetration of the nerve terminals by carbachol and subsequent exchange with endogenous acetylcholine (McKinstry and Koelle, 1967).

2. Pharmacology of the Postsynaptic Receptor

Confirmation that acetylcholine is the transmitter released by preganglionic terminals has come from electrophysiological experiments in which
it has been shown that exposure of ganglia to appropriate concentrations
of such classical "nicotinic" acetylcholine antagonists as hexamethonium
or curare results in a failure of ganglionic transmission in the absence of
alterations in the resting membrane potential. The possibility that additional functionally important "muscarinic" cholinergic receptor sites are
also present in mammalian sympathetic ganglia has been apparent since
Koppanyi (1932) demonstrated that pilocarpine excites the superior
cervical ganglion of the cat, and that this action can be abolished by
atropine.

The first demonstration that this second, "muscarinic", receptor can be
activated by synaptically released acetylcholine was by Eccles and Libet
(1961), who observed that the several components of the complex surface
potential evoked by preganglionic stimulation of a partially curarized
superior cervical ganglion are sensitive to blockade by various acetylcholine antagonists (Fig. 6.3). Increasing concentrations of dihydro-β-
erythroidine or curare in the bath decrease the amplitude of the initial
negative (N) potential and increase the amplitude of the late negative (LN)
potential. Low concentrations of atropine selectively abolish the P and
LN waves. As exposure to *botulinum* toxin, which is known to impair the
release of acetylcholine from nerve endings, caused a disappearance of all
three potentials, it was suggested that acetylcholine is involved in the
generation of each phase of the complex potential (Eccles and Libet, 1961).
The P and LN potentials were also blocked by dibenamine and reserpine
(Eccles and Libet, 1962), although dibenamine depressed the P potential in
concentrations which did not affect the LN potential.

As a result of these experiments, Eccles and Libet (1961) suggested that
acetylcholine released at the preganglionic terminals is able to cause
ganglionic depolarization by acting either at "nicotinic", curare-sensitive,
sites (N potential) or at atropine-sensitive "muscarinic" sites (LN potential). The hyperpolarizing P potential was thought to arise from an activation by acetylcholine of atropine-sensitive sites on chromaffin cells in the
ganglion with a subsequent release of catecholamines, which then hyperpolarized the ganglion cells. This hypothesis is illustrated in Fig. 6.4. Libet
(1967) has since demonstrated that both the P and LN potentials are

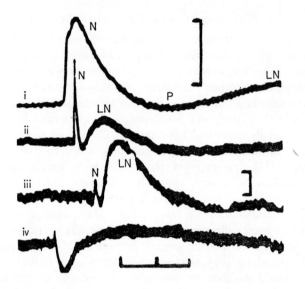

Fig. 6.3. Ganglionic action potentials set up by single preganglionic volleys, recorded from rabbit superior cervical ganglion. (i) synaptic potential after partial curarization (d-tubocurarine, $2 \cdot 5 \times 10^{-5}$ M). (ii) as in (i) but at 1/10th of sweep speed; (iii) after complete curarization $(8 \times 10^{-5}$ M); (iv) after addition of 3×10^{-6} M prostigmine to (iii). Voltage calibration $0 \cdot 1$ mV for (i) and (ii), $0 \cdot 02$ mV for (iii) and (iv). Time scale, 10/sec for (i) and 1/sec for (ii), (iii) and (iv) (Eccles, R. M. 1952).

subject to post-tetanic potentiation and can be augmented by inhibition of ganglionic acetylcholinesterase.

An involvement of muscarinic receptors in the responses to preganglion-ically released acetylcholine is suggested by the demonstration, in the cat, that treatment of the superior cervical ganglion with anticholinesterase agents evokes postganglionic firing which is resistant to d-tubocurarine and hexamethonium, although antagonized by atropine (Fig. 6.5A, B) (Takeshige and Volle, 1962; Volle, 1962). Since cholinesterase inhibitors do not evoke firing in denervated ganglia (Volle and Koelle, 1961, Take-shige and Volle, 1962), the firing can be attributed to acetylcholine released spontaneously from nerve endings and acting on muscarinic postsynaptic receptors.

The persistent depolarization and firing of sympathetic ganglion cells that follows tetanic preganglionic stimulation can also be prevented by atropine (Paton and Perry, 1953; Takeshige and Volle, 1962, 1964a; Libet, 1964). Similarly, the persistent depolarization produced in normal ganglia by cholinesterase inhibitors (Mason, 1962) is blocked by pretreatment with atropine (Takeshige and Volle, 1964a).

Acetylcholine is the only substance with a demonstrated ability to activate both types of excitatory cholinoceptive receptor in sympathetic

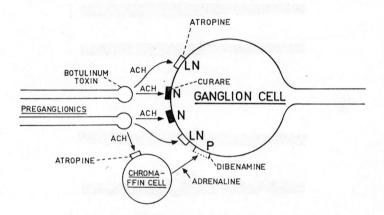

FIG. 6.4. Diagrammatic representation of the postulated production of N, P and LN waves of ganglion cells by presynaptically released transmitter. The receptor sites are shown on the surface of the ganglion and chromaffin cells. See further description in text. Modified from Eccles and Libet (1961).

ganglia (Takeshige and Volle, 1965). In untreated ganglia, the postganglionic response to acetylcholine is characterized by a single burst of firing, that is immediate in onset and sensitive to blockade by hexamethonium. However, after conditioning with anticholinesterase drugs, with repetitive preganglionic stimulation or by repeated injections of potassium ions, the response to acetylcholine is characterized by a bimodal pattern consisting of an initial period of discharge, followed in 1–2 sec by a later-occurring period of firing. The "early response" to injected acetylcholine is abolished by d-tubocurarine or hexamethonium and the "late response" by small doses of atropine (Fig. 6.5B). In ganglia conditioned by the above procedures, the threshold dose of acetylcholine required for activation of the

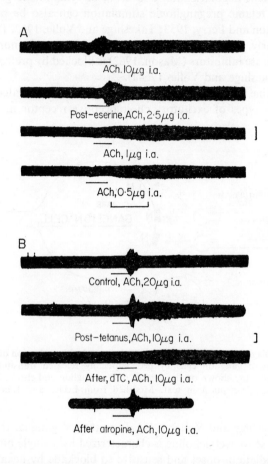

FIG. 6.5. A and B. Postganglionic discharges of cat superior cervical ganglion in response to intra-arterial injections of acetylcholine in the amounts indicated, and at times shown by horizontal lines. In A an intra-arterial injection of 100 μg of eserine greatly increases the effectiveness of acetylcholine in evoking a delayed discharge. In B after conditioning by a tetanus (60/sec for 10 sec) there is in the second record an increase in the delayed discharge. The third and fourth records show selective depression of the early and late discharges by *d*-tubocurarine and atropine respectively. Time scales 1 sec; voltage calibration, 10 μV (Takeshige and Volle, 1962).

atropine-sensitive late discharge is lower than that required for activation of the early response. This difference in the sensitivity of the two receptors to acetylcholine may account for the failure of anticholinesterase agents to cause hexamethonium-sensitive postganglionic firing. A bimodal response to acetylcholine occurs quite frequently in chronically denervated ganglia that have not otherwise been treated (Takeshige and Volle, 1963b). Superior cervical ganglion cells of the cat and rat do not exhibit denervation supersensitivity to acetylcholine or carbachol; indeed it has been reported

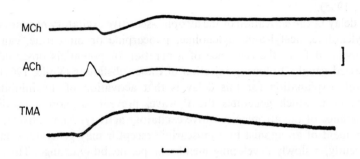

FIG. 6.6. Surface potentials of the superior cervical ganglion evoked by acetyl-β-methylcholine (MCh), acetylcholine (ACh), and tetramethylammonium (TMA). An upward deflection of the tracing indicates increasing negativity of the ganglion with respect to the crushed end of the post-ganglionic nerve and a downward deflection positivity. The vertical calibration is equal to 400 μV and the horizontal calibration to 4 sec (Takeshige and Volle, 1964b).

that sensitivity to carbachol is actually reduced by denervation (Volle and Koelle, 1961; Brown, 1966).

The potentials recorded from the surface of the superior cervical ganglion of the cat after an injection of acetylcholine are remarkably similar to those evoked by nerve stimulation in the curarized rabbit ganglion (Fig. 6.6) (Takeshige and Volle, 1964b). The triphasic ganglionic wave-form consisting of an initial period of negativity followed in turn by periods of positivity and negativity (Fig. 6.6) resembles the N, P and LN waves evoked by synaptic activation. Acetyl-β-methylcholine, a "muscarinic" receptor stimulant, produces only a biphasic potential, that is delayed in onset and consists of a period of positivity succeeded by a negativity (Fig. 6.6).

These studies, collectively, provide convincing evidence for the presence of both "nicotinic" and "muscarinic" cholinoceptive excitatory receptors in mammalian sympathetic ganglia. This conclusion cannot, however, be applied to all autonomic ganglia, for evidence obtained with the muscarinic stimulant, 4-(M-chloro-phenylcarbamoyloxy) 2-butynyltrimethylammonium chloride (McN-A-343), suggests that parasympathetic ganglia do not possess excitatory atropine-sensitive cholinoceptive receptors (Roszkowski, 1961; Smith, 1966). It has been reported, moreover, that the superior cervical ganglion of the frog is insensitive to muscarine-like drugs (Ginsborg, 1965).

A delay in the activation of the atropine-sensitive excitatory receptors by acetylcholine, acetyl-β-methylcholine, pilocarpine or muscarine, can be extrapolated from the sequence of generation of potentials observed in curarized ganglia following injection of these substances (Volle, 1966). A possible explanation for this delay is that activation of the inhibitory mechanism, which generates the P wave, prevents a more immediate appearance of the atropine-sensitive excitatory activity. Alternatively, the attachment of an agonist to a muscarinic receptor may generate, what is inherently, a slowly developing membrane permeability change. Thus the activation of muscarinic receptors on Betz cells in the cerebral cortex (Krnjević and Phillis, 1963b) or on Renshaw cells (Curtis and Ryall, 1966a) by iontophoretically applied cholinergic compounds results in a slowly-developing excitation of these neurones.

The function of this atropine-sensitive excitatory receptor may be that of acting as a modulating influence on the main pathway of transmission via the "nicotinic" receptor. Drugs such as pilocarpine, muscarine and acetyl-β-methylcholine, when administered in small doses, enhance the transmission of ganglionic action potentials. Libet (1964, 1967) has proposed that the persistent ganglionic depolarization resulting from the activation of the atropine-sensitive excitatory receptor represents a slow excitatory postsynaptic potential that contributes to the recruitment of cells.

The blockade of transmission in sympathetic ganglia by drugs related to acetylcholine has been attributed either to a curare-like action that does not involve a change in the polarization of the ganglion, or to sustained depolarization subsequent to a period of stimulation, such as occurs with nicotine (Paton and Perry, 1953). A notable addition to this classification of the types of ganglionic blockade is the finding that the depression of transmission produced by acetyl-β-methylcholine is associated with a

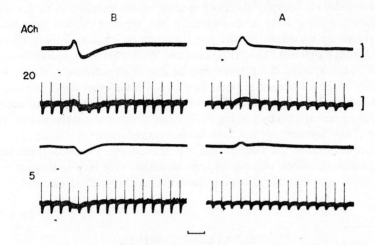

FIG. 6.7. The ganglion potentials and blockade produced in the superior cervical ganglion by acetylcholine before (B) and after (A) the administration of 1 μg of atropine. The top tracing of each pair shows the ganglion potentials of the unstimulated ganglion evoked by 5 or 20 μg of acetylcholine before and after atropine. The bottom tracing of each pair shows the effect on the stimulated ganglion of 5–20 μg of acetylcholine before and after atropine. Similar findings have been made with acetyl-β-methylcholine. The vertical calibrations are 400 μV (top) and 1 μV (bottom) and apply to the unstimulated and stimulated ganglion, respectively. The horizontal calibration is 4 sec (Takeshige and Volle, 1963).

phase of ganglionic hyperpolarization (Takeshige, Pappano, De Groat and Volle, 1963; Takeshige and Volle, 1964b). Like the ganglionic blockade produced by acetyl-β-methylcholine, that produced by moderate doses of acetylcholine is antagonized by small doses of atropine (Fig. 6.7) and occurs either during the falling phase of depolarization or during the period of hyperpolarization. This depression of ganglionic transmission, with the appearance of a hyperpolarization and the abolition of both responses by atropine, suggests the existence of an atropine-sensitive cholinoceptive site which participates in transmission as an inhibitory modulator mechanism. The available evidence does not allow a clear distinction to be made between the possible presence of an atropine-sensitive excitatory receptor on chromaffin cells or on adrenergic neurones and their terminals, excitation of which releases noradrenaline which subsequently inhibits ganglion cells and a direct cholinergic inhibitory synapse on the ganglion cells. A recent report that the P wave of an isolated rabbit superior cervical ganglion is increased by reductions in the potassium concentration of the perfusing fluid from 6 to 0 mM (Kosterlitz, Lees and Wallis, 1968), supports the view that in this species, the P wave may be due to an increase in the permeability of the membrane to potassium ions. On the other hand, the size of the hyperpolarization which follows exposure of the ganglion to acetylcholine is not altered by varying the external potassium concentration. The rate of development of the acetylcholine-induced hyperpolarization and its subsequent recovery are diminished in potassium-free solutions. It has been suggested, therefore, that the hyperpolarization may be a consequence of an active extrusion of sodium ions from the ganglion cells (Kosterlitz *et al.*, 1968).

B. CATECHOLAMINES

The effects of the catecholamines on the transmission of impulses through autonomic ganglia have been a matter of considerable controversy. In 1939, Marrazzi demonstrated a blocking action of adrenaline on transmission in the cervical ganglion of the cat. He was also able to demonstrate that endogenously liberated catecholamines impair transmission and extended these findings to include other autonomic ganglia (Marrazzi, 1939; Marrazzi and Marrazzi, 1947; Suden and Marrazzi, 1951). A period of post-inhibitory facilitation was ascribed to the vasoconstrictor effects of adrenaline rather than to an effect of adrenaline on ganglion cells. On the basis of these findings, Marrazzi was the first to postulate that adrenaline acted as an inhibitory modulator of ganglionic transmission.

Bulbring and Burn (1942b) and Bulbring (1944) observed facilitatory effects of small doses of adrenaline on ganglionic transmission and inhibitory effects with larger doses. Similar qualitative differences in effect, that depended on the dose of the amine, were described by Malmejac, (1955), Trendelenburg (1956) and Pardo, Cato, Gijon and Alonso De-Florida (1963). Konzett (1950) demonstrated that sympathomimetic amines potentiate the effects of acetylcholine injected into the perfusion of the superior cervical ganglion of the cat.

The effects of adrenaline on ganglia are further complicated by the fact that any given dose of this amine may cause inhibition of ganglionic transmission when low frequencies of preganglionic stimulation are used, while facilitation is observed with high rates of stimulation (Elliott, 1965).

In a recent systematic study of the ganglionic effects of sympatho-mimetic amines, De Groat and Volle (1966a) obtained good evidence for the presence of two different types of receptors which are both activated by adrenaline and noradrenaline. Interaction of the amines with α-receptors causes hyperpolarization of the ganglion cells accompanied by inhibition

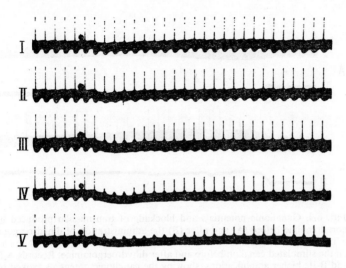

Fig. 6.8. Ganglionic potentials and blockade of transmission produced by graded doses of noradrenaline. Records I, II, III, IV and V: the ganglionic potentials and depression of transmission produced by the intra-arterial administration of 0·1, 0·25, 0·5, 2·0 and 8·0 μg of noradrenaline respectively. Ganglionic action potentials were evoked by submaximal preganglionic stimulation at a frequency of 0·5 cps. Injections were marked by a calibration signal of 200 μV. Horizontal calibration is 5 sec (De Groat and Volle, 1966a).

of ganglionic transmission (Fig. 6.8). These effects are antagonized by *alpha* but not *beta* adrenergic blocking compounds. *Alpha*-effects are prominent after noradrenaline, detectable after adrenaline and absent after isoprenaline. Activation of the β-receptors, on the other hand, was most pronounced after isoprenaline and was observed with noradrenaline only after block of the α-receptors (Fig. 6.9). Interaction of the amines with β-receptors caused depolarization of ganglion cells, which was accompanied by a facilitation of ganglionic transmission (Fig. 6.10). These actions of isoprenaline are unaffected by *alpha* blocking agents and are antagonized by *beta* adrenergic blocking compounds. The effect of catecholamines on the response of the ganglion to nicotinic and muscarinic drugs was the subject of a further study (De Groat and Volle, 1966b). The nicotonic postganglionic discharge observed after nicotine or acetylcholine was not affected by prior injection of the amines. However, administration of

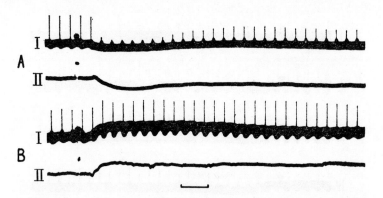

Fig. 6.9. Ganglionic potentials and blockade of transmission produced by noradrenaline before (A) and after (B) the administration of dihydroergota-mine (50 μg i.a.). Records A-I and B-I: the effects of noradrenaline (8 μg i.a.) on the stimulated ganglion before and after dihydroergotamine. Records A-II and B-II: higher amplifications, showing the ganglionic potentials evoked by noradrenaline (4 μg i.a.) in the unstimulated ganglion before and after dihydro-ergotamine. Ganglionic action potentials were evoked by submaximal pre-ganglionic stimulation at a frequency of 0·5 cps. (The peaks of some of the ganglionic action potentials went off the oscilloscope screen in record B-I). All calibrations are the same as those in Fig. 6.8 (De Groat and Volle, 1966a).

isoprenaline caused the appearance of a late, atropine-sensitive, post-ganglionic discharge in response to injections of acetylcholine (Fig. 6.11); or in other words, the catecholamine revealed the muscarinic actions of acetylcholine. Noradrenaline caused the appearance of the late, atropine-sensitive postganglionic discharge in response to acetylcholine, only after an α-receptor blocking agent had been given.

These observations of De Groat and Volle (1966a, b) have resolved most of the contradictions of the past and lead directly to the question of a possible physiological role of the catecholamines in modifying ganglionic transmission.

Histochemical techniques have revealed the presence of large numbers of adrenergic nerve terminals in the neighbourhood of the ganglion cells of the prevertebral ganglia of the cat (coeliac and inferior mesenteric ganglia). The superior cervical ganglion of the cat (like most of the paravertebral ganglia) has relatively few adrenergic nerve terminals (Hamberger, Norberg and Sjöqvist, 1964; Hamberger and Norberg, 1965a;

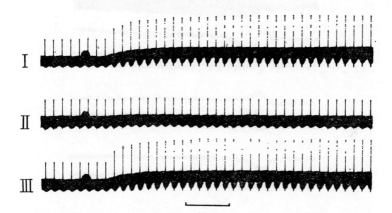

FIG. 6.10. Ganglionic potentials and enhancement of transmission produced by isoprenaline (0·2 μg i.a.) before and after the administration of dichloroisoproterenol (DCI) (300 μg i.a.). Record I: the ganglionic response to isoprenaline in the untreated ganglion. Record II: response to isoprenaline 10 min after the administration of DCI. Record III: response to ISO 40 min after the administration of DCI. Ganglionic action potentials were evoked by submaximal preganglionic stimulation at a frequency of 0·5 cps. Injections were marked by a calibration of 200μV. Horizontal calibration is 10 sec (De Groat and Volle, 1966a).

Hamberger, Norberg and Ungerstedt, 1965). Some of the fluorescent nerve terminals in this ganglion are derived from the axon collaterals of adrenergic nerve cells (Csillik, Kalman and Knyihár, 1967). In the rabbit, however, the superior cervical ganglion is rich in adrenergic nerve endings, associated with ganglion cells. Their number is not affected by preganglionic denervation (Hamberger et al., 1965).

There are several reports that pre- or postganglionic stimulation of the feline superior cervical ganglion causes a release of an adrenaline-like agent into the effluent of the perfused ganglion (Bulbring, 1944; Reinert,

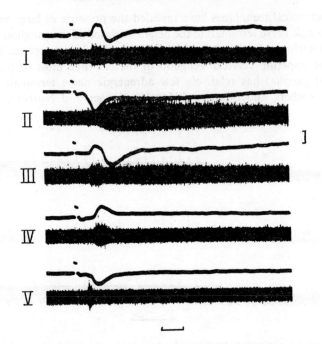

FIG. 6.11. Effect of isoprenaline (2 μg i.a.) on the ganglionic responses to acetylcholine (10 μg i.a.) before and after the administration of atropine (1 μg i.a.). Top and bottom tracings on each record are the ganglionic surface potentials and the postganglionic potentials, respectively. An upward deflection of the ganglionic response indicates depolarization. Each pair of records shows the responses produced by acetylcholine in (i), the untreated ganglion; (ii) and (iii) 20 sec and 10 min after an injection of isoprenaline; (iv) after atropine and (v) 20 sec after an injection of isoprenaline in a ganglion treated with atropine. Injections were marked by a 200 μV calibration signal in each of the top tracings. Vertical calibration for the bottom tracing in each pair is 10 μV. Time scale: 4 sec (De Groat and Volle, 1966b).

1963; Weir and McLennan, 1963). Bulbring (1944) postulated that the ganglion may contain chromaffin cells which release catecholamine and this suggestion was adopted by Eccles and Libet (1961) to account for their observation that the hyperpolarizing P potential in rabbit superior cervical ganglia is abolished by dibenamine and reserpine. It has now been established, however, that few or no chromaffin cells occur in the superior cervical ganglion (Norberg and Sjöqvist 1966) and that in the prevertebral ganglia they only occur in clusters adjacent to the capsule (Norberg and Sjöqvist, 1966). This localization throws serious doubt on their physiological importance, especially as an innervation of these cells has not been established. Small, non-chromaffin fluorescent cells of a special type have been observed in the superior cervical ganglia of several species (Eränkö and Härkönen, 1965; Norberg and Sjöqvist, 1966) and microspectrophotometric measurements have shown that they contain a catecholamine, and not 5-hydroxytryptamine as originally proposed (Eränko and Härkönen, 1965). These cells may be identical to the interneurones that recent electron microscopic investigations have revealed in sympathetic ganglia (Elfvin, 1963a, b; Grillo, 1966; Williams, 1967) and it cannot be excluded that they have a similar function to that ascribed to the chromaffin cells by Eccles and Libet (1961).

The effects on ganglia of drugs that affect the metabolism of catecholamines are extremely complex and the reports often contradictory. Inhibitors of monoamine oxidase have been reported to cause an increase in the noradrenaline content of ganglia either with (Gertner, 1961), or without (Reinert, 1963), an accompanying block of ganglionic transmission. Similarly reserpine has been reported to facilitate transmission in sympathetic ganglia by causing a depletion of catecholamines (Costa et al., 1961), although this has been questioned by Weir and McLennan (1963) and Reinert (1963). Reserpine causes a reduction in the amplitude of both the P and LN components of the ganglionic response to preganglionic stimulation (Libet, 1962). Dibenamine also blocks both the P and LN components, although it depresses the P potential preferentially (Eccles and Libet, 1961). However, other adrenergic *alpha* blocking agents do not have this action and dibenamine is known to possess many types of blocking action (Furchgott, 1954), including an action against acetylcholine.

In summary, it must be concluded that the evidence for an inhibitory transmitter action of noradrenaline in sympathetic ganglia is promising but not conclusive. Differences between ganglia, both within and between species, have complicated an assessment of the significance of many of the results. Recent evidence suggests that the slow inhibitory postsynaptic potential (P potential) in bullfrog sympathetic ganglion cells is due to electrogenic sodium pump, which removes sodium from the interior of the cell (Koketsu and Nishi, 1967; Nishi and Koketsu, 1967). This conclusion is supported by the observation that the P potential is depressed when the potassium concentration in the Ringers solution is reduced from 2 to

0·2mM and augmented during hyperpolarization of the ganglion cells. Further evidence in support of the concept of a sodium pump was obtained from experiments with metabolic inhibitors, such as ouabain. These results are difficult to reconcile with those obtained from the rabbit superior cervical ganglion (Kosterlitz *et al.*, 1968) and it appears that the two inhibitory processes may reflect species differences. An alternative possibility is that the two groups of investigators were observing different phenomena, since Kosterlitz *et al.* (1968) employed single pulses to evoke P potentials whilst Koketsu and Nishi used repetitive stimulation.

An adrenergic element has also been invoked in synaptic transmission in certain parasympathetic ganglia (Suden, Hart, Lindenberg and Marrazzi, 1951; McDougal and West, 1954; Kewenter, 1965). The generally accepted view has been that inhibition of peristalsis occurs through a direct effect of the adrenergic transmitter on the smooth muscle cells in the intestinal wall. Fluorescent microscopical studies have now shown that adrenergic nerves, other than the vasomotor nerves, in the gastrointestinal tract of several species invest and terminate around the intramural cholinergic ganglion cells and not in the muscle layers (Norberg, 1964; Norberg and Sjöqvist, 1966). It is therefore likely that nervous adrenergic inhibition of intestinal motility is exerted by an indirect effect on the parasympathetic ganglion cells. Exogenously administered catecholamines may also act directly on the smooth muscle cells. Adrenergic terminals surrounding non-fluorescent nerve cell bodies have also been observed in the ciliary ganglion and the intramural ganglia of the cat bladder (Hamberger and Norberg, 1965b; Norberg and Sjöqvist, 1966).

C. 5-HYDROXYTRYPTAMINE

The effects of 5-hydroxytryptamine on transmission of nerve impulses in the autonomic nervous system have been explored by several investigators. The first report on a ganglionic action of 5-hydroxytryptamine was misleading in so far as a large intra-arterial injection depressed the transmission of preganglionic impulses through the ciliary ganglion of the dog (Page and McCubbin, 1953). Stimulation of the perfused superior cervical ganglion of the cat by 5-hydroxytryptamine was initially demonstrated by Robertson (1954).

Trendelenburg (1956a) studied the ganglionic effects of 5-hydroxy-tryptamine by injecting it into the blood supply of the superior cervical ganglion and observing the responses of the nictitating membrane. Small doses of 5-hydroxytryptamine caused a contraction of the nictitating membrane which was blocked by nicotine or cocaine but not by hexamethonium. Low doses, which did not stimulate the ganglion themselves, potentiated the response of the nictitating membrane to submaximal preganglionic stimulation (Trendelenburg, 1956a, 1967). 5-Hydroxytryptamine also potentiated the ganglionic response to acetylcholine (Trendelenburg, 1956b).

Gertner and Romano (1961) reported that 5-hydroxytryptamine had only a slight potentiating effect on ganglionic transmission through the perfused superior cervical ganglion of the cat. Gertner (1962) has attributed the greater sensitivity to 5-hydroxytryptamine of ganglia with a normal circulation to the somewhat elevated concentration of calcium in the perfusion fluid. The ganglionic stimulating action of 5-hydroxytryptamine was prevented by morphine, methadone and cocaine (Gertner, 1962). Hertzler (1961) studied the effect of 5-hydroxytryptamine on transmission through the stellate ganglion of the rat both *in vivo* and *in vitro* and observed an increased amplitude of the postganglionic responses.

Gyermek and Bindler (1962a, b) have evaluated the effects of 5-hydroxytryptamine and a series of related indolealkylamines on the inferior mesenteric ganglion of the cat. Postganglionic activity was recorded from small bundles of fibres or single fibres in the hypogastric nerve. Close intra-arterial injections of various indolealkylamines produced a marked increase in postganglionic spontaneous activity, leaving preganglionic activity unchanged.

Rather different results were obtained on the superior cervical ganglion of the rat by Jéquier (1965). 5-Hydroxytryptamine caused an initial, brief depolarization of cells in this ganglion, which was associated with a small reduction in the response to preganglionic stimulation. After ganglia had been incubated for several hours in a Krebs solution containing either 5-hydroxytryptamine or 5-hydroxytryptophan, the effects of acetylcholine, carbachol and preganglionic stimulation were markedly depressed. Jéquier postulates that the amine has a brief depolarizing action as a result of its combination with receptors on the cell surface and then penetrates slowly into the ganglion cells to produce an inhibitory effect.

Sympathetic ganglia do not appear to contain measurable amounts of 5-hydroxytryptamine (Gaddum and Paasonen, 1955) although they are able to synthesize the amine from its precursor, 5-hydroxytryptophan

(Gaddum and Giarman, 1956). As 5-hydroxytryptophan decarboxylase and dihydroxyphenylanine (DOPA)-decarboxylase are now regarded as one and the same enzyme, this conversion of precursor to amine cannot be regarded as evidence in favour of a physiological role of 5-hydroxytryptamine in sympathetic ganglia. Observations on perfused ganglia have shown that there is no 5-hydroxytryptamine in the effluent, either under resting conditions or during preganglionic stimulation (Gertner, Paasonen and Giarman, 1959). The amine was, however, detectable in the effluent 2 hr after administration of the monoamine oxidase inhibitor, iproniazid. Preganglionic stimulation did not accelerate the appearance of the amine, nor did it increase its content in the effluent. Addition of both iproniazid and 5-hydroxytryptophan to the perfusion fluid resulted in a rapid appearance of 5-hydroxytryptamine in the effluent. The significance of these findings must await further evaluation.

The pharmacological findings, however, indicate that 5-hydroxytryptamine stimulates sympathetic ganglia and facilitates ganglionic transmission. The abolition of this effect by depolarizing agents, such as nicotine, but not by competitive ganglionic blocking substances suggests that the amine acts on ganglion cells at receptors which are different from those for acetylcholine.

D. HISTAMINE

A stimulating effect of histamine on ganglionic transmission has been described (Trendelenburg, 1954, 1955, 1957; Konzett, 1952). Histamine was able to potentiate the excitant action of nicotine-like substances in the perfused superior cervical ganglion (Konzett, 1952; Trendelenburg, 1956). These actions of histamine on sympathetic ganglia were abolished by the histamine antagonist, mepyramine and by nicotine but not by hexamethonium. A depressant action of histamine in transmission through the feline superior cervical ganglion has also been demonstrated (Gertner and Kohn, 1959).

The histamine-releasing compound 48/80 blocks transmission through the perfused superior cervical ganglion of the cat (Gertner, 1955). This effect is not due to a decrease in the release of acetylcholine in response to preganglionic nerve stimulation but to a decrease in sensitivity to acetylcholine. Histamine was present in the effluent after injections of 48/80 but there appeared to be no relationship between the degree of blocking and the amount of histamine released. However, as repeated injections of 48/80 caused increasing degrees of block it appears that there may be a relationship between histamine depletion and failure of transmission.

Sympathetic ganglia contain considerable amounts of histamine (Euler, 1949, 1966; Werle and Palm, 1950; Euler and Purkhold, 1951) of which some appears to be located in the mast cells. In a recent study Gertner (1965) demonstrated a 25% depletion of the histamine content of the superior cervical ganglion by the compound 48/80, which is known to release mast cell histamine. Preganglionic denervation, on the other hand, reduced the histamine content of the ganglion by 86% suggesting that most of the histamine is associated with the preganglionic fibres.

E. POLYPEPTIDES

The polypeptides angiotensin, bradykinin, oxytocin and substance P have been shown to influence transmission through the superior cervical ganglion of cats and in some instances similar effects have been observed in dogs and rabbits.

Angiotensin, the most potent ganglionic stimulant, has been studied in the greatest detail and its effects appear to be both complex and dose-dependent. In addition to directly stimulating ganglionic cells (Lewis and Reit, 1965) angiotensin may alter ganglionic transmission when injected into the ganglion at concentrations insufficient to elicit a direct response (Haefely, Hürlimann and Thoenen, 1965; Panisset, Biron and Beaulnes, 1966). In immediately substimulant doses, angiotensin greatly potentiated contractions of the nictitating membrane evoked by preganglionic stimulation of the superior cervical ganglion. In some preparations, this enhancement lasted for several hours (Panisset et al., 1966). Very low doses of angiotensin had the opposite effect, inhibiting the responses of the nictitating membrane to preganglionic stimulation. This depressant effect was abolished by dihydroergotamine, a finding which could implicate noradrenaline in the synaptic effects of angiotensin (Haefely et al., 1965; Panisset et al., 1966).

Substance P, although devoid of direct stimulant action of ganglionic elements (Lewis and Reit, 1966) may modify synaptic transmission through the ganglion. A potentiation of transmission was observed after small doses and a depression after injection of larger doses of this peptide (Beleslin, Radmanović and Varagić, 1960). This finding was not confirmed by Lewis and Reit (1966) who attributed the differences to the use of different preparations of Substance P.

The contractions of the nictitating membrane evoked by injections of angiotensin or bradykinin were not due to an action on preganglionic nerve terminals, as they occurred in chronically denervated ganglia and must therefore have been due to a direct effect on ganglion cells (Lewis and Reit, 1965). The receptors for the two peptides are different, as tachyphylaxis was readily produced by each peptide, but only to its own actions. When, as a result of tachyphylaxis, the ganglion cells had become insensitive to either peptide, their sensitivity to applied or synaptically released acetylcholine was unimpaired. Conversely, after hexamethonium and atropine blockade of the cholinergic receptors, ganglion cells continued to respond to the peptides indicating that they act on different receptors to those activated by acetylcholine (Lewis and Reit, 1965). Of interest is the finding that the tachyphylaxis of ganglion cells produced by histamine extended to angiotensin, but not to bradykinin. Furthermore, the histamine antagonist, mepyramine, decreased ganglionic responses to histamine and angiotensin but not to bradykinin. As the tachyphylaxis produced by angiotensin did not extend to histamine, it appears that the receptors for histamine are not the same as those for angiotensin. Lewis and Reit (1965) have suggested that angiotensin, through an interaction with its specific receptor, initiates a sequence of events which subsequently involves the histamine receptor in order to cause a stimulation of ganglion cells.

Angiotensin appears therefore, to have at least three actions on sympathetic ganglia, including a direct stimulant action on postsynaptic receptors; a facilitatory action on acetylcholine release from the presynaptic terminals (to account for the potentiation of transmission by concentrations of angiotensin below those necessary for direct stimulation) and a depressant action on transmission, which may be related to the release of noradrenaline.

A stimulant action of oxytocin on feline superior cervical ganglion cells has also been reported (Lewis and Reit, 1966).

F. AMINO ACIDS

Gamma-aminobutyric acid has been shown to possess weak ganglionic blocking activity in that it depressed transmission through the superior cervical and inferior mesenteric ganglia of the cat (De Groat, 1966; Matthews and Roberts, 1961).

An inhibitory action of various *alpha* amino acids, including glycine and alanine, on impulse transmission through the superior cervical ganglion was described by Damjanovich, Fehér, Halasz and Mechler (1960), who had to use high concentrations before a weak depressant action became evident. Depression of the excitant actions of acetylcholine and potassium was more marked. The depressant actions of γ-aminobutyric acid on feline superior cervical ganglia are antagonized by picrotoxin, but not by strychnine (De Groat, 1966).

CONCLUSIONS

1. The identification of acetylcholine as a transmitter in sympathetic ganglia furnishes a classic example of the fulfilment of the criteria described in Chapter 1.

2. Two receptors for acetylcholine are present on ganglion cell membranes. A "nicotinic" receptor mediates the short latency, direct effects of preganglionic volleys and a "muscarinic" receptor is responsible for slower effects. Between them, these receptors are responsible for the early junctional potential (N wave) and late depolarizing (LN) wave evoked in sympathetic ganglia by an orthodromic volley.

3. The N wave and transmission through the ganglion are blocked by "nicotinic" acetylcholine antagonists, such as nicotine, hexamethonium and *d*-tubocurarine. The LN wave is abolished by "muscarinic" antagonists, such as atropine and hyoscine.

4. Muscarinic antagonists also abolish the positive (P) potential, that can be recorded from the surface of sympathetic ganglia after orthodromic stimulation. As the P wave is also blocked by the α-adrenergic antagonist, dibenamine, it has been proposed that catecholamines are involved in its generation.

5. Transmission through the ganglion is not markedly influenced when cholinesterase is inhibited. In the presence of anticholinesterases, however, tetanic orthodromic stimulation initiates prolonged repetitive discharges, which are blocked by atropine and hyoscine and must therefore be mediated by the muscarinic receptors. This depolarization is associated with a reduction in the LN wave and a potentiation of the P wave.

6. The functional significance of the late junctional potential (LN wave) may be to contribute to the recruitment of cells by subsequent orthodromic volleys.

7. There is evidence that acetylcholine and acetyl-β-methylcholine hyperpolarize ganglion cells. It has not yet been established whether this is a direct action or whether it involves the release of an inhibitory transmitter from chromaffin cells or adrenergic nerve terminals.

8. Catecholamines both facilitate and depress impulse transmission through sympathetic ganglia. The facilitatory response results from depolarization of ganglion cells and is mediated by receptors which are blocked by β-adrenergic antagonists. β-effects are most pronounced with isoprenaline.

The inhibitory effects of the catecholamines are due to a hyperpolarization and result from an interaction with α-receptors. They are most prominent with noradrenaline. Inhibitory actions are blocked by α-adrenergic antagonists.

9. There is evidence that the P wave results from activation of a sodium pump in the membrane, which hyperpolarizes the cell by extruding sodium. Catecholamine-induced hyperpolarization may also result from activation of the sodium pump.

10. 5-Hydroxytryptamine and histamine stimulate sympathetic ganglia and facilitate ganglionic transmission. These effects are not blocked by drugs such as hexamethonium, which suggests that they do not act by releasing acetylcholine or on acetylcholine receptors.

11. The polypeptides, angiotensin and substance P, modify transmission through sympathetic ganglia. Their action appears to be rather complex and may involve several sites.

CHAPTER 7

PHARMACOLOGICAL STUDIES ON NEURONES IN THE BRAIN AND SPINAL CORD.
PART I. CHOLINERGIC MECHANISMS

IN the next two chapters the pharmacology of possible synaptic transmitter agents in the central nervous system is discussed. Neuropharmacological investigations can be carried out at several levels, depending on the type of information required. For some purposes, the drug may be administered orally to an intact animal and changes in its responses to its environment observed. Alternatively, the effects of drugs administered by a variety of routes on the spontaneous or evoked activity of areas of the nervous system can be measured. However, although these techniques may yield valuable information about the effects of drugs on whole populations of neurones, they rarely permit the actual site and mode of action of a particular substance to be determined.

Even when the responses of single neurones within various areas of the central nervous system are studied with a microelectrode, it is impossible to be certain of the effects of systemically or topically applied drugs. Diffusional barriers may prevent the access of the compound to the recording site or the effect observed may be secondary to actions of the drug on neurones elsewhere in the nervous system. Other factors which have to be considered when interpreting observations obtained from systemic application of drugs include the possibility of localized or generalized vascular changes induced directly or indirectly by the drug, or that the agent may rapidly be inactivated enzymatically in the circulation or tissues.

The development of techniques for the application of drugs directly into the extracellular environment of single nerve cells has greatly contributed to the progress in this field during the past decade. The methods used are based upon those of Nastuk (1953), the substances being applied

149

by iontophoresis from fine glass micropipettes (Curtis, 1964). Multi-barrel micropipettes permit intra- or extracellular recording of potentials from cells, whilst substances are ejected into the immediate extraneuronal environment. Electrical records are obtained from neurones within the volume of tissue affected by the injected agent and thus any observed alterations in nerve cell behaviour are unlikely to be due to impulses relayed from other cells. Micropipette assemblies of four, six or eight tubes fused around a centre barrel have been used extensively. In most instances the centre barrel is used for recording the extracellular spike responses and the surrounding barrels contain aqueous solutions of salts of the compounds to be tested. In this fashion, up to eight different agents can be tested upon a particular neurone, the active ions being ejected by means of suitably polarized currents. Intracellular recording, whilst drugs are applied into the immediate proximity of the neurone, is possible with co-axial or side-by-side electrode assemblies (Fig. 7.1). In each instance, the hyperfine microelectrode for intracellular recording projects some 40–50μ beyond the tip of the other micropipette.

A variety of techniques have been developed for locating the position from which electrical recordings have been obtained by making small, but histologically detectable, marks or lesions at the electrode tip. Intracellular marks have been made by ejecting a dye, such as Fast Green, into the cell from an intracellular recording electrode (Thomas and Wilson, 1965). The passage of small amounts of hydrogen ion from one barrel of a multiple barrelled micropipette results in the formation of small (50–$150\,\mu$) lesions in nervous tissue. These can readily be identified after histological preparation of the tissue (McCance and Phillis, 1965). An example of several "acid-lesions" is presented in Fig. 7.11.

In the sections to follow, the results obtained by these pharmacological micromethods are discussed in some detail, supplemented by accounts of results obtained with other methods.

The complexity of the synaptic junction is such, however, that several possible mechanisms of drug action must be considered before the actions of a substance upon a neurone can be evaluated. For example, the substance may interfere with the synthesis, transport or release of transmitter from presynaptic terminals, or may prevent the released transmitter from affecting specific receptors on the subsynaptic membrane.

Postsynaptically, a drug may act on subsynaptic or nonsynaptic membrane receptors to effect alterations in membrane permeability or alterna-

tively interfere with the electrogenic components of the membrane to prevent spike initiation.

Drug actions on adjacent capillaries and neighboring glial cells must also be considered. Actions of the monoamines on capillaries in the brain are unlikely to influence neuronal excitability to a marked extent, for as it is reasonable to assume a degree of pharmacological homogeneity of brain capillaries, it would be anticipated that modifications in neuronal excitability as a result of actions on capillaries would be uniform. However, the effects of the monoamines on neuronal excitability vary considerably. Krnjević and Schwartz (1967a) have recently demonstrated that γ-aminobutyric acid and acetylcholine depolarize some glial cells in the cerebral cortex. The result of such an effect on the adjacent neurones can only be conjectured at.

For these reasons, the mass of information which has been obtained by the iontophoretic technique must be interpreted with caution. The mere demonstration of an effect of an iontophoretically administered compound on either spontaneous or induced cellular activity does not indicate which of the many possible sites of drug action in the microenvironment of the cell are involved. The failure of a substance to produce a demonstrable effect on neurones in a particular structure does not necessarily indicate that it is without effect, for potentially reactive neurones may have been overlooked on account of their size or infrequency of occurrence. The effects of localized "synaptic" barriers and high concentrations of catabolic enzymes must also be considered. Moreover, it has been established that anaesthetic agents commonly employed in neuropharmacological investigations may reduce or abolish the effects of various compounds. The effects of substances on neurones in the brain and spinal cord to be discussed in this section are presented in Table 7.

A. CHOLINERGIC EXCITATORY SYNAPSES IN THE CENTRAL NERVOUS SYSTEM

Until comparatively recently, evidence that acetylcholine was a transmitter in the central nervous system was based mainly on the results of studies on the distribution of choline acetyltransferase or acetylcholinesterase, on changes in the acetylcholine content of the brain under various conditions, on the release of acetylcholine from the central nervous system either into the blood stream or into the ventricular or subarachnoidal spaces and on the central effects of systemically applied acetylcholine, anticholinesterases and acetylcholine-antagonists such as atropine. There was little direct evidence, however, that acetylcholine either excited or depressed particular central neurones by an interaction with subsynaptic transmitter receptors.

With the development of micropharmacological techniques it has been possible to analyse the chemical idiosyncrasies of neurones in many areas of the central nervous system. Neurones that are excited by iontophoretically applied acetylcholine have now been observed in spinal cord, medulla, pons, cerebellum, colliculi, medial and lateral geniculate bodies, thalamus, hypothalamus, basal ganglia, hippocampus and cerebral cortex of the cat.

1. Effects of Acetylcholine on the Spinal Cord

(a) *Renshaw cells*. The most extensively investigated cholinergic synapses within the central nervous system are those on Renshaw cells in the spinal cord, and these are of particular interest because they are the neurones in the vertebrate central nervous system for which there is the best evidence that acetylcholine is an excitatory synaptic transmitter. It is now generally accepted that acetylcholine is released by the synaptic terminals of motor axon collaterals upon Renshaw cells, although all of the evidence for this is pharmacological in nature. The initial experiments on the pharmacological specificity of the cholinergic synapses on these neurones were carried out using either intravenously or intra-arterially administered drugs (Eccles, Fatt and Koketsu, 1954; Eccles, Eccles and Fatt, 1956) and in some cases, anomalous features between the pharmacology of peripheral neuromuscular cholinoceptive synapses and those on Renshaw cells were due to the presence of the blood–brain barrier within the spinal cord. However, when compounds were applied by iontophoretic injection into the immediate environment of the Renshaw cells under observation, the pharmacology of the excitation by impulses in axon collateral fibres was shown to be practically identical to that of the "nicotinic" type of cholinergic synapse at the neuromuscular junction (Curtis and Eccles, 1958a, 1958b; Curtis, Phillis and Watkins, 1961a; Curtis and Ryall, 1966a, b, c).

The terms "nicotinic" and "muscarinic" were originally introduced by Dale (1914) to describe peripheral actions of various choline derivatives and have since been applied to the receptors with which these combine (Barlow, 1955; Waser, 1961, 1963). The receptors have been characterized on the basis of the activities of substances that either mimic or antagonize the action of acetylcholine. Neuropharmacological investigators have considered that "nicotinic" characteristics are exhibited when neurones are excited by carbachol or nicotine (*inter alia*) and that this excitation and that of acetylcholine can be antagonized by dihydro-β-erythroidine (Unna, Kniazuk and Greslin, 1944). On the other hand, the possession of "muscarinic" characteristics implies that a neurone is susceptible to excitation by acetyl-β-methylcholine (*inter alia*) and that the excitation is antagonized by atropine (Dale, 1914; Henderson and Roepke, 1937; Ambache, 1955). Renshaw cells are readily excited by acetylcholine, related choline esters and by nicotine (Fig. 7.2). This action of acetylcholine can be potentiated by a prior application of anticholinesterases and both the action of acetylcholine and the initial phase of the orthodromic excitation of Renshaw cells by stimulation of the ventral root are blocked by the acetylcholine antagonists, dihydro-β-erythroidine and d-tubocurarine. Of the various cholinomimetic substances tested as excitants of Renshaw cells, nicotine, carbachol and tetramethylammonium are more active than acetylcholine, whereas butyrylcholine and propionylcholine are less active. Although this would suggest that the receptors for acetylcholine are nicotinic in nature, the potencies of DL-muscarine and of acetyl-β-methylcholine are higher (Fig. 7.2) than would be expected if nicotinic receptors were the only sites for interaction with these excitants (Curtis and Ryall, 1966a). An intensive investigation has revealed that there are at least three types of acetylcholine receptor on the Renshaw cell. The excitatory actions of acetylcholine, nicotine, and carbachol are due predominantly to an interaction with nicotinic receptors and can be blocked by dihydro-β-erythroidine (Fig. 7.3). Acetyl-β-methylcholine and DL-muscarine interact with muscarinic receptors and can be blocked by atropine (Fig. 7.3). In the presence of dihydro-β-erythroidine and atropine, cholinomimetics may depress Renshaw cells. A third type of receptor has been proposed to account for this depression (Curtis and Ryall, 1966b). It has been shown that the response to ventral root stimulation consists of an early high frequency discharge which is blocked by dihydro-β-erythroidine, indicating that it is mediated by nicotinic receptors and a subsequent late discharge which is specifically depressed by atropine (Curtis and Ryall, 1966c). An example of the synaptic responses of a Renshaw cell to ventral root stimulation is shown in Fig. 7.4. It can be seen that the initial high frequency response is followed by a pause which may have a duration

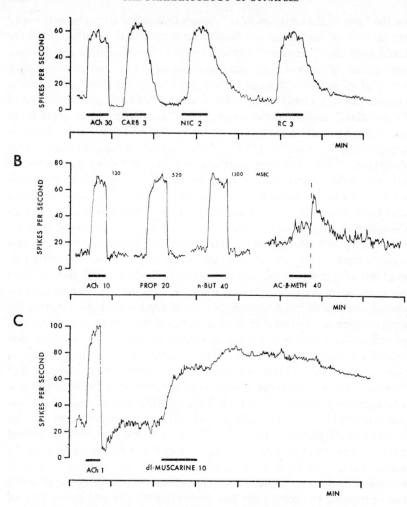

FIG. 7.2. Patterns of firing of three Renshaw cells in response to the iontophoretic administration of various cholinomimetric agents. These records and those in subsequent figures of this type, represent cell discharge frequencies recorded extracellularly by a sodium chloride-filled barrel of the multiple-barrel electrode and are plotted by means of a rectilinear ink-writing paper recorder. The periods of drug application are indicated by horizontal bars above or below the traces. Ordinates: spikes per second. Abscissae: time in minutes. A. Acetylcholine (ACh, 30 nA); carbachol (CARB, 3nA); nicotine (Nic, 2 nA) and β-carbomethoxyethyl-trimethylammonium (RC, 3 nA).

of over 100 msec. Curtis and Ryall have suggested that this pause is the result of a desensitization of the nicotinic excitatory receptors and an unmasking of the inhibitory effects of acetylcholine. Activation of the muscarinic receptors then produces the late synaptic response which lasts for several hundred milliseconds. The rate and pattern of firing during the initial response is determined by the intensity of the acetylcholine depolarization and the ability of the cell to fire at high frequencies. Since administration of anticholinesterases does not change the firing frequency during the early part of the initial response (Eccles et al., 1954, 1956), it is likely that the frequency attained is limited by the refractory period of the neurones. The relative insensitivity of the first few spikes to dihydro-β-erythroidine (Curtis et al., 1961a) suggests that the concentration of acetylcholine during this period is considerably in excess of the threshold amount required for excitation.

There are certain similarities between the synaptic responses of Renshaw cells and those of neurones in sympathetic ganglia. The response of a sympathetic ganglion to an orthodromic volley consists of an initial spike discharge followed by a positive wave (P wave) and subsequent late negative potential (LN wave). The P wave corresponds to a slow inhibitory postsynaptic potential and the LN wave to a late excitatory postsynaptic potential (see p. 123). Whereas the initial short latency excitatory postsynaptic potential can be depressed by "nicotinic" antagonists, the late excitatory potential is specifically depressed by "muscarinic" antagonists (Eccles and Libet, 1961; Volle, 1962a; Libet, 1964). Furthermore, there is pharmacological evidence for the presence of both nicotinic and muscarinic receptors within sympathetic ganglia (Trendelenburg, 1955, 1967; Ambache, Perry and Robertson, 1956; Takeshige and Volle, 1962, 1963, 1964; Takeshige, Pappano, de Groat and Volle, 1963).

A similar Renshaw-type cell may also exist in the spinal cord of amphibians. Antidromic impulses in ventral root fibres of the frog or toad spinal cord initiate a depolarization of the dorsal root fibres and generation of a dorsal root potential (Barron and Matthews, 1938; Eccles and Malcolm, 1946; Koketsu, 1956). This dorsal root potential is readily blocked

---

B. Acetylcholine (ACh. 10nA); propionylcholine (PROP, 20 nA) n-butyrylcholine (n- BUT, 40 nA) and acetyl-β-methylcholine (AC-β-METH, 40 nA). The vertical broken line indicates the termination of the current used to eject acetyl-β-methylcholine. The figures above each tracing indicate the recovery time in msec after the ejection. C. Acetylcholine (ACh, 1nA) and dl-muscarine (10 nA) (Curtis and Ryall, 1966a).

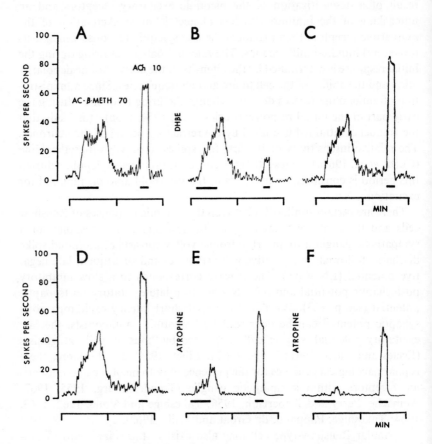

FIG. 7.3. Firing of a Renshaw cell by electrophoretic administration of acetyl-β-methylcholine (AC-β-METH 70 nA) and acetylcholine (ACh, 10 nA) during times indicated by lower horizontal bars. A. Control responses. B. 3 min after a current of 10 nA began to eject dihydro-β-erythroidine (DHβE) from a pipette containing 50 mM DHβE hydrobromide and 165 mM NaCl. C, D. 2 min after DHβE application. E. 5 min after intravenous atropine sulphate (0·1 mg/kg). F. 11 min after a further dose of atropine sulphate (0·5 mg/kg). Ordinates: spikes per second. Abscissae: time in minutes (Curtis and Ryall, 1966b).

by dihydro-β-erythroidine and other acetylcholine antagonists (Fig. 7.5) (Koketsu, 1956; Kiraly and Phillis, 1961; Mitchell and Phillis, 1962; Grinnell, 1966), suggesting that the synaptic pathway leading to dorsal root depolarization begins with the release of acetylcholine by moto-neurone axon collaterals, the existence of which has been shown by Sala Y Pons (1892) and Silver (1942). The antidromically produced dorsal root potential is sometimes large enough to produce firing of the dorsal root fibres, which in turn may cause orthodromic depolarization and firing of

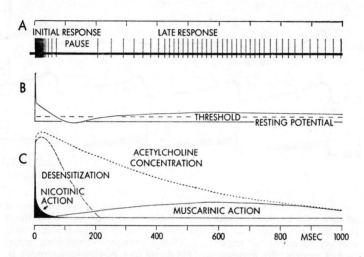

FIG. 7.4. Diagrammatic representation of the response of a Renshaw cell to a maximal ventral root volley. A. Firing pattern. B. Intracellularly recorded excitatory postsynaptic potential. C. Analysis of nicontinic and muscarinic actions of acetylcholine (Curtis and Ryall, 1966c).

motoneurones (Katz and Miledi, 1963). A direct, short latency effect of antidromically firing motoneurones on adjacent motoneurones has also been described. Washizu (1960), recording intracellularly from an isolated toad spinal cord, found that 20% of the motoneurones could be fired by stimulation of either of two adjacent ventral roots. The responses were not identical, however, as there was always a latency difference of 0·6 msec or more between the two routes of excitation. There was no prepotential associated with excitation from either ventral root and Washizu concluded that the later response was probably the result of ephaptic transmission through dendritic junctions between motoneurones. Kubota and Brook-hart (1962), Katz and Miledi (1963) and Grinnell (1966) on the other hand have observed a graded postsynaptic depolarization in frog motoneurones after stimulation of a ventral root. This ventral root excitatory postsynaptic potential has been extensively studied by Kubota and Brookhart (1963), who made the observation that succinylcholine, decamethonium or curare reduced the magnitude of the potential and as a result, suggested that the

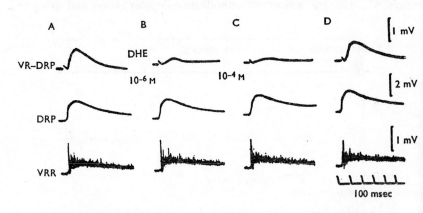

FIG. 7.5. Responses recorded from the dorsal and ventral roots of 9th segment of an amphibian (toad) spinal cord. VR-DRP and DRP are the potentials recorded from dorsal root following stimulation of corresponding ventral root and 8th dorsal root respectively. VRR is response recorded from ventral root of segment after stimulation of 8th dorsal root. A. Control responses. B. Responses after 10 min exposure to 10^{-6} M dihydro-β-erythroidine hydrobromide (DHE). C. After a further 10 min exposure to 10^{-4} M dihydro-β-erythroidine hydrobromide. D. Responses 3 hr after washing when VR-DRP had recovered. Time, 100 msec. Voltage calibrations, VR-DRP, 1 mV; DRP, 2 mV; VRR, 1 mV (Kiraly and Phillis, 1961).

potential was generated at a chemical synapse between recurrent axon collaterals and distal portions of the motoneurone dendrites. This finding has not been confirmed by Grinnell (1966) who was unable to affect the magnitude of the potential with a wide variety of transmitter blocking agents, which included curare, dihydro-β-erythroidine, atropine and hexamethonium. Grinnell's findings suggest that the potential is a result of current passage from adjacent dendrites and thus may be an example of an electrically transmitting junction in the amphibian spinal cord. Similar electrotonic junctions have been postulated in the teleost spinal cord, as a result of electrophysiological and ultrastructural investigations (Bennet, Aljure, Nakajima and Pappas, 1963).

(b) *Motoneurones and interneurones.* Many experimental investigations on the actions of acetylcholine have been undertaken since Feldberg and Minz (1932) described the muscular fibrillations produced by an intravenous injection of relatively high doses of acetylcholine, which could be abolished by mechanical destruction of the central nervous system. Bülbring and Burn (1941), using a method of perfusing the lower part of the spinal cord of a dog and of perfusing by a separate second circulation the muscles of the hind limb, found that the injection of small doses of acetylcholine into the spinal cord circulation elicited a discharge of motor impulses. Discharge from spinal motoneurones was also detected by Calma and Wright (1944) after injection of acetylcholine into the central end of the subclavian artery in a decerebrate cat. These experiments, and many of a similar nature, have been criticized because following the intra-arterial or intravenous administration of acetylcholine, the site of action of this substance cannot be determined with any precision, and effects observed may have arisen because of alterations in the behaviour of peripheral sensory receptors, or neurones elsewhere in the nervous system, having synaptic connections with the cells under observation. In later experiments precautions were taken to ensure that the injected acetylcholine was limited in its distribution to the spinal cord by using the technique of close intra-arterial injection. Sectioning of the dorsal roots further limits the possibility of afferent impulses from the periphery reaching the spinal cord. Under these conditions acetylcholine has been shown to have excitant effects on neurones within the spinal cord (Feldberg, Gray and Perry, 1953; de Molina, Gray and Palmer, 1958). Kennard (1953) recorded muscle contractions when minute amounts of acetylcholine were injected through fine capillary glass tubes inserted into the grey matter of the cord in the region of the anterior horn cells. In another series of experiments, however, Curtis, Eccles and Eccles (1957) observed a depression of spinal reflexes by intra-arterially injected acetylcholine, which was presumed to be the result of an activation of Renshaw cells with a consequent inhibition of motoneurones.

An initial survey of hundreds of spinal cord interneurones and motoneurones in cats anaesthetized with pentobarbitone sodium failed to reveal an action of iontophoretically applied acetylcholine on neurones other shaw cells (Curtis *et al.*, 1961a). In more recent experiments aesthetized or gas anaesthetized cats, however, both excitant and nt actions of acetylcholine on interneurones in the spinal cord have served (Salmoiraghi and Stefanis, 1965; Curtis, Ryall and Watkins, Weight and Salmoiraghi, 1966). Since dorsal roots contain only e amounts of acetylcholine and choline acetyltransferase (Mac-Intosh, 1941; Feldberg, 1945, 1957; Feldberg and Vogt, 1949; Hebb, 1957, 1961), it is generally agreed that most primary afferent fibres do not form cholinergic synapses on spinal cord neurones. It is unlikely, therefore, that monosynaptic responses to dorsal root stimulation, such as the monosynaptic ventral root reflexes or the monosynaptic excitation of interneurones, are cholinergic. Histochemical studies of the distribution of acetylcholinesterase in fibres within the spinal cords of cats or rats suggest that both descending and ascending cholinergic fibres are present in the spinal cord (Gwyn and Wolstencroft, 1966; Waldron, 1967). For the present, however, the presence of cholinoceptive receptors on interneurones in the spinal cord can be regarded as no more than suggestive that acetylcholine or a related substance plays a transmitter role at certain synapses in the spinal cord. There are many other excitatory pathways converging onto these neurones other than those from dorsal root afferent fibres and these have yet to be tested pharmacologically. The results obtained to date suggest the presence of cholingeric terminals on interneurones within the spinal cord and the passage of the next few years will doubtless produce more convincing evidence that this is, in fact, the case.

2. *Effects of Acetylcholine on the Brain*

Neurones that are either excited or inhibited by iontophoretically applied acetylcholine have been observed in almost all regions of the brain which have been explored with this technique and in several regions such as the cerebellum and cerebral cortex, thalamus, lateral and medial geniculate nuclei and caudate nucleus, there is reasonable evidence to suggest that the acetylcholine receptors are involved in cholinergic synaptic transmission. In some areas of the brain, a high proportion of specific types of neurone are excited by acetylcholine. Such neurones may be identified by their characteristic responses to a given form of stimulus. For instance, 87% of the 93 thalamic neurones excited monosynaptically by brachium conjunctivum stimulation were found to be excited by acetylcholine (Mc-

Cance, Phillis and Westerman, 1966a, b). Other groups of neurones have been identified by the invasion of an antidromic spike following the stimulation of their axons at a remote point in the central nervous system. The deep pyramidal or Betz cells in the peri-cruciate area of the cerebral cortex in cats can be activated antidromically when the pyramidal tracts are stimulated in the medulla. Eighty-three percent of 168 Betz cells tested were excited by acetylcholine (Krnjević and Phillis, 1963a) and a comparable percentage of acetylcholine-excited Betz cells has been recorded by Crawford and Curtis (1966). Acetylcholine-excited cells, however, constituted only a small proportion (approximately 15%) of all the cells examined in this area of the cerebral cortex.

(a) *Receptor pharmacology*. The pharmacological specificity of acetylcholine receptors on cortical Betz cells and on acetylcholine-excited neurones in the caudate nucleus are characteristically "muscarinic" in nature (Krnjević and Phillis, 1963b; Crawford and Curtis, 1966; McLennan and York, 1966). Characteristic features of the receptors on these neurones are their insensitivity to an excitant action of nicotine and the effectiveness of hyoscine and atropine as acetylcholine antagonists, whereas dihydro-β-erythroidine is ineffective. The action of acetylcholine on Betz cells is typically of slow onset, with delays of up to 60 sec being not infrequent and the after-discharge continues for considerably longer than is observed when acetylcholine is applied to Renshaw cells. This time-course of action, with a slow onset and prolonged duration, appears to be characteristic of muscarinic synapses including those on Renshaw cells, in the central nervous system.

On yet another group of neurones, including those in the lateral and medial geniculate nuclei (Phillis, Tebēcis and York, 1967; Tebēcis, 1968), the ventrobasal complex of the thalamus (Andersen and Curtis, 1964; McCance, Phillis, Tebēcis and Westerman, 1968) and brainstem (Salmoiraghi and Steiner, 1963; Bradley and Wolstencroft, 1965) the acetylcholine receptor appears to be of an intermediate type. This conclusion is derived from the results obtained with various cholinomimetic drugs such as carbachol and acetyl-β-methylcholine, which have comparable actions on these neurones, as well as the finding that both "muscarinic" and "nicotinic" acetylcholine-blockers were effective antagonists. The time-course of the acetylcholine excitation of such neurones also appears to be intermediate between those recorded for Renshaw cells and deep pyramidal cells. The excitant effects of acetylcholine on neurones in this intermediate category may ultimately prove to be a result of its interaction with several different types of receptor.

(b) *Medulla and pons.* The pharmacology and distribution of acetyl-choline-excited cells in the medulla and pons have been studied by several groups of investigators (Salmoiraghi and Steiner, 1963; Bradley and Wolstencroft, 1965; Bradley, Dhawan and Wolstencroft, 1966; Steiner and Meyer, 1966; Yamamoto, 1967; Gallindo, Krnjević and Schwartz, 1967). Neurones in different brainstem nuclei differed markedly in their sensitivity to acetylcholine and in some areas, such as the paramedian reticular nucleus, almost all of the neurones were excited by acetylcholine. Excitatory responses had both nicotinic and muscarinic properties, whereas the inhibitory responses were only muscarinic (Bradley *et al.*, 1966).

(c) *Cerebellum.* Acetylcholine-excited neurones have been observed in both the cortex and deep nuclei of the cerebellum, although there has been some disagreement over the identity of the acetylcholine-sensitive neurones in the cerebellar cortex. According to Crawford, Curtis, Voorhoeve and Wilson (1966), these are exclusively Purkinje cells, whereas McCance and Phillis (1964, 1968) have identified them as being both granule layer cells and Purkinje cells. In the investigations of McCance and Phillis, acetyl-choline-excited cells were found with increasing frequency as the electrode penetrated more deeply into the cerebellar cortex. An analysis of the relative activities of the various cholinomimetics and acetylcholine antagonists tested, indicated that the receptors on these cells were "nicotinic" in type. By employing a technique for making small lesions within the cortical tissue to define the recording site at which acetylcholine-sensitive cells were encountered, and by examining serial sections of the cortical area, McCance and Phillis (1968) established beyond doubt that cells within the granular layer are excited by acetylcholine. It is thus possible to refute the suggestion (Crawford *et al.*, 1966) that the electrical activity recorded in these experiments was, in fact, due to adjacent Purkinje cells. Purkinje cells were undoubtedly excited during the application of acetylcholine into the vicinity of their cell bodies, but did not respond when acetylcholine was applied in the molecular layer. The question arises therefore, as to whether Purkinje cell excitation was the result of a direct action of acetylcholine on the cell soma or was secondary to an excitation of cells in the adjacent granule cell layer, with subsequent synaptic excitation of Purkinje cells by parallel fibres. There appears to be, at the moment, no way of resolving this question satisfactorily and hence the presence of acetylcholine receptors of Purkinje cells soma cannot be excluded. It appears more likely, however, that Purkinje cell excitation was a consequence of prior granule cell excitation.

Histochemical studies on the distribution of acetylcholinesterase in the cerebellar cortex and peduncles, described in Chapter 2, suggest that a proportion of the mossy afferent fibres to the cerebellum may be cholinergic in nature. The region of origin of these fibres has been ascertained by placing bipolar, coaxial stimulating electrodes stereotaxically in various nuclei in brainstem and pons, including the lateral reticular nucleus, the nucleus reticularis tegmenti pontis or the mesencephalic reticular formation/nucleus reticularis pontis oralis complex, and the inferior olive. The small size of the extracellularly recorded spike potentials of individual neurones in the granular layer made it difficult to study the synaptic activation of individual cells. A ratemeter was therefore used to assess changes in the discharge frequency of groups of adjacent cells during brief (5–15 sec) periods of repetitive stimulation (10 per sec) of the pontine and medullary nuclei.

Repetitive stimulation of nuclei in the medulla and pons frequently initiated an increased frequency of discharge of granular neurones. If these neurones were also excited by acetylcholine, the discharge frequencies evoked by both brain stem and chemical stimulation were compared before and after the application of dihydro-β-erythroidine. Increases in the firing of granular neurones induced by stimulation of the lateral reticular nucleus or the nucleus reticularis tegmenti pontis were not affected by dihydro-β-erythroidine, even though the action of acetylcholine was abolished, indicating that few cholinergic mossy afferent fibres are likely to originate in these areas. The effects of stimulation in the mesencephalic reticular formation/nucleus reticularis pontis oralis complex were more susceptible to antagonism by dihydro-β-erythroidine. Stimulation of this area caused an increased discharge frequency of several acetylcholine-excited neurones in the posterior vermal cortex, and iontophoretically applied dihydro-β-erythroidine abolished both the actions of acetylcholine and those of pontine stimulation (Fig. 7.6). The synaptically evoked discharges of other acetylcholine-sensitive neurones were, however, unaffected by dihydro-β-erythroidine and this finding, together with the observation that stimulation of the mesencephalic reticular formation/nucleus reticularis pontis oralis complex sometimes excited acetylcholine-insensitive neurones in the granular layer, suggests that not all of the mossy afferents arising in this area are cholinergic in nature.

Histochemical and manometric studies on the distribution of acetylcholinesterase in the feline cerebellar cortex had indicated that the presence of only 30% of the enzyme is dependent on the integrity of the afferent connections to the cerebellum (Austin and Phillis, 1965; Phillis, 1965, 1968). This is in contrast to the rat cerebellum, where the presence of

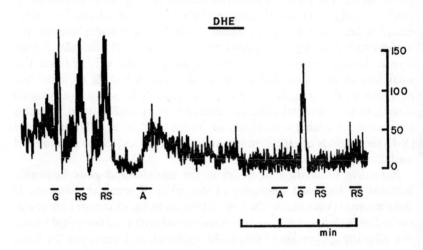

FIG. 7.6. Firing frequency record from cerebellar granule layer cells. L-glutamate (G, 40nA), acetylcholine (A, 50nA) and mesencephalic reticular formation stimulation (RS) increased the rate of firing. After dihydro-β-erythroidine (DHE, 80 nA) the effects of acetylcholine and reticular formation stimulation were abolished. Firing frequencies are indicated by the vertical scale (spikes/sec) (McCance and Phillis, 1968).

acetylcholinesterase in the neocerebellar cortex is largely dependent on the integrity of the afferent fibres (Sperti and Sperti, 1959; Mead and van der Loos, 1964; Kása, Csillik, Joó and Knyihár, 1966). Some cells in the granular layer of the feline cerebellar cortex contain acetylcholinesterase (Phillis, 1965, 1968), and it has been suggested that the enzyme may be located within intracortical association fibres as well as mossy afferent fibres.

Acetylcholine, choline acetyltransferase and acetylcholinesterase are also present in the feline molecular layer (Austin and Phillis, 1965; Phillis and Chong, 1965; Goldberg and McCaman, 1967; Phillis, 1965, 1968) suggesting that a proportion of the fibres in this layer may be cholinergic. Dihydro-β-erythroidine and atropine, however, failed to modify either the magnitude or duration of the negative potentials generated near the surface of the molecular layer by "in-line" stimulation of the surface of a folium (Crawford et al., 1966; McCance and Phillis, 1968). As the generation of these potentials has been attributed to synaptic excitation of Purkinje cell dendrites by parallel fibres (Eccles, Llinás and Sasaki, 1966a), it appears unlikely that many parallel fibres are cholinergic.

Stimulation of the inferior olive excites climbing fibres, which also synapse with Purkinje cell dendrites (Szentágothai and Rajkovits, 1959; Eccles et al., 1966b). The failure of intravenously administered atropine or dihydro-β-erythroidine to alter the configuration of the negative–positive potentials recorded by electrodes on the molecular layer during inferior olive stimulation, suggests that climbing fibres are unlikely to be cholinergic (Crawford et al., 1966; McCance and Phillis, 1968).

Acetylcholine-excited neurones have been identified in all three cerebellar deep nuclei, the proportion of sensitive cells tending to be greater in the more lateral nuclei (Chapman and McCance, 1967). The receptors on these cells appear to be more muscarinic in character than those on neurones in the cerebellar cortex, as excitation frequently has long latency of onset and a considerable duration. Atropine and hyoscine, but not dihydro-β-erythroidine, readily antagonize the actions of acetylcholine. The involvement of acetylcholine as a synaptic transmitter in the deep nuclei has not yet been established. Possible pathways include cholinergic fibres from the pons and medulla and the presence of acetylcholinesterase in many cells in the deep nuclei (Phillis, 1965, 1968) suggests that intra- or internuclear pathways may also be cholinergic.

(d) *Thalamus.* The axons of acetylcholinesterase-containing cerebellar deep nuclear neurones can be followed into the brachium conjunctivum and may project to the ventrolateral nucleus of the thalamus (Phillis, 1965, 1968). Pharmacological studies on the responses evoked in the thalamus by brachium conjunctivum stimulation indicate that a proportion of the fibres in this system are cholinergic. Intracarotid administration of atropine has been shown to depress the focal potentials evoked in the ventrolateral nucleus by brachium conjunctivum stimulation (Frigyesi and Purpura, 1966; McCance, Phillis and Westerman, 1968a, b). The reduction in amplitude of these focal potentials was rarely complete, suggesting that

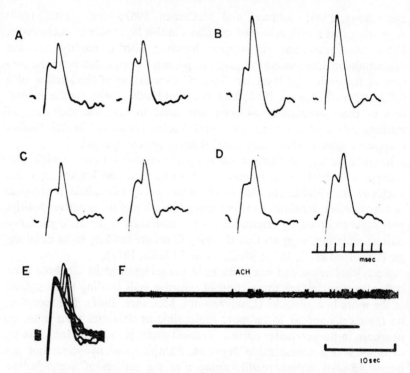

FIG. 7.7. Focal potentials with a superimposed orthodromic spike evoked in the nucleus ventralis lateralis of the thalamus by brachium conjunctivum stimulation. A. Control responses. B. During application of acetylcholine (40 nA) the amplitude of both focal potentials and action potentials was augmented. C. 2 min after acetylcholine application. D. After dihydro-β-erythroidine (120 nA for 60 sec). E. Responses during repetitive stimulation of the brachium conjunctivum at 15/sec showing latency fluctuations in orthodromic response. F. Acetylcholine (ACh, 80 nA) induced excitation of this cell (McCance, Phillis and Westerman, 1968a).

only a limited number of the cerebellar efferents to this nucleus are cholinergic in nature. This conclusion is supported by the finding that many of the efferent fibres in the brachium conjunctivum do not stain for acetylcholinesterase (Phillis, 1968).

An example of action potentials evoked in a thalamic neurone by brachium conjunctivum stimulation is demonstrated in Fig. 7.7. The neurone was activated monosynaptically by stimulation of the brachium

and failed to follow repetitive stimulation at 15/sec (Fig. 7.7 E). This particular neurone was relatively insensitive to acetylcholine, a current of 80 nA
being necessary to initiate firing (Fig. 7.7.F). Acetylcholine (40 nA) had a
subthreshold action on the neurone, reducing the latency of the evoked
spike and significantly increasing its amplitude. This increase in spike
amplitude was probably a result of facilitation of invasion of the action
potential into the soma and dendritic processes of the neurone and suggests
that acetylcholine receptors were present on the dendrites. Acetylcholine
also increased the amplitude and duration of focal potentials evoked by
brachium conjunctivum stimulation.

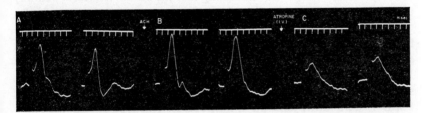

Fig. 7.8. Action potentials of a thalamic neurone (in nucleus ventralis lateralis)
evoked by brachium conjunctivum stimulation. A. Controls. B. Application of
acetylcholine (60 nA) excited neurone and increased amplitude of the evoked
response. C. After an intravenous injection of atropine (1 mg/kg) the synaptically evoked spike failed (McCance, Phillis and Westerman, 1968a).

Dihydro-β-erythroidine and atropine, applied iontophoretically, were
effective antagonists of the excitant actions of acetylcholine on thalamic
neurones but failed to block the excitant effects of brachium conjunctivum
stimulation (Fig. 7.7D). When administered intravenously, atropine had a
more pronounced action, reducing the magnitude of evoked potentials
and abolishing the monosynaptically evoked responses of some thalamic
neurones, but not of others. An example of an atropine-sensitive response
is illustrated in Fig. 7.8. This neurone was excited by acetylcholine, which
also increased the spike amplitude (Fig. 7.8B). After atropine (1 mgm/kg,
intravenously) the brachium conjunctivum-evoked spike response failed,
exposing the underlying atropine-resistant component of the field potential
(Fig. 7.8C).

Reticular formation stimulation excites some thalamic and geniculate
neurones and inhibits others (Phillis and Tebēcis, 1967b; Phillis, Tebēcis

and York, 1967b; Tebēcis, 1967; McCance *et al.*, 1968a). The facilitatory effects of reticular formation stimulation on some neurones in these areas are likely to be mediated by acetylcholine, as they can be abolished by acetylcholine antagonists. Facilitatory responses to reticular formation stimulation which were unaffected by acetylcholine antagonists have also been observed and the possibility that these are mediated by noradrenaline or 5-hydroxytryptamine will be discussed in the relevant sections of Chapter 8.

The synaptic responses of neurones in the ventrobasal complex of the thalamus evoked by limb nerve stimulation were consistently resistant to acetylcholine antagonists, indicating that the medial lemniscal pathway to the thalamus is non-cholinergic. A comparison of the responses of a thalamic neurone to stimulation of the triceps nerve and the reticular formation can be seen in Fig. 7.9A (1) and (2). Triceps nerve stimulation evoked a typical burst of three to four spikes, with a minimal latency of 12 msec and a total duration of approximately 16 msec. The responses to a single stimulating pulse in the brain stem (at stereotaxic coordinates A3, L3, D-1) were rather different in time-course. This type of response had a variable latency and a duration of several hundred milliseconds, the inter-spike interval being of the order of 100 msec. This cell was excited by acetylcholine and after an application of atropine (120 nA) for 90 sec, the acetylcholine sensitivity was abolished and the response to reticular stimulation blocked, while the responses evoked by triceps nerve stimulation remained unaltered. Dihydro-β-erythroidine also abolished this type of excitant action of reticular formation stimulation (Fig. 7.9B).

The facilitatory effects of reticular formation stimulation on thalamic neurones could be most readily demonstrated when the reticular formation was stimulated repetitively. Excitation was then evident either as a direct increase in cell firing frequency (Fig. 7.10) or as an enhancement of the responses to L-glutamate. After application of an acetylcholine antagonist to such neurones, the effects of reticular formation stimulation were frequently reduced or abolished (Fig. 7.10), indicating that transmission had been mediated entirely or in part by acetylcholine.

Acetylcholine-excited neurones were found in all areas of the thalamus tested; the highest proportions being located in the ventrobasal complex (Fig. 7.11). This area contains the thalamocortical relay neurones, of which a high proportion are excited by acetylcholine (Andersen and Curtis, 1964; McCance *et al.*, 1968a). Thalamocortical relay neurones varied

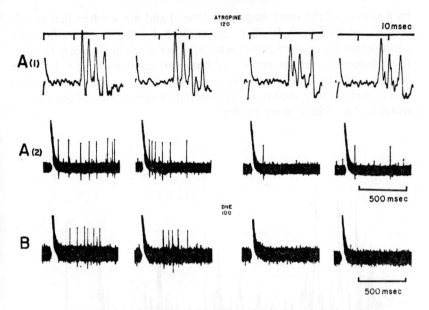

FIG. 7.9. A. Orthodromic responses of an acetylcholine-excitable thalamic neurone evoked by triceps nerve (A(i)) and reticular formation stimulation (A(2)). After an application of atropine (120 nA for 90 sec) the response to triceps stimulation was still present but the response to reticular stimulation had been largely abolished. B. response of another acetylcholine—sensitive neurone in the ventro-basal thalamus to reticular formation stimulation. Dihydro-β-erythroidine (DHE, 100 nA, for 60 sec) abolished these synaptic effects (McCance, Phillis and Westerman, 1968a).

in their sensitivity to acetylcholine; the more sensitive cells responding to acetylcholine applications with a short latency of onset and rapid termination of firing after the cessation of application. On the less responsive relay cells, large amounts of acetylcholine evoked a discharge after latencies of 30⁻45 sec and firing usually continued for a comparable period of time after its application had been terminated.

The relative activities of various cholinomimetic substances as excitants of thalamic neurones are presented in Table 8. The use of nine-barrelled electrodes, containing seven choline esters or related compounds, greatly facilitated an assessment of these relative potencies. An example of the actions of acetylcholine and six other cholinomimetic agents on a thalamic neurone is illustrated in Fig. 7.12. All of these compounds were applied by a current of the same magnitude (60nA) and it is evident that acetyl-choline, acetyl-β-methylcholine and carbachol, were considerably more effective than the other compounds tested. After an application of carbachol, the subsequent excitant actions of both carbachol itself and the other cholinometics were frequently depressed (Fig. 7.12). A comparable reduction in excitability was also observed to follow applications of muscarone, which had no initial excitant action.

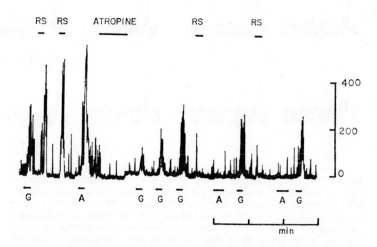

FIG. 7.10. Ink-recorder of discharge frequency of a neurone in the nucleus ventralis lateralis of the thalamus. Reticular formation stimulation (RS, 5/sec for 10 sec), L-glutamate (G, 40 nA) and acetylcholine (A, 40 nA) excited the cell. After atropine (60 nA for 60 sec) the effects of reticular formation stimulation and acetylcholine were abolished, but L-glutamate excitation was unaltered (McCance, Phillis and Westerman, 1968a). Ordinate—spikes per sec.

The conclusion that acetylcholine is released in the thalamus by synaptic terminals of pathways from the brain stem reticular formation and cerebellum is consistent with the presence of acetylcholine (MacIntosh 1941), choline acetyltransferase (Hebb and Silver, 1956) and acetylcholinesterase (Phillis, Tebēcis and York, 1967b; McCance et al., 1968a) in the feline thalamus. Cholinergic pathways from the brain stem reticular formation to the thalamus have been postulated as a result of studies on the distribution of acetylcholinesterase in normal and operated rats

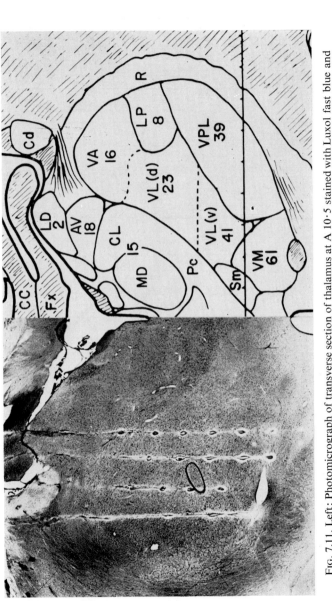

FIG. 7.11. Left: Photomicrograph of transverse section of thalamus at A 10·5 stained with Luxol fast blue and neutral red. Four parallel electrode tracks with numerous acid lesions are visible. Right: A 10·5 (diagram and abbreviations after Jasper & Ajmone-Marson (1954). Numbers represent percentages of cells excited by acetylcholine in various thalamic nuclei. Data from N. centralis lateralis (CL) and N. medialis dorsalis (MD) and also from N. ventralis postero-medialis (VPM) and N. ventralis medialis (VM) have been combined. A broken line 1·5 mm above the Horsley-Clark zero has been used to divide the N. ventralis lateralis (VL). Percentages are based on the following total numbers of cells in each case: N. lateralis dorsalis (LD), 58; N. ventralis anterior (VA), 140; N. lateralis posterior (LP), 84; CL/MD, 193; VL (d) (above line), 287; VL (v) (below line), 270; N. ventralis posterolateralis (VPL), 170; VPM/VM,135 (McCance, Phillis and Westerman, 1968a).

TABLE 8.

RELATIVE ACTIVITIES OF CHOLINOMIMETIC SUBSTANCES AS
EXCITANTS OF THALAMIC NEURONES.

(McCance, Phillis, Tebēcis and Westerman, 1968)

Potencies expressed relative to that of acetylcholine ($+++$)	
Carbachol (carbamyl-choline chloride)	$++++$
Acetylcholine chloride	$+++$
Acetyl-β-methylcholine chloride	$+++$
Arecoline hydrobromide	$++$
Nicotine hydrogen tartrate	$++$
d,1-Muscarine iodide	$++$
Succinylcholine chloride	$++$
Propionylcholine chloride	$+$
Butyrylcholine iodide	$+$
Pilocarpine hydrochloride	$+$
d,1-Muscarone iodide	0

(Shute and Lewis, 1963, 1967). Furthermore, a release of acetylcholine from the ventrobasal thalamus during reticular formation stimulation has been described (Phillis, Tebēcis and York, 1968b).

(e) *Lateral geniculate nucleus.* In the lateral geniculate nucleus, acetyl-choline satisfies most of the criteria that have been developed for the identification of synaptic transmitters. It is present in moderate amounts in the nucleus (Cobbin, Leeder and Pollard, 1965) as are choline acetyltransferase and acetylcholinesterase (Feldberg and Vogt, 1948; Hebb and Silver, 1956; Burgen and Chipman, 1951; Phillis *et al.*, 1967b). The low content of these substances in the optic nerve and tract suggests that acetylcholine is not the transmitter released by the majority of optic nerve terminals upon lateral geniculate neurones. This conclusion is supported by the observation that intracarotid injections of atropine cause only a small reduction in the magnitude of visually evoked fields in the lateral geniculate nucleus (David, Murayama, Machne and Unna, 1963) and that iontophoretically applied acetylcholine antagonists are without action upon the synaptic firing of geniculate neurones evoked by impulses in the optic nerves (Curtis and Davis, 1962; Phillis *et al.*, 1967b). Nevertheless, many neurones in the lateral geniculate, including geniculocortical relay neurones (Fig. 7.13A, B) are powerfully excited by acetylcholine (Phillis *et al.*, 1967b; Satinsky, 1967). This action of acetylcholine, as well as the excitant effects of reticular formation stimulation on geniculate neurones can be abolished by various antagonists, including benzoquinonium (Phillis *et al.*, 1967b). Histochemical investigations have shown that acetylcholinesterase-containing nerve fibres project from the mesencephalic reticular formation to the lateral geniculate nucleus (Shute and Lewis, 1963, 1967) and these may constitute the acetylcholine-releasing pathway.

(f) *Medial geniculate nucleus.* Studies on the feline medial geniculate

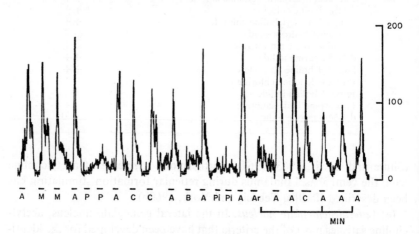

FIG. 7.12. Excitant effects of a number of cholinomimetics applied to a thalamic neurone recorded at a depth of 4,810 μ below the dorsal surface of thalamus. All applications are at currents of 60 nA. Acetylcholine (A), acetyl-β-methyl choline (M) and carbachol (C) were approximately equieffective and were much more active than propionylcholine (P), butyrylcholine (B), pilocarpine (Pi) and arecoline (Ar) on this unit. After the second, longer, application of carbachol, excitation induced by acetylcholine was significantly reduced. (McCance, Phillis, Tebēcis and Westerman, 1968).

nucleus (MGN) (Tebēcis, 1968; and unpublished observations) indicate that ACh is a transmitter in this structure.

Iontophoretically applied ACh has excitatory and inhibitory effects on many medial geniculate neurones, as well as dual excitatory inhibitory effects on a small proportion. Both the excitatory and inhibitory effects of ACh are potentiated by the cholinesterase inhibitors, neostigmine, eserine and edrophonium, and antagonized by the cholinergic blocking agents, atropine, hyoscine, hexamethonium, dihydro-β-erythroidine and curare.

ACh excites a large proportion of geniculocortical relay units. In particular, a proportion of the excitatory synaptic responses evoked by stimulation of the auditory cortex and inferior colliculus are potentiated by eserine and neostigmine, and blocked by atropine. Similar results also suggest the presence of cholinergic pathways from the brain stem to the MGN. The cholinoceptive receptors on medial geniculate neurones are either muscarinic, nicotinic or intermediate in type.

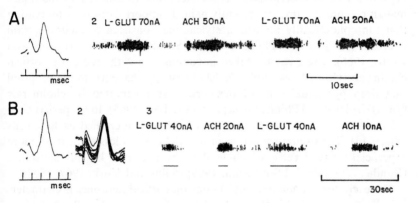

FIG. 7.13. A_1, B_1. Responses recorded from two neurones in the dorsal lateral geniculate nucleus upon antidromic stimulation of optic radiation fibres in the ipsilateral visual cortex. B_2. Ability of an antidromic response to follow a frequency of 100/sec. A_2, B_3. Comparisons of the excitant actions of acetylcholine, (ACh) and L-glutamate (L-Glut) on these neurones. (Phillis, Tebēcis and York, 1967b).

(g) *Basal ganglia*. The caudate nucleus contains high concentrations of acetylcholine, choline acetyltransferase and acetylcholinesterase (Mac Intosh, 1941; Feldberg and Vogt, 1948; Hebb and Silver, 1956; Burgen and Chipman, 1951) and acetylcholine release from the nucleus has been demonstrated (Mitchell and Szerb, 1962; McLennan, 1964). Acetylcholine excited and inhibited neurones are present in the caudate nucleus (Bloom, Costa and Salmoiraghi, 1965) and a remarkable correlation has been observed between the effects of acetylcholine and those of stimulation of the nucleus ventralis anterior in the thalamus (McLennan and York, 1966). Both types of acetylcholine effect and the responses to nucleus ventralis anterior stimulation are prevented by atropine, suggesting that the final synapse in this thalamo-caudate pathway may be cholinergic in nature. Iontophoretically applied acetylcholine excited 60% of the neurones tested in a survey of the globus pallidus–putamen complex and inhibited 13%. Both the excitant and depressant effects of acetylcholine, which were duplicated by a variety of cholinomimetic compounds, were blocked by atropine, dihydro-β-erythroidine and benzoquinonium (York, 1968).

(h) *Cerebral cortex.* The considerable amount of indirect evidence which favours a role of acetylcholine as an excitatory transmitter in the mammalian cerebral cortex, has recently gained support from the observation that iontophoretically applied acetylcholine consistently excites certain neurones (Krnjević and Phillis, 1963a, b; Spehlmann, 1963; Crawford and Curtis, 1966). These results, taken in conjunction with studies on cortical choline acetyltransferase and acetylcholinesterase have led to the proposal that deep pyramidal cells of the cortex are innervated by cholinergic fibres (Krnjević and Phillis, 1963a; Krnjević, 1964, 1965). In the pericruciate area, many of the ACh sensitive cells have been identified as Betz cells (Fig. 7.14). The excitatory action of acetylcholine is less evident on more superficial cortical cells, which tend to be inhibited by this substance (Randić, Siminoff and Straughan, 1964; Phillis and York, 1967, 1968).

The excitatory action of acetylcholine on cortical neurones is characteristically "muscarinic" in nature, with a slow onset and prolonged afterdischarge. Two other characteristic features are the insensitivity of these neurones to nicotine, and the effectiveness of atropine and hyoscine as blocking agents, whereas dihydro-β-erythroidine and d-tubocurarine are ineffective (Krnjević and Phillis, 1963b). There is no obvious association between acetylcholine-sensitivity and the ability of deep cortical neurones to give short latency responses to stimulation from the periphery or the thalamic relay nuclei (Krnjević and Phillis, 1963a). Similarly, although some of these neurones respond to transcallosal volleys or activation of the midline thalamic nuclei (recruiting responses) other, non-cholinoceptive cells are also excited by these pathways and the synaptic responses of both types of neurone are insensitive to atropine or hyoscine (Krnjević and Phillis, 1963a). Repetitive stimulation in the mesencephalic reticular formation excites Betz cells but this response also appears to be insensitive to acetylcholine antagonists (Phillis and York, unpublished observations).

The main types of activity that appear to be significantly related to acetylcholine-excitation are irregular spontaneous discharges ("projection activity") and prolonged repetitive responses to single pulse stimulation

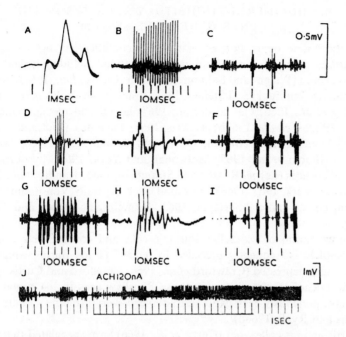

FIG. 7.14. Two Betz cells found at depth of 1·1 mm in lateral precruciate cortex and identified by antidromic activation from medullary pyramid (A); large and small spikes had latencies of 0·7 and 2·0 msec respectively. Both were driven at 300/sec antidromically (B) and fired spontaneously in the absence of stimulation (C). They gave early responses to peripheral (contralateral fore-paw) stimulation (D), and fired after a short latency when stimulating specific afferent nucleus in thalamus (E). There were also marked late repetitive discharges after peripheral and specific thalamic excitation with single shocks (F and G). Similar early firing and later repetitive responses were evoked by transcallosal stimulation in H and I. Both units were strongly excited by ACh applied iontophoretically during period indicated by white line in J. (Note lower amplification). Cat under Dial. (Krnjević and Phillis, 1963a).

of thalamic relay nuclei (Adrian, 1941; Morison and Dempsey, 1943). In the light of the widespread nature of cholinergic inhibition in the cerebral cortex (Phillis and York, 1967a, 1968a, b), it is possible that the action of ACh on deep pyramidal cells is in fact, a disinhibition, brought about by inhibition of inhibitory neurones within the cortex.

B. CHOLINERGIC INHIBITORY SYNAPSES IN THE CENTRAL NERVOUS SYSTEM

Acetylcholine depression of neuronal excitability has been observed in various areas of the central nervous system, including spinal cord interneurones (Weight and Salmoiraghi, 1966; Curtis *et al.*, 1966) medulla and pons (Salmoiraghi and Steiner, 1963; Bradley and Wolstencroft, 1965; Bradley *et al.*, 1966; Galindo *et al.*, 1967) lateral and medial geniculate nuclei (Phillis *et al.*, 1967b; Tebēcis, 1968) thalamus (McCance *et al.*, 1968a) hypothalamus (Bloom, Oliver and Salmoiraghi, 1963), caudate nucleus (Bloom *et al.*, 1965; McLennan and York, 1966), pyriform and cerebral cortices (Legge, Randić and Straughan, 1966; Randić *et al.*, 1964; Phillis and York, 1967, 1968) and rabbit olfactory bulb (Von Baumgarten, Bloom, Oliver and Salmoriaghi, 1963; Salmoiraghi, Bloom and Costa, 1964).

The excitation of cerebellar Purkinje cells and cortical Betz cells by acetylcholine is frequently preceded by a brief period during which the firing rate is depressed (Crawford *et al.*, 1966; Crawford and Curtis, 1966) and acetylcholine also depresses those Renshaw cells in the spinal cord that have previously been exposed to dihydro-β-erythroidine and atropine (Curtis and Ryall, 1966b).

Curtis and his colleagues (Curtis *et al.*, 1966) have speculated that until cholinergic pathways can be found to account for these depressant effects of acetylcholine, the possibility that they are mediated by a nonsynaptic mechanism must be considered. Acetylcholine may interact either with postsynaptic membrane components which are distinct from transmitter receptors, or influence intracellular metabolic processes, or even glial cells. The interaction of cholinomimetics with membrane receptor sites in close proximity to the synaptic transmitter receptors could also affect subsequent synaptic effects. Such an effect may account for the reduction in acetylcholine excitation of thalamic neurones after prior applications of carbachol or dl-muscarone (McCance *et al.*, 1968).

In two instances, however, accumulated evidence suggests that acetylcholine functions as an inhibitory transmitter in the brain. A correlation between the atropine-sensitive inhibitory effects of acetylcholine and nucleus ventralis anterior stimulation on caudate neurones has been described in the previous section and constitutes one of the examples of cholinergic inhibition.

The concept of a cholinergic inhibitory mechanism in the cerebral cortex was originally proposed to account for the augmentation of primary cortical responses by topically applied atropine (Chatfield and Purpura, 1954; Chatfield and Lord, 1955). Topically applied tubocurarine also enhances cortical responses (Chang, 1953; Feldberg, Malcolm and Sherwood, 1956) and this has been interpreted as a blockade of inhibitory transmission, though not necessarily of cholinergic inhibitory synapses (Morlock and Ward, 1961). Recurrent inhibition of cortical neurones by impulses in pyramidal tract axon collaterals may be depressed by dihydro-β-erythroidine and strychnine (Morrell, 1959) although these findings have not been confirmed (Brooks and Asanuma, 1965; Crawford, Curtis, Voorhoeve and Wilson, 1963).

Most stimuli which elicit cortical activity also evoke some inhibition of cortical neurones, reducing neuronal excitability for periods of 100–300 msec (Phillips, 1956a, b, 1959; Branch and Martin, 1958; Lux and Klee, 1962; Krnjević, Randić and Straughan, 1966). However, short duration cortical inhibitions evoked by single stimuli applied directly to the cortical surface or to underlying structures are resistant to a variety of acetylcholine antagonists and strychnine (Crawford et al., 1963; Krnjević et al., 1966).

Cortical neurones that are depressed by acetylcholine have been located in the primary sensory motor, auditory and visual areas and in a non-visual part of the lateral gyrus. Such cells are most frequently found in cortical layers II, III and IV and the receptors on these cells appear to be intermediate in type between nicotinic and muscarinic receptors. Carbachol, nicotine and acetyl-β-methylcholine are potent depressants of acetylcholine-depressed cortical neurones (Fig. 7.15A) and their actions, as well as those of acetylcholine are antagonized by a variety of "nicotinic" and "muscarinic" blockers and strychnine (Phillis and York, 1967a, b, 1968a, b). Anticholinesterases also have powerful depressant effects and potentiate the action of acetylcholine (Fig. 7.15B).

By repetitively stimulating the adjacent cortex (Fig. 7.16B) pyramidal tracts, mesencephalic reticular formation or lateral hypothalamus (Fig. 7.16A) (10–15 pulses/sec for 10 sec), it has been possible to demonstrate inhibition of the spontaneous or L-glutamate-induced excitation of acetylcholine-depressed cortical neurones. Inhibitions of this type may have a duration of over 1 min. These inhibitory effects of repetitive stimulation are potentiated by prior application of a cholinesterase inhibitor (Fig.

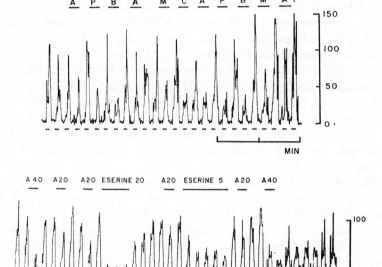

FIG. 7.15. *Above.* Responses of a precruciate cortical cell to constant duration (7 sec) pulses of L-glutamic acid (50 nA) applied iontophoretically every 15 sec (indicated by horizontal bars below the trace in all figures). These responses were used as a measure of cell excitability. The iontophoretic application of the various cholinomimetic drugs, acetylcholine (A), propionylcholine (P), butyrylcholine (B), acetyl-β-methylcholine (M) and carbachol (C) (all 40 nA) is indicated by horizontal bars above the trace. The scale on the right is cell firing frequency in spikes per second.

Below. Acetylcholine (A) caused a marked depression of this cortical neurone at 40 nA whereas at 20 nA a smaller depression was evident. Iontophoretically applied eserine (20 nA) had a potent depressant action followed by a slow recovery. A second application at 1/4 the previous dose (5 nA) still had strong depressant action. After eserine the depressant response of this cell to ACh (40 nA) was considerably prolonged in its timecourse. (Phillis and York, 1968b)

7.17A) and the depressant effects of both neural stimulation and acetyl-choline are antagonized by "nicotinic" and "muscarinic" blockers or strychnine (Fig. 7.17B) (Phillis and York, 1967a, b; 1968a, b). Comparable inhibitions during direct surface stimulation have been observed in isolated cortical slabs, suggesting that cholinergic inhibitory interneurones may be present in the cerebral cortex.

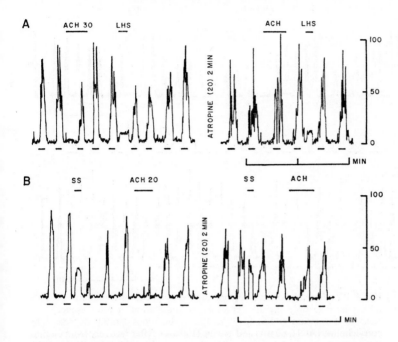

FIG. 7.16. A. and B. Records from precruciate cortical neurones illustrating the depressant effect of acetylcholine (ACH), lateral hypothalamic (LHS) and direct cortical (SS) stimulation on L-glutamate evoked firing. Periods of drug application or stimulation are indicated by horizontal bars. Atropine abolished the inhibitory effects of both acetylcholine and nervous stimulation. (Phillis and York, 1968a).

The presence of both strychnine-antagonized and resistant inhibitions of cortical neurones suggests that more than one inhibitory transmitter is present in the cerebral cortex. Krnjević and Schwartz (1967) have shown that the actions of γ-aminobutyric acid on cortical neurones would qualify it to act as the inhibitory transmitter responsible for generating the short latency, short duration, strychnine-resistant inhibitions evoked by single pulses. Various monoamines, as well as acetylcholine, may be involved in the generation of the long duration, strychnine-susceptible inhibitions evoked by repetitive stimulation. Noradrenaline, 5-hydroxytryptamine and histamine also depress the excitability of many cortical neurones and are

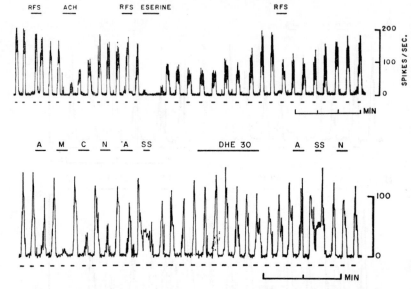

FIG. 7.17. *Above.* A cortical neurone excited by pulses of L-glutamic acid (20 nA) is initially only slightly depressed by stimulation of the mesencephalic reticular formation (RFS) (5·5 V, 10/sec) but considerably depressed by acetylcholine (ACH, 60 nA) and eserine (100 nA). After recovery from eserine, RFS caused a marked depression. Depth of cell below cortical surface −300 μ (Phillis and York, 1967a).

Below. Depressant effects of acetylcholine (A), acetyl-β-methylcholine (M), carbachol (C), nicotine (N), and cortical surface stimulation (SS) on this precruciate cortical neurone were abolished by dihydro-β-erythroidine (DHE, 30 nA) (Phillis and York, unpublished observations).

antagonized by strychnine (Phillis and York, 1967b; Phillis, Tebēcis and York, 1968a). The system in the feline cerebral cortex may be comparable to that observed in certain neurones of *Aplysia californicans* (Kehoe, 1967), in which a dual system of short and long duration inhibitions, evoked by single and repetitive stimuli respectively occurs. The reversal potentials for these two inhibitory processes have been shown to differ, although both can be simulated by acetylcholine.

C. ACETYLCHOLINE RELEASE FROM THE BRAIN

A relationship between the acetylcholine content and the level of activity in the brain has been described by a number of investigators. Variations in the concentration of acetylcholine have been correlated with physiological changes in nervous activity, such as those occurring in the transition from sleep to wakefulness or during the administration of anaesthetics or convulsants (Elliot, Swank and Henderson, 1950; Richter and Crossland, 1949; Tobias, Lipton and Lepinat, 1946). In general, states of activation of the nervous system are associated with a decrease in its acetylcholine content.

Investigations of the rate of release of acetylcholine into pools of eserinized saline on the surface of the cerebral cortex support the interpretation that increased cortical activity results in a release of acetylcholine from its storage sites in the nerve terminals. Experiments of this type, originally conceived by MacIntosh and Oborin (1953), have since been employed to study the nature and distribution of cholinergic pathways to the cerebral cortex (Mitchell, 1963; Kanai and Szerb, 1965; Celesia and Jasper, 1966, Phillis, 1968b). Acetylcholine release occurs from both the primary and association areas of the cerebral cortex. A comparison of the mean rates of acetylcholine release from several cortical areas of cats anaesthetized with different anaesthetics is presented in Table 9. Although the animals were assessed as being at comparable depths of anaesthesia, it is evident that the highest rates of release from the sensori-motor area were recorded when volatile anaesthetics were used. With the exception of pentobarbitone sodium-anaesthetized animals, the differences were less marked when the other cortical areas were compared. The rate of release from the sensori-motor cortex was invariably higher than that from other areas.

An extensive survey of the effects of different modalities and frequencies of stimulation on the rates of release of acetylcholine from the cerebral cortex has furnished some interesting findings (Phillis, 1968b). The most striking feature of the results was the discovery that peripheral stimulation causes comparable increases in the acetylcholine output from all the cortical areas tested (Table 9), regardless of the type of stimulation employed. Thus stimulation of the left forepaw caused marked increases in the rate of acetylcholine release in both the ipsi -and contralateral sensori-motor areas, as well as from the auditory, visual and parietal cortices. Auditory and visual stimulation evoked an increased rate of release in other areas as well as in the auditory or visual areas. An optimal increase in the rate of acetylcholine release was found to coincide with stimulation frequencies of about 1 per sec. Marked increases or decreases in the frequency of

T.P.O.S.—G

TABLE 9.

A. MEAN RATES OF ACETYLCHOLINE RELEASE FROM UNSTIMULATED CORTEX[a]

Anaesthetic	Area of cortex											
	Sensorimotor			Auditory			Visual			Parietal		
	No. of cats	Mean rate of release	S.D.	No. of cats	Mean rate of release	S.D.	No. of cats	Mean rate of release	S.D.	No. of cats	Mean rate of release	S.D.
Diethylether	5	3·04	1·61	5	0·98	0·74	5	0·65	0·42	5	1·37	1·1
Halothane	6	2·27	2·12	6	0·62	0·36	3	0·44	—	2	0·60	—
Pentobarbitone sodium	13	0·45	0·54	9	0·18	0·18	6	0·18	0·17	5	0·34	0·2
Dial	5	1·92	2·14	5	0·65	0·45	3	0·84	—	4	0·51	0·46
Chloralose	7	0·88	0·77	7	0·60	0·42	6	0·37	0·073	6	0·62	0·51
Encéphale isolé	3	0·45	—	—	—	—	—	—	—	3	0·20	—

[a] Rates of release are expressed in ng/min per cm^2

B. MEAN PERCENTAGE INCREASE IN RATE OF RELEASE OF ACh INDUCED BY VARIOUS MODES OF STIMULATION (PENTOBARBITONE SODIUM ANAESTHETISED CATS·

Cortical area	Left forepaw	Left hindpaw	Left facial	Auditory	Visual	Reticular formation	Direct cortical[c]
Right sensori-motor	230(25–650)[b]	120(20–260)	170(30–280)	100(20–170)	160(40–220)	—	120(80–170)
Left sensori-motor	250(0–650)	50(0–100)	190(30–350)	110(0–300)	100(10–180)	180(40–320)	140(100–210)
Auditory	320(80–650)	—	130(10–250)	85(·0–190)	120(30–200)	210(80–320)	100(50–160)
Visual	90(25–150)	—	70(20–130)	80(65–100)	110(30–200)	70(30–160)	30(10–60)
Parietta	30(5–60)	—	—	—	—	—	—

[a] Rate of release immediately before and after stimulation used to calculate baseline for these figures.
[b] Ranges.
[c] Stimulation of left sensorimotor cortex within the cup. ACh release was determined simultaneously.

stimulation were associated with a reduction in the amount of acetylcholine released (Mitchell, 1963; Phillis, 1968b).

Stimulation in areas of the brain stem which evoked a desynchronization of the electrocorticogram, also caused an increase in the rate of acetylcholine release (Kanai and Szerb, 1965; Phillis, 1968b) and it has therefore been suggested that the acetylcholine-releasing pathways may be associated with the "reticular arousal system". This would be consistent with the diffuse nature of the acetylcholine-releasing system described in this section. As acetylcholine has an inhibitory action on many cells in the cerebral cortex, it is possible that desynchronization of the electrocorticogram is a result of inhibitory rather than excitatory actions of acetylcholine on cortical neurones.

Other investigations have been concerned with acetylcholine release from the feline caudate nucleus (Mitchell and Szerb, 1962, McLennan, 1964) and thalamus (Phillis, Tebēcis and York, 1968b). "Push–pull" cannulae were employed in these experiments, in which an increased release of acetylcholine during stimulation of the nucleus ventralis anterior (caudate nucleus experiments) or reticular formation, forepaw and visual system (thalamic experiments) was demonstrated.

The use of push–pull cannulae has recently been criticized by Chase and Kopin (1968), who have established that the release of labelled inulin from the olfactory bulb is increased during olfactory stimulation. As inulin, injected into the cerebrospinal fluid, remains largely in the "extracellular" space, the odour-induced alterations in its efflux suggest that local changes within this compartment may attend neural stimulation. These authors have suggested that during perfusion with a push–pull cannula, a steep concentration gradient may be created in the artificial extracellular space surrounding the cannula tip. Relatively small variations in hydrostatic pressure or in the transport or diffusion rates of extracellular components might produce substantial changes in the concentrations of substances in the push–pull cannula perfusate. However, these considerations may not be as important when the push–pull cannula is used to study the release of endogenous substances, such as the acetylcholine release from the caudate nucleus and thalamus. Collier and Murray-Brown (1968) were unable to demonstrate an increased release of labelled urea into cups on the cerebral cortex during stimulation of the reticular formation, even though the rate of acetylcholine release was augmented.

CONCLUSIONS

1. Some of the techniques that have been used to study synaptic transmission in the central nervous system and their limitations are described. Iontophoresis of drugs from fine glass micropipettes is undoubtedly the most satisfactory technique available, but even with this method the results must be interpreted with caution.

2. Motor-axon collateral-Renshaw cell synapses in the mammalian spinal cord are the best known example of a cholinergic junction in the central nervous system. Recent investigations have shown that the Renshaw cell has three cholinergic receptors; a "nicotinic" receptor mediating short-latency excitation, a "muscarinic" receptor giving slower excitatory responses and an inhibitory receptor. All three receptors appear to be involved in the response to motor-axon collateral stimulation. The presence of non-cholinergic excitatory and inhibitory synapses in Renshaw cells has also been described.

3. Excitatory or depressant actions of acetylcholine on interneurones in the spinal cord have been described. There is currently no indication as to whether these effects are mediated by synaptic receptors.

4. Acetylcholine has either excitatory or depressant actions on neurones in many areas of the brain (see Table 7). In certain structures there is convincing evidence for cholinergic synaptic transmission. These include the cerebral and cerebellar cortices, thalamus, lateral and medial geniculate nuclei and caudate nucleus.

5. Cholinergic excitatory transmission in the cerebellar cortex occurs between mossy fibres and some granule layer cells. Excitatory cholinergic pathways project from the brain stem to the thalamus and geniculate nuclei, from the thalamus to the caudate nucleus and from the cerebellum to the thalamus. There is also evidence for cholinergic projections from the inferior colliculus and cerebral cortex to the medial geniculate nucleus.

6. Inhibitory cholinergic transmission has been established in the cerebral cortex and caudate nucleus. In the cortex, these inhibitions have a longer duration than the non-cholinergic inhibitions and are most evident after repetitive stimulation of the adjacent cortical surface.

7. Acetylcholine receptors on cortical deep pyramidal cells are classically "muscarinic" in nature. On many other cells in the central nervous system, the receptors appear to be intermediate between the nicotinic and muscarinic types of receptor.

8. Acetylcholine release has been demonstrated in the spinal cord, cerebral and cerebellar cortices, thalamus and caudate nucleus. The rate of release can be augmented by various forms of stimulation. The pattern of the increases in release from the cerebral cortex during stimulation indicates that the cholinergic fibres are part of a diffuse projection system, rather than the specific afferent pathways.

CHAPTER 8

PHARMACOLOGICAL STUDIES ON NEURONES IN THE BRAIN AND SPINAL CORD. PART 2. MONOAMINES AND OTHER SUBSTANCES

A. ADRENERGIC MECHANISMS IN THE CENTRAL NERVOUS SYSTEM

Investigations of the central nervous actions of the catecholamines have been complicated by the presence of a blood–brain barrier in most areas of the central nervous system other than the hypothalamus (Weil-Malherbe, Axelrod and Tomchick, 1959; Weil-Malherbe, Whitby and Axelrod, 1961). The vascular effects of noradrenaline and adrenaline may also complicate the interpretation of experimental results when these compounds are administered into the blood stream. For instance, careful studies by Baust and his collaborators (Baust and Katz, 1961; Baust, Niemczyk and Vieth, 1963; Baust and Niemczyk, 1963) have shown that the changes in discharge rate of neurones in the reticular formation and hypothalamus, evoked by an intravenous injection of adrenaline, are a result of the elevation in blood pressure produced by this substance. Similar changes could be induced by a mechanically produced rise in blood pressure, caused by compression of the descending aorta. When blood pressure was kept constant artificially, no changes in electrical activity could be demonstrated following the administration of adrenaline.

1. *Spinal Cord*

Noradrenaline appears to be the only catecholamine normally present in the mammalian spinal cord, where it has been detected in descending fibres from the brain (Vogt, 1954; Anderson and Cudia, 1962; Magnusson and Rosengren, 1963; Carlsson, Falck, Fuxe and Hillarp, 1964; Dahlström and Fuxe, 1965; Anderson and Holgerson, 1966). Significant amounts of dopamine were detected in the rat and ox spinal cord by McGeer and McGeer (1962), but these results have not been confirmed by other workers (Magnusson and Rosengren, 1963; Andén, 1965; Laverty and Sharman, 1965).

The effects of catecholamines on spinal cord reflexes have not been entirely consistent, although indicative of some influence on neuronal excitability. Intravenous administration of large doses of adrenaline (200–400 μg) caused a long-lasting depression of the knee-jerk reflex in cats, which was preceded by an enhancement during the period of blood pressure elevation (Schweitzer and Wright, 1937). These results have been confirmed by other investigators (Sigg, Ochs and Gerard, 1955; Ten Cate, Boeles and Biersteker, 1959; McLennan, 1961). The depressant effect of adrenaline may be replaced by one of facilitation if the level of anaesthesia is reduced (Sigg et al., 1955).

Intra-arterial injection or topical application of adrenaline in spinal cats caused an augmentation of the monosynaptic extensor reflex, whilst flexor reflexes were depressed. This was associated with an increased positivity of the ventral root (recorded against an electrode on the cord dorsum) (Bernhard, Skoglund and Therman, 1947; Bernhard and Skoglund, 1953). The possibility that changes in blood pressure were responsible for increases in excitability of extensor motoneurones was eliminated by Stavraky (1947), who used a valve to control pressure fluctuations whilst he recorded the tension developed by quadriceps muscle. The observation, by Sigg et al. (1955), that the effects of adrenaline and noradrenaline on spinal reflexes were dependent on the level of anaesthesia has been confirmed in more recent studies (Wilson, 1956; Kissel and Domino, 1959). These authors have also reported a facilitation of extensor reflexes in unanaesthetized animals.

The potency of catecholamines as depressants of the patellar reflex in anaesthetized animals was dependent on the route of administration (McLennan, 1961). Intravenously administered adrenaline had a more marked effect than noradrenaline, and dopamine was almost inactive. The effects of adrenaline and noradrenaline administered in this manner were antagonized by the α-blocking agents, dibenzyline and chlorpromazine. However, when the drugs were applied topically on to an exposed spinal cord, the order of potency was reversed, with dopamine proving to be the most effective depressant of patellar reflexes. These effects could be prevented by the beta receptor blocking agent, dichloroisopropylnoradrenaline and by strychnine, but not by dibenzyline or chlorpromazine.

The failure of Curtis *et al.* (1957) to observe effects of adrenaline and noradrenaline on monosynaptic reflexes was probably due to their use of barbiturate anaesthetized animals. These authors attributed the occasional slight potentiation of reflexes observed in their experiments to local vascular effects, although Schweitzer and Wright (1937) and Stavraky (1947) have provided evidence to exclude this possibility.

Skoglund (1961) has described an action of small doses of noradrenaline on the excitability of individual spinal interneurones, recorded with a microelectrode. The commonest effect seen with a threshold dose of 1 μg/kg of intra-arterially administered noradrenaline was an increase in cell excitability, with potentiated synaptic responses and spontaneous firing. Evidence that noradrenaline is an excitatory transmitter in the pathway from the thoracic spinal cord to gastrocnemius fusimotor neurones has recently been obtained (Ellaway and Pascoe, 1958). Fusimotor neurone discharges evoked by spinal cord stimulation were blocked by phenoxybenzamine and chlorpromazine and potentiated by substances which block the re-uptake of noradrenaline into nerve terminals, such as cocaine and desmethylimipramine. Inhibition of catechol-O-methyltransferase with catechol caused a marked increase in fusimotor neurone discharges. Depletion of catecholamine stores with reserpine or tetrabenazine reduced or abolished the effects of cord stimulation. All these effects are compatible with the concept that the pathway from the thoracic spinal cord to gastrocnemius fusimotor neurones contains a noradrenergic link.

The initial experiments in which iontophoretically applied adrenaline, noradrenaline and dopamine were tested on spinal interneurones were conducted with barbiturate anaesthetized animals (Curtis *et al.*, 1961a; Curtis, 1962), which may explain the negative results obtained. In more recent experiments on unanaesthetized or diethyl ether anaesthetized cats, both depressant and excitant effects of noradrenaline on various spinal interneurones have been observed (Engberg and Ryall, 1966; Weight and Salmoiraghi, 1966a). Depressant effects of iontophoretically applied noradrenaline on motoneurones and Renshaw cells have also been observed (Biscoe and Curtis, 1966; Engberg and Ryall, 1966; Weight and Salmoiraghi, 1966b, 1967; Phillis, Tebēcis and York, 1968c).

Intracellular records of motoneuronal responses and the changes in membrane potential during the application of noradrenaline into their immediate extracellular environment have recently been obtained in this laboratory. A side-by-side combination of a multiple barrelled electrode and a hyperfine microelectrode was used in these experiments and some typical responses are presented in Fig. 8.1. Noradrenaline (applied by a current of 100 nA) blocked the invasion of an antidromic spike into the soma-dendritic area of the motoneurones in Fig. 8.1A. Invasion of the spike into the initial segment area was also depressed. A comparison between the membrane potential changes induced by γ-aminobutyric acid and noradrenaline is presented in Fig. 8.1B. The hyperpolarization associated with γ-aminobutyric acid had a more rapid onset and decline than that induced by noradrenaline. During the application of both substances, inhibitory post-synaptic potentials were depressed (Fig. 8.1C). Excitatory postsynaptic potentials were also reduced.

Noradrenaline-containing nerve terminals are present in the dorsal and ventral horns and form close contacts with the cell bodies and processes of some α-motoneurones (Dahlström and Fuxe, 1965). The presence of noradrenaline in the spinal cord is dependent on the integrity of descending pathways from the brain stem (Andén, Häggendal, Magnusson and Rosengren, 1964; Dahlström and Fuxe, 1965) and electrical stimulation of descending tracts in the upper cervical region of isolated spinal cords causes a release of noradrenaline (Andén, Carlsson, Hillarp and Magnusson, 1965). The terminals containing noradrenaline are probably derived from small, unmyelinated nerve fibres (Dahlström and Fuxe, 1965) and little is known about the properties of terminals of this type. Biscoe and Curtis (1966) have argued that noradrenaline is unlikely to be an inhibitory transmitter for Renshaw cells as its action is unaffected by doses of strychnine which block postsynaptic inhibitions. Antagonism between noradrenaline and strychnine has been observed in the thalamus, geniculate nuclei and cerebral cortex (Phillis and Tebēcis, 1967; Tebēcis, 1967; Phillis and York, 1967) and it is conceivable that such an effect has been overlooked in the spinal cord. It is also possible that Renshaw cells are influenced by more than one inhibitory transmitter.

The concentration of catecholamines in the central nervous system can be augmented by administration of their amino acid precursor L-3,4-dihydroxyphenylalanine (DOPA), which passes the blood–brain barrier to enter the tissues of brain and spinal cord. DOPA is then transformed into dopamine by the action of DOPA-decarboxylase which is present at all

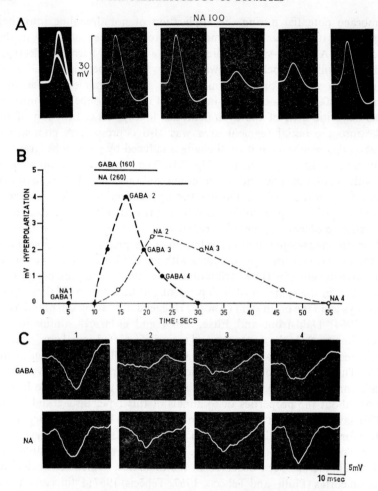

FIG. 8.1. Intracellular records showing inhibitory effects of noradrenaline (NA) and γ-amino-butyric acid (GABA). A. Antidromic spike of a biceps-semitendinosus (BST) motoneurone evoked by stimulation of ventral root L7. The first record shows partial failure of the soma-dendritic (SD) spike during repetitive stimulation at 20/sec. An application of NA (100 nA) blocked the SD spike and reduced the size of the initial segment (IS) spike within a few sec. Recovery occurred within 60 sec after the application was terminated. B. Graph showing changes in membrane potential of another BST moto-neurone (resting potential 50 mV) during the application of γ-amino-butyric acid (GABA) and NA. The latter was applied 1 min. after the end of GABA application. C. NA and GABA depression of IPSPs evoked by stimulation of the sural nerve in the same motoneurone represented in B. The relative times of recording of each IPSP shown in C are indicated by the corresponding numbers in graph B (Phillis, Tebēcis and York, 1968c).

sites where endogenous dopamine is formed and at many other sites as well (Vogt, 1965).

Carlsson, Magnusson and Rosengren (1963) found that DOPA increased the flexor reflex in acute spinal animals. Further experiments on the effects of DOPA on spinal reflexes have indicated that there is a noradrenergic descending pathway in the spinal cord, which inhibits transmission of short latency effects from flexor reflex afferents. Increases in the flexor reflex, such as those described by Carlsson *et al.* (1963) are due to a long latency, long lasting discharge of flexor motoneurones evoked by repetitive activity in the flexor reflex afferents (Andén, Jukes, Lundberg and Vyklicky, 1966a, b; Andén, Jukes and Lundberg, 1966). Certain objections have been raised against the use of the monoamine precursors, DOPA and 5-hydroxytryptophan (5-HTP), from which 5-hydroxytryptamine is formed (Gessa, Costa, Kuntzman and Brodie, 1962). Their decarboxylation appears to be brought about by one and the same enzyme, which suggests that after an injection of DOPA, dopamine would accumulate at 5-hydroxytryptaminergic synapses and might produce some unusual responses on liberation by presynaptic nerve impulses.

2. *The Arousal System*

The effects of catecholamines upon various parameters of brain function vary with the dose and route of administration. Many investigators have attempted to relate cerebral cortical activity to the concentration of circulatory adrenaline or noradrenaline in the blood. Intravenous injection of these catecholamines leads to an arousal in the cortical electroencephalogram (Bonvallet, Dell and Hiebel, 1954; Bonvallet, Hugelin and Dell, 1956; Rothballer, 1956; Longo and Silvestrini, 1957; Jasper, 1958; Capon, 1958; Mantegazzini, Poeck and Santibanez, 1959; Bradley, 1960; Dell, 1960), which can be abolished by coagulation of the mesencephalic reticular formation (Rothballer, 1956). Some investigators (Bonvallet *et al.*, 1954; Bonvallet *et al.*, 1956; Bradley and Mollica, 1958; Rothballer, 1959; Dell, 1960) have suggested that adrenaline acts directly on cells of the mesencephalic reticular formation. However adrenaline injected directly into the cerebral circulation does not produce an arousal until the drug has had time to recirculate and induce a rise in blood pressure (Longo and Silvestrini, 1957; Capon, 1960) and the effects of intravenous adrenaline on the cortical electroencephalogram can be reproduced by elevating the blood pressure to a comparable extent (Albe-Fessard and Hesse, 1953; Baust *et al.*, 1963). It is therefore difficult to accept the conclusion that the arousal response to injections of adrenaline is entirely due to an action of this substance on cells in the reticular formation.

Support for the concept of an arousal system in the brain stem, operating through an adrenergic mechanism has been forthcoming from experiments in which catecholamines were administered by micro-injection of small volumes of concentrated solution, or by direct application of crystalline substance, into the brain stem of freely moving, unanesthetized cats (Cordeau, Moreau, Beaulnes and Laurin, 1963; Yamaguchi, Ling and Marczynski, 1964). Injections of adrenaline into the pontine and medullary reticular formation produced behavioural and electroencephalographic arousal in sleeping cats. Doses of d-amphetamine, a sympathomimetic agent, elicit strong and long lasting electroencephalographic activation and behavioural excitement when administered into the mesencephalic reticular formation.

3. *Intra-ventricular Administration*

Application of drugs into the cerebral ventricles through implanted cannulae has been extensively utilized as an experimental technique. The results obtained with this method, and their implications in the control of body temperature have been described in a monograph by Feldberg (1963) and a recent review by Feldberg and Fleischhauer (1965). On injection into the cerebral ventricles of cats, noradrenaline and adrenaline (25–100 μg) lowered rectal temperatures for several hours and caused a cessation of the shivering which accompanied the fever produced by an intraventricular injection of bacterial pyrogens (Feldberg and Fleischhauer, 1965). 5-Hydroxytryptamine (200 μg intraventricularly) had the opposite effect, causing a long lasting rise in temperature accompanied by shivering. These hypothermic and hyperthermic effects could be reproduced when the amines were applied by microinjection into the anterior hypothalamus in microgram amounts, suggesting that their action was on this region of the brain. Injections into the posterior or ventromedian hypothalamus did not affect body temperatures (Feldberg and Fleischhauer, 1965). Kulkarni (1967) has recently reported rather different results when monoamines are injected into the lateral cerebral ventricles and it is, therefore, possible that small variations in the cannula position influence the site of action of perfused drugs and thus affect the results. Injections of adrenaline and noradrenaline into the cerebral ventricles have a marked depressant and analgesic effect; the general state of the animal resembling that of light anaesthesia (Leimdorfer and Metzner, 1949; Feldberg and Sherwood, 1954). When injected into the nucleus centralis medialis of the thalamus, noradrenaline produced unmistakable deep sleep, characterized by long lasting phases of desynchronized electrocortical activity, hippocampal theta rhythm and the disappearance of electromyographic potentials (Yamaguchi et al., 1964). Diametrically opposite reactions have been produced by the injection of noradrenaline and acetylcholine into the "hypogenic" forebrain area constituted by the medial and lateral preoptic regions. In this area, noradrenaline always induced electroencephalographic and behavioural arousal, motor hyperactivity and non-directed rage behaviour, whereas acetylcholine administered through the same cannula produced behavioural and electroencephalographic sleep (Hernandez-Peon and Chavez-Ibarra, 1963; Hernandez-Peon, Chavez-Ibarra, Morgan and Timo-Iaria, 1963; Hernandez-Peon, 1965; Yamaguchi et al., 1964).

4. Actions of Iontophoretically Applied Catecholamines on Brain

(a) *Brain stem.* Iontophoretically applied noradrenaline excites or inhibits many neurones in the pons and medulla (Bradley and Wolstencroft, 1962, 1965; Meyer, 1965; Yamamoto, 1967). Dopamine and adrenaline frequently had no action on units which responded to noradrenaline, and when they did, their effects were of the same kind, though often weaker (Bradley and Wolstencroft, 1965). An examination of the pharmacological properties of twenty-two rostrally projecting neurones in the nucleus reticularis gigantocellularis revealed that noradrenaline excited eight and inhibited thirteen, whereas in the nearby paramedian reticular nucleus an almost uniform inhibitory action was observed (Bradley, Wolstencroft, Hösli and Avanzino, 1966). Some of the rostrally projecting neurones in the nucleus reticularis gigantocellularis may belong to the ascending reticular activating system and would therefore account for the "arousal" effect observed with catecholamines. Dopamine had a purely depressant action on neurones in the cuneate and gracile nuclei (Meyer, 1965).

(b) *Cerebellum.* Dopamine, noradrenaline and adrenaline depress the excitability of cells in the neocerebellar cortex, while noradrenaline exerts excitatory effects upon neurones in the flocculus (Phillis, 1965; Yamamoto, 1967). The histochemical evidence for a noradrenergic innervation of the cerebellar cortex has already been discussed (Andén, Fuxe and Ungerstedt, 1967).

(c) *Thalamus.* An extensive study of the pharmacological properties of catecholamine receptors on thalamic neurones has shown that these are clearly different from those of peripheral adrenergic receptors (Phillis and Tebēcis, 1967b). Peripheral adrenergic receptors have been divided into α- and β-categories on the basis of their responses to various sympathomimetic amines (Ahlquist, 1948). Adrenaline is the most potent of the amines on α-receptors, with isoprenaline having the least effect. Isoprenaline is the most potent on β-receptors, and noradrenaline is the least effective. In general the effects on α-receptors are excitatory and those on β-receptors inhibitory.

Noradrenaline, adrenaline, isoprenaline and dopamine, applied iontophoretically, were tested on thalamic neurones and with the exception of dopamine which depressed nearly all the cells tested none of these sympathomimetic amines proved to be significantly more potent as either a depressant or excitant than the others (Table 10).

The magnitude and duration of the depressant actions of noradrenaline and adrenaline varied considerably. More sensitive neurones, which occurred most frequently in the dorsal thalamus, responded to extremely small amounts of catecholamine and recovery often took several minutes. Recovery after a dopamine application was always rapid. Excitatory responses to noradrenaline and adrenaline were most marked in the ventrobasal complex of the thalamus (Fig. 8.2) and frequently involved neurones that were also excited by acetylcholine. Desensitization occurred when either substance was applied repeatedly and this tachyphylaxis lasted for several minutes (Fig. 8.2). After desensitization to the excitatory effects, some of these cells were inhibited by the catecholamines, suggesting the presence of at least two types of membrane receptor on the same neurone (Phillis and Tebēcis, 1967b).

The monoamine oxidase inhibitor, iproniazid, also depressed neurones that were sensitive to noradrenaline depression and occasionally potentiated the action of noradrenaline. It was concluded that the depressant effects of iproniazid were unlikely to be due to a potentiation of endogenously released noradrenaline as recovery occurred within a few minutes (Phillis and Tebēcis, 1967b). The inhibitory effects of iproniazid on mono-

TABLE 10.

ACTIONS OF VARIOUS MONOAMINES ON THALAMIC NEURONES

Substance	Action	Position of neurone in thalamus[a]		
		Superficial	Intermediate	Deep
Dopamine	No effect	4 (14%)	0	1 (11%)
	Depression	24 (86%)	11 (100%)	8 (89%)
	Excitation	0	0	0
Noradrenaline	No effect	26 (34%)	31 (45%)	27 (33%)
	Depression	48 (63%)	24 (35%)	30 (37%)
	Excitation	2 (3%)	14 (20%)	25 (30%)
Adrenaline	No effect	22 (36%)	19 (34%)	7 (30%)
	Depression	35 (55%)	32 (57%)	14 (61%)
	Excitation	6 (9%)	5 (9%)	2 (9%)
Isoprenaline	No effect	8 (53%)	6 (26%)	6 (43%)
	Depression	6 (40%)	14 (61%)	5 (36%)
	Excitation	1 (7%)	3 (13%)	3 (21%)
5-Hydroxy-tryptamine	No effect	3 (11%)	1 (6%)	0
	Depression	24 (86%)	15 (83%)	8 (73%)
	Excitation	1 (3%)	2 (11%)	3 (27%)

[a] Neurones are grouped into three depth categories; *superficial group* cells at depths of 0–3 mm; *intermediate group* at depths of 3–6 mm; *deep group* cells at depths of 6–9 mm. Position of cells was determined by acid-lesioning. The figures indicate numbers and percentages of neurones tested in each depth group and the responses observed. (Phillis and Tebécis, 1967b).

amine oxidase are largely irreversible (Zeller, 1959). *Alpha-* and *beta-*adrenergic antagonists have pronounced depressant actions on thalamic neurones that are inhibited by noradrenaline and frequently excite cells that were excited by the catecholamines (Fig. 8.3). These actions were attributed to the sympathomimetic activity of the antagonists. With the exception of D-INPEA, which reduced the excitant actions of noradrenaline, the adrenergic antagonists did not appear to produce a specific block of the catecholamines. These results are described in more detail in a late section of this chapter.

Picrotoxin and strychnine antagonized the inhibitory effects of both the catecholamines and reticular formation stimulation on thalamic neurones

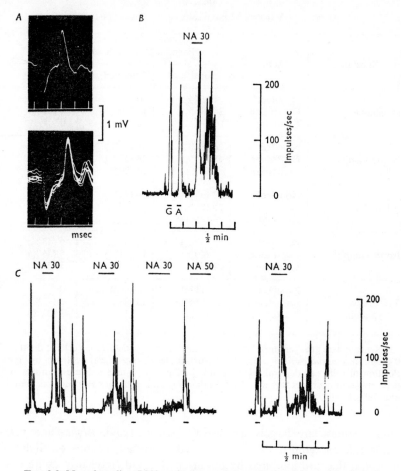

FIG. 8.2. Noradrenaline (NA) excitation and an example of desensitization of a thalamo-cortical neurone as a result of repeated applications of NA (30 and 50 nA). A (top record); antidromic spike evoked by stimulation of ipsilateral sensori-motor cortex; (bottom record): same response at stimulation of 100/sec. B. Same unit firing to L-glutamate (40 nA). ACh (20 A) and NA (30 nA). Excitation by NA had a long latency of onset and offset. C. A series of applications of L-glutamate (40 nA) and NA, illustrating a decreasing excitatory effect of NA with each successive application. The fourth application of NA evoked no firing. After a 10 min rest, NA (30 nA) again had a potent excitatory action on the cell. Firing induced by L-glutamate (40 nA) remained virtually at the same level throughout this series (Phillis and Tebēcis, 1967b).

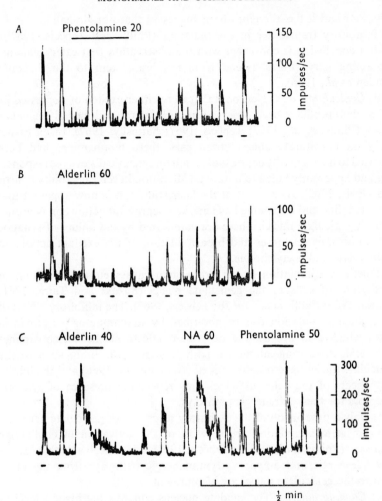

FIG. 8.3. Examples of responses of thalamic neurones to phentolamine and alderlin. A (1890 μ): phentolamine (20 nA) gradually depressed firing evoked by L-glutamate (70 nA). Recovery took 5 min. B (5580 μ): alderlin (60 nA) depressed L-glutamate (60 nA) firing and recovery was slow. C (7100 μ): alderlin (40 nA) had an initial excitatory action followed by a depression of L-gluta-mate (50 nA) firing. NA (60 nA) also caused a marked increase in firing rate. Phentolamine (50 nA) exhibited slight excitatory activity, manifested as an increase in rate of background firing and a potentiation of L-glutamate (50 nA) firing (Phillis and Tebēcis, 1967b).

(Fig. 8.4) and it has therefore been suggested that noradrenaline may be an inhibitory transmitter in the thalamus (Phillis and Tebēcis, 1967b). Such a conclusion is consistent with the observation that catecholamine-containing nerve fibres ascend from the brain stem to the thalamus (Andén *et al.*, 1966).

(d) *Geniculate nuclei.* Neurones that were either excited or depressed by catecholamines have been observed in both lateral and medial geniculate nuclei (Phillis *et al.*, 1967; Tebēcis, 1967; Satinsky, 1967). In an earlier study on barbiturate anaesthetized cats, these monoamines had been reported to have a mildly depressant action on synaptically evoked responses and had apparently failed to induce an alteration in cell excitability (Curtis and Davis, 1962). As a result of the later studies, it is now apparent that noradrenaline and dopamine have marked depressant actions on neurones in both geniculate nuclei. These are manifested by the failure of synaptic and antidromic responses and by a reduction of the excitant actions of L-glutamate and acetylcholine.

Repetitive stimulation in the brain stem causes either depression or facilitation of cells in the geniculate nuclei (Suzuki and Taira, 1961; Ogawa, 1963; Phillis *et al.*, 1967b; Tebēcis, 1967). The inhibitory effects of brain stem stimulation can be abolished by strychnine or picrotoxin in doses which also abolish the depressant effects of the catecholamines (Fig. 8.5). Ascending adrenergic pathways from the brain stem to the geniculate nuclei have been described (Andén *et al.*, 1966) and the inhibitory effects of the catecholamines may reflect the presence of synaptic receptors for these adrenergic pathways.

As only a proportion of the excitatory responses of geniculate neurones to brain stem stimulation are a result of the activation of cholinergic pathways (Phillis *et al.*, 1967b; Tebēcis, 1968), it is conceivable that excitatory adrenergic and 5-hydroxytryptaminergic pathways from the brain stem to the geniculate nuclei are also present.

(e) *Caudate nucleus.* The caudate nucleus contains the highest level of dopamine of any area in the nervous system (Bertler and Rosengren, 1959) and is virtually devoid of noradrenaline, which is surprising as the corpus striatum contains as much dopamine-β-oxidase as the hypothalamus, a noradrenaline-rich area of the brain (Udenfriend and Creveling, 1959). The levels of dopamine in the caudate nucleus are markedly reduced by lesions affecting certain ascending pathways to the striatum (Bertler *et al.*, 1964), particularly those emanating from the substantia nigra (Andén *et al.*,

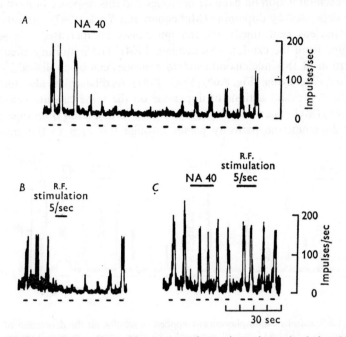

Fig. 8.4. Inhibitory effects of intravenous picrotoxin on depression induced by NA and stimulation of reticular formation on a thalamic cell in the superficial layer. A. NA (40 nA) caused an almost complete depression of firing induced by L-glutamate (40 nA) and recovery took several min. B. R.F. stimulation (5/sec) also caused a complete depression of L-glutamate (40 nA) firing. C. Records of the same cells 2 min after an intravenous injection of picrotoxin (1 mg/kg). NA (40 nA) and R.F. stimulation (5/sec) had no depressant action on L-glutamate (40 nA) firing (Phillis and Tebécis, 1967b).

1964; Poirer and Sourkes, 1965). Retrograde changes in the dopamine content of cells of the substantia nigra occur as a result of the removal of the ipsilateral caudate nucleus (Andén, Dahlström, Fuxe and Larsson, 1965), and it appears therefore, that dopamine in the caudate nucleus is in the terminals of nigro-neostriatal fibres (Andén et al., 1966).

Dopamine has an inhibitory action on some cells of the caudate nucleus ($\simeq 60\%$) and excites others ($\simeq 10\%$) (Bloom et al., 1965; McLennan and York, 1967). Attempts to relate these actions to synaptic transmission have yielded somewhat confusing results. Stimulation of the substantia nigra

has an excitant action on caudate neurones and this response in most cells
can be depressed by dopamine (McLennan and York, 1967). Stimulation
of the nucleus centromedianus thalami causes an increased release of
dopamine from the caudate (McLennan, 1964). The inhibitory effects of
stimulation of this nucleus on caudate neurones can be abolished by the
α-blocker, dibenzyline (Fig. 8.6B) (York, 1967). As dibenzyline also antagonizes the depressant actions of dopamine on the same caudate neurones
(Fig. 8.6A) (McLennan and York, 1967; York, 1967), it has been suggested
that a dopaminergic pathway passes through this area to the caudate

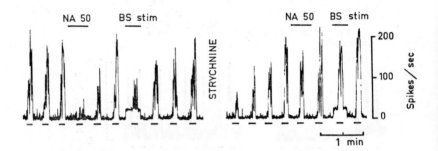

FIG. 8.5. Effect of iontophoretically applied strychnine on the depression of
L-glutamate (50 nA) firing of a medial geniculate neurone by noradrenaline
(NA, 50 nA) and brain stem reticular formation (BS, 9V at 30/sec). Strychnine
(60 nA) was applied for 1 min (during gap in trace). The record following the
gap was recorded 2 min after the end of the strychnine application. The inhibitory effects of both noradrenaline and nervous stimulation were markedly
reduced after strychnine (Tebēcis, 1967).

nucleus. The existence of such a pathway has, however, to be established
histochemically. Dibenzyline has antagonistic effects on the depression of
cerebral cortical neurones by amines other than dopamine, as well as by
acetylcholine and it may not, therefore, be a specific antagonist of dopamine in the caudate nucleus.

Noradrenaline also inhibits and excites many neurones in the caudate
nucleus (Bloom et al., 1965). It is conceivable therefore, that this compound
is actually released from the dopamine-containing nerve terminals, although
the low levels of noradrenaline in the nucleus (Vogt, 1954; Bertler and
Rosengren, 1959) suggest that noradrenaline would have to be synthesized
as required by the presynaptic terminals. This may be the function of the
dopamine-β-oxidase in the caudate nucleus.

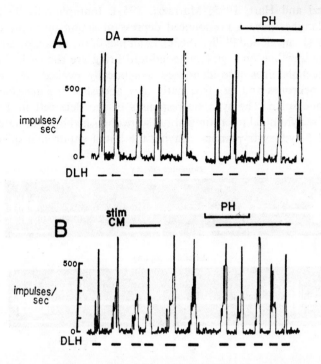

FIG. 8.6. A. Inhibitory action of dopamine (DA, 80 nA) on responses of a caudate nucleus neurone induced to fire by intermittent applications of DL-homocysteic acid (DLH, 40 nA). The inhibitory action is blocked by phenoxybenzamine (PH, 100 nA). B. Recording from the same cell in which stimulation of the nucleus centromedianus thalami (CM, 7V, 0·1 msec, 3/sec) also caused an inhibition which was blocked by phenoxybenzamine (80 nA) (York, 1967).

(f) *Cerebral cortex.* The noradrenaline content of the cerebral cortex is significantly reduced by destruction of the medial forebrain bundle in the lateral hypothalamus (Heller *et al.*, 1966) and as cortical noradrenaline appears to be located in fine nerve terminals (Fuxe, 1965b; Fuxe, Hamberger and Hökfelt, 1968), there is reason to suggest that it may be involved in synaptic transmission. Intracarotid injections of small amounts of adrenaline and noradrenaline have been shown to cause a reduction in the amplitude of transcallosally evoked potentials in the cerebral cortex, which was interpreted as a manifestation of cerebral synaptic inhibition

(Marrazzi and Hart, 1955; Marrazzi, 1957). Iontophoretically applied catecholamines have a pronounced depressant action on many cortical neurones (Krnjević and Phillis, 1963c). Examples of the action of dopamine and noradrenaline on L-glutamate-induced firing are shown in Fig. 8.7. The catecholamines also depressed synaptically evoked responses of cortical neurones and less frequently they abolished the invasion of an antidromic spike. The synaptic responses of the Betz cell in Fig. 8.8, evoked by pyramidal tract stimulation, were abolished by both noradrenaline and 5-hydroxytryptamine, leaving the initial antidromic spike. With

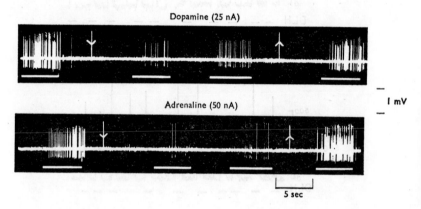

Fig. 8.7. Comparison of the blocking action of dopamine and of adrenaline on the excitation of a cerebral cortical unit by L-glutamate (30 nA); applications of glutamate are shown by the horizontal white lines below traces. The catechol amines were released from other barrels of same micropipette during the periods between arrows. The cat was anaesthetized with allobarbitone (Krnjević and Phillis, 1963c).

larger applications of the monoamines it was possible to depress the antidromic response. These depressant effects were antagonized by iontophoretically applied strychnine (Phillis and York, 1967).

Excitant actions of noradrenaline on cortical neurones have also been observed (Phillis, Tebēcis and York, 1968a; Roberts and Straughan, 1968). The inhibitory actions of these compounds usually have a rapid onset and short duration, whereas the excitant effects are frequently slow in onset, require triggering with L-glutamate, and often continue for 2–3 min after the application has terminated (Fig. 8.9.). Desensitization of the

excitant response has sometimes been observed after application of noradrenaline with large iontophoretic currents. On some cells, microelectro-
phoretic application of dibenamine, an α-blocker, for prolonged periods
is able to selectively antagonize noradrenaline excitation (Roberts and
Straughan, 1968).

(g) *Olfactory bulb*. Antidromic stimulation of mitral cell axons in the
lateral olfactory tract of rabbits produces inhibition of mitral cells in the
ipsilateral olfactory bulb, which is thought to be mediated via recurrent

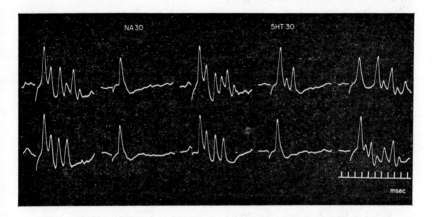

FIG. 8.8. The response of this cerebral cortical Betz cell to pyramidal tract
stimulation consisted of an antidromically invading action potential followed
by a series of synaptically evoked responses. Noradrenaline (NA, 30 nA) and
5-hydroxytryptamine (5HT, 30 nA) abolished the synaptic responses but failed
to block the antidromically evoked action potential (Phillis, Tebēcis and York,
unpublished observations).

axon collaterals (Green, Mancia and Von Baumgarten, 1962; Phillips,
Powell and Shepherd, 1963). In decerebrate rabbits, iontophoretically
applied noradrenaline decreases the discharge rate of mitral cells and both
the recurrent inhibition and actions of noradrenaline are depressed by the
α-blocker, dibenamine (Salmoiraghi *et al.*, 1964). Recurrent inhibition is
also reduced by reserpine and α-methyl-metatyrosine, which deplete brain
noradrenaline stores. This evidence suggests that noradrenaline or a closely
related compound may be an inhibitory transmitter for mitral cells or may
cause presynaptic inhibition of mitral cells (Salmoirgahi *et al.*, 1964). The

alternative possibility, that noradrenaline excites adjacent neurones which then inhibit transmission at terminals on mitral cells, was considered to be unlikely, as noradrenaline excitation was never observed in unanaesthetized rabbits. Histochemical studies, however, have shown that the catechol-amine-containing nerve terminals are around cells in the adjacent inner granular layer and not the mitral cells (Dahlström, Fuxe, Olson and Un-gerstedt, 1965) and these authors have suggested that the inhibition of mitral cells by iontophoretically applied noradrenaline is due to an effect on cells in the inner granular layer.

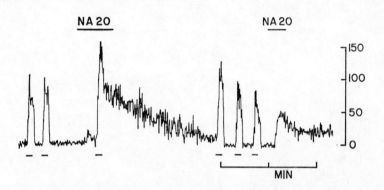

FIG. 8.9. Noradrenaline (NA, 20 nA) excitation of a cortical neurone. Hori-zontal bars below the record denote applications of L-glutamate (30 nA). The initial response to noradrenaline commenced before the subsequent applica-tion of L-glutamate and potentiated the amino-acid excitation. The second response to noradrenaline is less pronounced, indicating a certain degree of desensitization. Subsequent applications of noradrenaline were without an effect (Phillis, Tebēcis and York, unpublished observations).

5. Dihydroxyphenylalanine—the Dopamine Precursor

Brief mention will be made of the effects of the catecholamine precursor, L-3,4 dihydroxyphenylalanine (DOPA). The actions of DOPA on the activity of the central nervous system in different animals have been studied by several investigators (see reviews by Sourkes, 1964; Carlsson, 1964; Vogt, 1965; Hornykiewicz, 1966). Most authors agree that doses of DOPA ranging from 100 mg to 1 g/kg produce marked stimulation of locomotor activity, accompanied by behavioural and electroencephalo-graphic arousal changes in the treated animal. Animals show increased irritability and aggressiveness, fight with one another and prefer isolated positions. With high doses (500 mg/kg or more) of DOPA, autonomic signs such as piloerection, salivation, hyperpnea, pupillary dilatation, urination, defecation and ejaculation may be observed, "Catatonic" postures and "fear" reactions have also been described. The varied phenomena following administration of DOPA to animals suggest that it has an action at multiple sites in the body and it is likely that at least some of these effects are due to the actions of amines synthesized from it at various points in the central nervous system. It has been assumed that DOPA is pharmacologically inert, but this concept may have to be reassessed in the light of the demonstration that iontophoretically applied DOPA has an excitant action on cortical neurones (Krnjević and Phillis, 1963c). Such an action may explain the previously observed effects of DOPA on electrocorticograms (Dagirmanjian et al., 1963).

6. Adrenergic Antagonists

Adrenergic blocking drugs have been developed which are selective in their actions on the two types of peripheral receptor, some acting only on α-receptors (e.g. dibenzyline, dibenamine and phentolamine) and others on β-receptors (e.g. alderlin, dichloroisoproterenol). So specific are these blocking agents that it has become customary to identify the type of receptor on the basis of the effects of blocking drugs on the responses to sympathomimetic amines (Innes and Nickerson, 1965; Nickerson, 1965). However, when tested on thalamic neurones both α- and β-blockers exhibited sympathomimetic activity, duplicating the effects of noradrenaline or adrenaline on particular neurones. On thalamic neurones, D-INPEA (D-1-(4-nitrophenyl)-2-isopropylaminoethanol hydrochloride), a β-blocker, was the only compound which appeared to antagonize the excitant effects of noradrenaline. Antagonism of noradrenaline excitation in the lateral vestibular nucleus by dichloroisoproterenol (a β-blocker, Yamamoto, 1967), in the medulla by chlorpromazine (an α-blocker, Bradley et al., 1966) and in the cerebral cortex by dibenamine (an α-blocker, Roberts and Straughan, 1968) has also been described. Noradrenaline depression of neurones in the geniculate nuclei, thalamus and cerebral cortex is antagonized by strychnine (Tebēcis, 1967; Phillis and Tebēcis, 1967b; Phillis and York, 1967). Intravenously administered picrotoxin blocks the inhibitory effects of noradrenaline and caudate nucleus or reticular formation

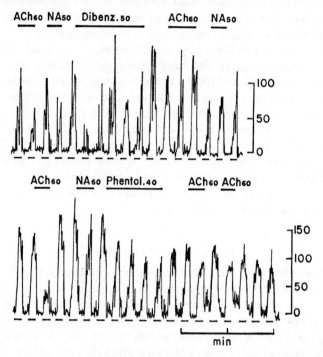

FIG. 8.10. The α-adrenergic antagonists, dibenzyline (50 nA) and phentolamine (40 nA), both antagonized the depressant effects of acetylcholine (ACH,
60 nA) on the L-glutamate evoked firing of these two cerebral cortical
neurones. Noradrenaline (NA, 50 nA) depression of the responses of the
neurone in the upper trace were only partially antagonized by dibenzyline
(Phillis, Tebēcis and York, unpublished observations).

stimulation on thalamic neurones (Phillis and Tebēcis, 1967b; Collins and
Simonton, 1967).

The depressant effects of noradrenaline and dopamine on some neurones
in the cerebral cortex can be antagonized by the α-blockers, dibenamine,
phentolamine and dibenzyline (Fig. 8.10), but a comparable simultaneous
reduction in the depressant action of acetylcholine was frequently observed
(Phillis, Tebēcis and York, unpublished observations). It is therefore
unlikely that the effect of these compounds was selective for catecholamine
depression. The depressant effects of noradrenaline on cerebral cortical

neurones were antagonized by the antihistamine compounds, tripelenammine, mepyramine and chlorcyclizine (Phillis, Tebēcis and York, 1968a), which also depressed the inhibitory actions of acetylcholine as well as of histamine on cortical neurones. It is obvious from studies in this laboratory that careful testing is essential before any antagonist can be considered to act selectively against its designated agonist.

B. 5-HYDROXYTRYPTAMINE AND CENTRAL SYNAPTIC TRANSMISSION

After the isolation and identification of serotonin by Rapport, Green and Page (1948), it became evident that it was identical with the "enteramine" which Erspamer and Asero (1952) had found to be widely distributed in the animal kingdom. The finding that the hallucinogenic indole, lysergic acid diethylamide could specifically inhibit the action of 5-hydroxytryptamine in mammalian smooth muscle, led Gaddum and Hameed (1954) and Woolley and Shaw (1954) to postulate that lysergic acid diethylamide owes its central actions to interaction with 5-hydroxytryptamine. These speculations have stimulated many investigations on the central actions of 5-hydroxytryptamine.

5-Hydroxytryptamine is found in the highest concentrations in the hypothalamus and midbrain (Udenfriend, Bogdanski and Weissbach, 1957). Histochemical investigations have revealed that ascending 5-hydroxytryptamine-containing nerve fibres to the diencephalon and telencephalon emanate mainly from nerve cells in the nucleus raphé dorsalis, nucleus raphé medianus and reticular formation of the mesencephalon (Andén et al., 1966).

1. Spinal Cord

In the spinal cord, 5-hydroxytryptamine is found in the grey matter, with much lower concentrations in white matter (Carlsson et al., 1963; Andén, 1965; Anderson and Holgerson, 1966). Histochemical and degeneration studies indicate that the amine is localized in descending nerve fibres emanating from the brain stem reticular formation (Carlsson et al., 1963; Carlsson et al., 1964; Andén et al., 1964; Dahlström and Fuxe, 1965). Stimulation of descending tracts in mouse and frog spinal cords has been shown to induce a release of 5-hydroxytryptamine (Andén, Carlsson, Hillarp and Magnusson, 1964).

5-Hydroxytryptamine does not readily enter the central nervous system (Udenfriend, Weissbach and Bogdanski, 1957; Costa and Aprison, 1958; Bulat and Supek, 1957) and many investigators have therefore studied the effects of administration of its precursor, 5-hydroxytryptophan, or of related compounds, such as tryptamine, which are able to penetrate the blood–brain barrier. There are a number of reports in the literature of the effects of intravascularly administered 5-hydroxytryptamine on spinal reflexes (Slater, Davis, Leary and Boyd, 1955; Curtis, Eccles and Eccles, 1955; Little, Distefano and Leary, 1957; Weidmann and Cerletti, 1957, 1960; Kissel and Domino, 1959; Voorhoeve, 1960). In general, an initial potentiation followed by a secondary decrease in the magnitude of flexor reflexes and an early inhibition and later potentiation of monosynaptic extensor reflexes was observed.

5-Hydroxytryptophan depresses dorsal root potentials and reflexes, depresses transmission from flexor reflex afferents to motoneurones and ascending pathways and causes an increased excitability in flexor and extensor motoneurones, with an increase in monosynaptic reflexes and often a spontaneous discharge in the ventral root (Andén, Jukes and Lundberg, 1964; Lundberg, 1965; Anderson and Shibuya, 1966). The effects of tryptamine, α-methyltryptamine and related α- or N-alkyl-tryptamines and their 5-methoxy derivatives on spinal reflexes have been described by Vane *et al.* (1961) and Marley and Vane (1967). These compounds facilitated a monosynaptic extensor reflex (knee jerk) and increased the basal tension and peak twitch tensions of a polysynaptic reflex. On the other hand, however, Marczynski (1962) has observed a depression of the knee jerk and flexion reflexes following administration of several tryptamine derivatives.

Although Angelucci (1956) was unable to demonstrate an action of 5-hydroxytryptamine on flexor reflexes of the frog spinal cord, Carels (1962) concluded that it depressed the monosynaptic activation of motoneurones in this species. Since the invasion of an antidromically propagating spike into motoneurones was not affected, Carels concluded that 5-hydroxytryptamine was acting presynaptically and depressing the release of transmitter. Further studies have shown that 5-hydroxytryptamine has an excitant action on amphibian motoneurones, causing a ventral root discharge which is associated with a sustained motoneuronal depolarization (Fig. 8.11) (Tebēcis and Phillis, 1967). Under these conditions, the short latency reflex response from an isolated toad spinal cord is depressed and polysynaptic reflexes augmented. 5-Hydroxytryptamine application also resulted

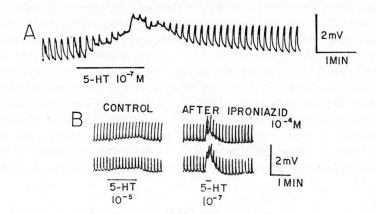

FIG. 8.11. A. Direct-coupling record of the responses of 9th ventral root of an isolated toad spinal cord evoked by dorsal root stimulation, showing changes in polarization level and evoked response size during an application of 5-hydroxytryptamine (5-HT, 10^{-7} M). B. Dorsal (upper) and ventral root (lower) d.c. records of 9th lumbar segment of an isolated toad spinal cord. Stimulation of adjacent dorsal root. The dorsal and ventral root responses were recorded simultaneously. After recording the control response to 5-HT, the preparation was treated with the monoamine oxidase inhibitor, iproniazid (10^{-4} M), for 30 min. The action of 5-HT was greatly potentiated, as it caused a more pronounced depolarization in both roots at 1/100 of the previous concentration. The d.c. records in this figure were plotted with an ink-recorder (negativity upwards) (Tebēcis and Phillis, 1967).

in a depolarization of dorsal root terminals (Fig. 8.11), with a consequent reduction in the magnitude of the dorsal root potential. The effects of 5-hydroxytryptamine were potentiated by the monoamine oxidase inhibitor, iproniazid. Various antagonists, such as lysergic acid diethylamide, had comparable effects to 5-hydroxytryptamine. When 5-hydroxytryptamine was applied to a preparation that was already responding to one of these compounds, its effect was reduced. However, it is doubtful whether such an interaction should be classified as an antagonism rather than an occlusion.

Iontophoretically applied 5-hydroxytryptamine excites or depresses many interneurones in the spinal cord of unanaesthetized or diethyl ether anaesthetized cats (Engberg and Ryall, 1966; Weight and Salmoiraghi, 1966). The failure of a previous investigation (Curtis et al., 1961a) to reveal these effects was probably a result of the use of barbiturate anaesthetized animals. Renshaw cells are depressed by 5-hydroxytryptamine (Engberg and Ryall, 1966). Many sympathetic preganglionic neurones in the lateral horn of the spinal cord are excited by 5-hydroxytryptamine (de Groat and Ryall, 1967). Fluorescent microscopy has revealed that many moto-neurones are surrounded by 5-hydroxytryptamine-containing nerve ter-minals (Dahlström and Fuxe, 1965) and it is therefore significant that this substance depresses orthodromic and antidromic excitation of moto-neurones. Excitatory and inhibitory postsynaptic potentials are also reduced and a hyperpolarization with a comparable time course to that illustrated for noradrenaline was frequently observed (Phillis *et al.*, 1968c).

2. Brain

The effects of 5-hydroxytryptamine on higher centres of the nervous system have been extensively investigated. Brodie and Shore (1957) suggested that this substance might be the transmitter for the "parasym-pathetic centre" of the brain, with noradrenaline occupying the correspond-ing role for the "sympathetic centre". Their hypothesis was based on several findings, some of which have since been modified. These included the characteristic pattern of distribution of noradrenaline and 5-hydroxytrypt-amine in the brain, and the psychogenic effects of lysergic acid diethyl-amide, a 5-hydroxytryptamine antagonist. Lysergic acid diethylamide also produced the marked symptoms of central sympathetic activation which would be expected if the parasympathetic transmitter was prevented from acting. The sedative effects of reserpine, which releases endogenous stores of 5-hydroxytryptamine, were compatible with this hypothesis. However, reserpine has since been shown to release endogenous stores of catechola-mines (Karki and Paasonen, 1959), histamine (Adam and Hye, 1964) and γ-aminobutyric acid (Balzer, Holtz and Palm, 1961) and results obtained from reserpinized cats, some of which had also been treated with mono-amine oxidase inhibitors have, therefore, become subject to interpreta-tional difficulties. Although lysergic acid diethylamide abolishes the lethargy induced by injection of 5-hydroxytryptamine into the cerebral ventricles of cats, other 5-hydroxytryptamine inhibitors do not antagonize this lethargy and substances such as morphine and amphetamine evoke an arousal. These results have shed doubt on the original findings which supported the Brodie and Shore hypothesis. It must also be pointed out that although lysergic acid diethylamide is both an hallucinogen and an antagonist of 5-hydroxytryptamine, some antagonists, such as 2-bromo-d-lysergic acid, are not hallucinogenic (Cerletti and Rothlin, 1955). Furthermore, lysergic acid diethylamide does not always appear to be an effective antagonist of 5-hydroxytryptamine (Phillis *et al.*, 1967a, Tebēcis and Phillis, 1967), nor is it specific, for it has been found to be a more effective antagonist of noradrenaline than of 5-hydroxytryptamine in the olfactory bulb (Salmoiraghi *et al.*, 1964).

Behavioural changes have been observed in rabbits, cats and dogs given 5-hydroxytryptophan (Udenfriend *et al.*, 1957; Costa, 1960). In dogs, depression follows small doses, whereas excitation characterizes the behaviour of animals injected with doses in excess of 20 mg/kg. Excitation was usually preceded by an initial phase of depression and was evident from symptoms such as postural incoordination, muscle tremors, salivation, lacrimation and piloerection. Administration of tryptamine and related compounds to unrestrained cats and mice causes a brief period of excitement followed by a prolonged phase of depression (Vane *et al.*, 1961). Microgram quantities of crystalline 5-hydroxytryptamine and related compounds have been observed to produce behavioural and electro-encephalographic arousal when administered directly into the mesencephalic reticular formation, the nucleus centralis medialis in the thalamus and the preoptic nucleus region. The effects are therefore similar to those evoked by acetylcholine (Yamaguchi, Marczynski and Ling, 1963; Yamaguchi *et al.*, 1964).

Injection of 5-hydroxytryptamine into the lateral ventricle of the cat causes ataxia, sleepiness and muscular weakness (Feldberg and Sherwood, 1954): the effects of intraventricularly administered amines on temperature control are discussed in the preceeding section on catecholamines (Feldberg and Fleischhauer, 1965).

The effects of intravascularly or topically administered 5-hydroxytryptamine or lysergic acid diethylamide have been ascertained on various structures of the brain including the lateral geniculate nucleus (Evarts, Landau, Freygang and Marshall, 1955; Evarts, 1958; Bishop, Burke and Hayhow, 1959, Bishop, Field, Hennessy and Smith, 1958), the hippocampus and related structures in the limbic system (Brucke, Gogolák and Stumpf, 1961; Eidelberg, Goldstein and Deza, 1967) and cerebral cortex (Purpura, 1957; Marrazzi, 1957; Ochs, Booker and Aprison, 1960; Koella, Smythies, Bull and Levy, 1960). As pointed out by Koella and his collaborators

(Koella *et al.*, 1960; Koella and Czicman, 1966), the effects of intravascularly administered 5-hydroxytryptamine may be mediated through a variety of systems which influence the monitored response. It is therefore surprising that, in spite of this fact and the relative impermeability of the blood-brain barrier to 5-hydroxytryptamine, many of the conclusions from these experiments have been confirmed in later experiments using the iontophoretic technique. Studies on the ability of drugs to pass through the blood–brain barrier involve the measurement of its tissue concentrations before and after administration of the substance into the blood stream. Although it is clear that the monoamines do not penetrate the barrier in amounts which lead to an alteration in tissue levels, it appears that the concentrations attained in the extracellular spaces may be sufficient to alter cell excitability.

(a) *Lateral geniculate nucleus*. Among the higher structures of the central nervous system with which 5-hydroxytryptamine has been implicated is the lateral geniculate nucleus. The postsynaptic responses of neurones in this nucleus produced by optic nerve impulses are reduced by an intracarotid injection of either lysergic acid diethylamide or bufotenine (Evarts *et al.*, 1955; Evarts, 1958). The action of lysergic acid diethylamide on these cells was confirmed by Bishop, Field, Hennessy and Smith (1958) using both intracarotid and intravenous injection. These investigators suggested that the failure of this compound to affect the spike potentials of presynaptic fibres and the increase it produced in synaptic delay as well as the finding that repetitive stimulation of the optic nerve overcomes the block produced by lysergic acid diethylamide (Bishop *et al.*, 1959) indicates that the compound interferes with the attachment of the natural excitatory transmitter to its appropriate subsynaptic receptors. As lysergic acid diethylamide was known to be an antagonist for 5-hydroxytryptamine, it appeared that the excitatory transmitter might be related to 5-hydroxytryptamine. However, 5-hydroxytryptamine itself had little effect on the potentials evoked in the lateral geniculate nucleus by optic nerve stimulation (Evarts, 1958; Bishop, Burke, Davis and Hayhow, 1960). The failure of previous investigations to reveal the presence of 5-hydroxytryptamine in the lateral geniculate nucleus (Bogdanski *et al.*, 1957) also made it unlikely that this substance was involved.

However, recent investigations have demonstrated that 5-hydroxytryptamine is present in the lateral geniculate nucleus (Deffenu, Bertaccini and Pepeu, 1967) and is located in nerve terminals (Fuxe, 1965), raising the possibility that 5-hydroxytryptamine could be a transmitter in this area.

Iontophoretically applied 5-hydroxytryptamine blocked the orthodromic activation of lateral geniculate neurones in barbiturate anaesthetized cats, but failed to influence antidromic or L-glutamate evoked activation (Curtis and Davis, 1962). Curtis and Davis concluded that, as antidromic responses were unaffected, 5-hydroxytryptamine was not reacting with inhibitory synapses, and was most probably interfering with the attachment of the excitatory transmitter to its subsynaptic receptor, or alternatively preventing the release of excitatory transmitter from optic nerve terminals. However, when tested on lateral geniculate neurones in unanaesthetized or gas-anaesthetized cats, iontophoretically applied 5-hydroxytryptamine depresses several types of excitation, including spontaneous firing, orthodromic, antidromic, L-glutamate and acetylcholine induced firing (Fig. 8.12) (Phillis *et al.*, 1967a; Satinsky, 1967). An excitant action on some cells in the lateral geniculate nucleus has also been described (Satinsky, 1967).

(b) *Thalamus.* 5-Hydroxytryptamine has both inhibitory and excitant actions on thalamic neurones (Phillis and Tebēcis, 1967b). Seventy-three to eighty-six percent of the neurones tested at various depths of the thalamus were inhibited by this substance, the responses to synaptic, antidromic and chemical stimulation being depressed or abolished (Fig. 8.13). An excitant action was observed on 27% of the neurones in the deeper thalamic nuclei. Whereas the inhibitory actions of 5-hydroxytryptamine had a short latency and short duration, excitation frequently developed over several seconds and often continued for periods of 2–3 min (Fig. 8.13). Bufotenine had a more marked inhibitory action than 5-hydroxytryptamine on cells in both the lateral geniculate nucleus and thalamus.

(c) *Hippocampus.* Many investigators have been interested in the effects of 5-hydroxytryptamine, 5-hydroxytryptophan and lysergic acid diethylamide on hippocampal activity. Intravenously administered 5-hydroxytryptamine caused a flattening of both neocortical and hippocampal activity with disappearance of the theta rhythm (Costa and Rinaldi, 1958; Monnier and Tissot, 1958). However Revzin and Costa (1960) in studying the effect of intravenously administered 5-hydroxytryptamine on the hippocampal response to amygdaloid stimulation in the cat, found that the effects were abolished by vagotomy and concluded that 5-hydroxytryptamine was not acting within the central nervous system. Intracarotid injection of 5-hydroxytryptophan in rabbits caused a biphasic response in the neocortical electroencephalogram, synchronization being succeeded by desynchronization, which was associated with the development of irregular

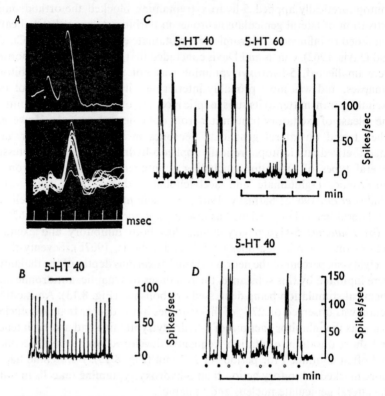

FIG. 8.12. Responses from the feline lateral geniculate nucleus. (A)-(D) are the responses of one neurone. A. Antidromic spikes evoked by single and repetitive (100/sec) stimulation of ipsilateral visual cortex. B. Bursts of firing evoked by light flashes in left eye at 10 sec intervals and recorded with electronic counter. 5-HT (40 nA) applied during period indicated. C. Depression of L-glutamate (40 nA) firing by 5-HT (40, 60 nA). D. Comparison of depression of acetylcholine (40 nA, open circles) and L-glutamate (40 nA, filled circles) firing by 5-HT (40 nA) (Phillis, Tebēcis and York, 1967a).

activity and then the appearance of a theta rhythm in the hippocampus (Costa, Pscheidt, Van Meester and Himwich, 1960). The firing rate of single neurones in the hippocampus and amygdala decreased sharply following intravenous administration of 5-hydroxytryptophan (Eidelberg et al., 1967). Lysergic acid diethylamide caused an abolition of slow wave activity and disappearance of the theta rhythm in the hippocampus (Sailer and Stumpf, 1957; Long, 1962; Stumpf, 1965). Stumpf (1965) concludes his review on hippocampal pharmacology by postulating that the results with lysergic acid diethylamide may be due to a direct interference with transmission between septo-hippocampal fibres and pyramidal neurones, thereby raising the possibility of 5-hydroxytryptaminergic transmission in the hippocampus.

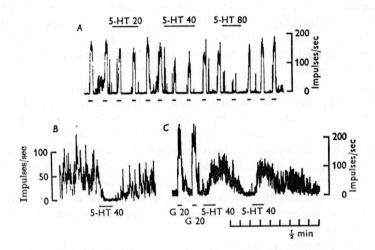

FIG. 8.13. Inhibitory and excitatory effects of 5-HT on neurones in the feline thalamus. A (5430 μ): L-glutamate (40 nA firing was slightly depressed by 5-HT (20 nA), markedly depressed by 5-HT (40 nA and almost completely blocked by 5-HT (80 nA). Recovery was typically rapid. B (4960 μ): this unit was firing spontaneously. 5-HT (40 nA) completely depressed this firing and recovery was rapid after termination of the drug. C (3970 μ): L-glutamate (20 nA) induced rapid firing. 5-HT (40 nA), on two subsequent applications induced marked firing with a longer latency of onset and offset (Phillis and Tebēcis, 1967b).

The hippocampal cortex contains relatively high concentrations of this amine (Paasonen, MacLean and Giarman, 1957) and its probable localization within nerve terminals (Fuxe, 1965) supports the concept that it might be a neurotransmitter in this area. Iontophoretic studies have shown that 5-hydroxytryptamine depresses many hippocampal neurones (50%) and excites a few (15%) (Stefanis, 1964; Herz and Nacimiento, 1965; Biscoe and Straughan, 1966). Further information concerning the significance of these actions will doubtless be the object of future investigations on hippocampal pharmacology.

(d) *Cerebral cortex*. The accumulated evidence strongly suggests that 5-hydroxytryptamine is a synaptic transmitter in the cerebral cortex, where it is present in fine nerve terminals. Interruption of the medial forebrain bundle in the lateral hypothalamus of rats and cats has been shown to produce a significant decrease in the 5-hydroxytryptamine content of the telencephalon (Andén *et al.*, 1965; Moore *et al.*, 1965). Electrical stimulation of the midbrain raphé, an area in which neuronal perikarya containing 5-hydroxytryptamine are aggregated, produces a decrease in the forebrain content of this amine in rats and an increase in its principal metabolite, 5-hydroxyindole acetic acid. Interruption of the medial forebrain bundle prevents the release of the 5-hydroxytryptamine remaining in the telencephalon (Aghajanian, Rosecrans and Sheard, 1967).

A desynchronization of electrocortical activity in cat *encéphale isolé* and *cerveau isolé* preparations after injection of 5-hydroxytryptamine into the cerebral circulation has been described (Mantegazzini, 1957; Glasser and Mantegazzini, 1960). 5-hydroxytryptophan, however, had a synchronizing effect in electrocortical activity in the *cerveau isolé* preparation (Glasser and Mantegazzini, 1960) which led these authors to conclude that the actions of exogenously administered and endogenously released 5-hydroxytryptamine differ.

Small quantities (1–10 μg/kg) of 5-hydroxytryptamine, bufotenine and lysergic acid diethylamide, administered intra-arterially, depress transcallosally evoked responses in the cerebral cortex (Marrazzi, 1957; Hart, Rodriguez and Marrazzi, 1961) and topically applied 5-hydroxytryptamine (0·5–1% solution) inhibits direct cortical responses (Ochs *et al.*, 1960). It was not unexpected therefore to find that iontophoretically applied 5-hydroxytryptamine depresses the excitability of many cortical neurones, including Betz cells (Krnjević and Phillis, 1963c; Phillis and York, 1967b; Roberts and Straughan, 1967). Synaptic, L-glutamate and acetylcholine-induced firing of cortical neurones was readily depressed by iontophoretically applied 5-hydroxytryptamine. Antidromic invasion of a spike into Betz cells was abolished only when the neurones belonged to the population of Betz cells with slower-conducting axons. An example of 5-hydroxytryptamine and noradrenaline induced depression of the synaptically evoked firing of a Betz cell is shown in Fig. 8.8. The responses were evoked by pyramidal tract stimulation and the initial spike in each response is the antidromically invading action potential. This was not abolished by either noradrenaline or 5-hydroxytryptamine. The inhibitory effects of 5-hydroxytryptamine on cortical neurones are duplicated by tryptamine and several of its derivatives.

Lysergic acid diethylamide and other derivatives of lysergic acid also depressed the excitability of cortical neurones but their actions, unlike those of the tryptamine derivatives had a slow onset and longer duration (Krnjević and Phillis, 1963). It has not been possible to demonstrate an effective specific antagonism between lysergic acid diethylamide and the

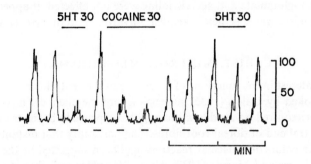

FIG. 8.14. Cocaine (30 nA) block of 5-hydroxytryptamine (5-HT, 30 nA) depression of L-glutamate (30 nA) firing of a cerebral cortical neurone (Phillis, Tebēcis and York, unpublished observations).

inhibitory action of 5-hydroxytryptamine in the cerebral cortex (Krnjević and Phillis, 1963c; Roberts and Straughan, 1967).

5-Hydroxytryptamine depression of cortical neurones was blocked by strychnine (Phillis and York, 1967b). Cocaine, another antagonist on peripheral tissues (Gyermek, 1961) also abolished the inhibitory effects of this amine on several cortical neurones (Fig. 8.14).

In unanaesthetized (*encéphale isolé*) animals, a high proportion of neurones (30%) in the cerebral cortex may be excited by 5-hydroxytryptamine (Roberts and Straughan, 1967), though in another investigation on unanaesthetized *cerveau isolé* preparations only depression was observed (Crawford and Curtis, 1966). However, as both excitation and depression of the same cortical cell with 5-hydroxytryptamine has been observed (Roberts and Straughan, 1967), it is possible that small fluctuations in the environmental conditions pertaining to the experiment may influence the type of response to this drug. In cats anaesthetized with nitrous oxide and methoxyflurane, 5-hydroxytryptamine depressed 89% of the 131 cortical neurones tested (Phillis and York, 1967b) and excitation was only observed on two occasions. The excitant actions of 5-hydroxytryptamine on cortical neurones could be prevented by prior applications of lysergic acid diethylamide, 2-bromo lysergic acid diethylamide and methysergide. As these compounds had depressant actions of their own, it was necessary to pass them with small currents for periods of several minutes to achieve a block of 5-hydroxytryptamine (Roberts and Straughan, 1967). Since the excitant actions of L-glutamate and acetylcholine were not affected, it appears that the antagonism was specifically against 5-hydroxytryptamine excitation.

C. HISTAMINERGIC MECHANISMS

Early interest in the functions of histamine in the central nervous system was provoked by Dale's (1935) suggestion that the chemical mediator of cutaneous axon-reflex vasodilatation might also prove to be the transmitter at the central end of dorsal root fibres. The possibility that histamine was involved in cutaneous vascular reactions had been suggested by the experiments of Lewis and Marvin (1927) whose "H-substance" shared many of the properties of histamine. Kwiatkowski (1943) pointed out that nerves which are known to give rise to vasodilatation in response to antidromic stimulation have a high histamine content and it was therefore proposed that histamine was the mediator of the axon-reflex vasodilatation.

The presence of histamine in various areas of the central nervous system, originally described by Kwiatkowski (1943), has been confirmed by subsequent investigators (Harris, Jacobsohn and Kahlson, 1952; Adam, 1961; McGeer, 1964; White, 1966; Adam and Hye, 1966). Although its distribution in mammalian brain is comparable in many respects to that of the biogenic monoamines, noradrenaline and 5-hydroxytryptamine, histamine has not been as favourably regarded as a potential neurotransmitter. This situation arose in part from the discovery that, in many parts of the body, histamine is primarily located in mast cells (Riley, 1959, Juhlin and Shelley, 1966).

However, the grey and white matter of the brain do not contain mast cells (Riley, 1959; Adam, 1961). Further evidence that brain histamine is not present in mast cells has come from experiments with the compound

48/80 (Adam and Hye, 1964). In doses that deplete the histamine content of mast cells in the skin, this compound reduces the concentration of histamine in the posterior lobe and stalk of the hypophysis but not in the anterior, lobe of the hypophysis or the brain.

Histamine synthesis from its amino acid precursor, histidine, occurs rapidly in the feline brain as does its degradation to methylhistamine by the enzyme histamine N-methyltransferase (White, 1959). It has recently been demonstrated that histamine is present in the nerve terminal and synaptic vesicle fractions of homogenates of hypothalamus, thalamus and cerebral cortex (Michaelson and Coffman, 1967; Kataoka and de Robertis, 1967). Brain histamine levels in the cat and rabbit are depleted by reserpine (as are the levels of the other biogenic monoamines) and high concentrations of chlorpromazine have the opposite effect (Green, 1964). Some of the behavioural changes induced by these compounds may therefore be a result of their actions on histamine metabolism in the brain.

There is evidence that histamine has potent effects on neuronal activity when administered into the carotid artery (Crossland and Mitchell, 1956), into the cerebral ventricles (Kohn and Millichap, 1958, Feldberg and Sherwood, 1954) or by direct injection into discrete areas of the brain (Heath and de Balbian Verster, 1961). Histamine also stimulates the rhinecephalon (Sawyer, 1955) and inhibits transcallosally evoked cortical potentials (Marrazzi, 1961). Intravascular histamine has been shown to produce an immediate arousal reaction (Goldstein, Pfeiffer and Munoz, 1963) which can be blocked by the histamine antagonist, promethazine.

1. *Spinal Cord*

Histamine has been reported to have excitatory actions on motoneurones in the frog spinal cord (Häusler and Sterz, 1952; Häusler, 1953) although this was not confirmed in a subsequent investigation (Angelucci, 1956). Kissel and Domino (1959) observed a depressant action of intravenously administered histamine on mammalian spinal reflexes. Iontophoretically applied histamine depresses the excitability of many interneurones and motoneurones in the spinal cord of cats anaesthetized with nitrous oxide and methoxyflurane or of decerebrate unanaesthetized animals. The depression of motoneurones is associated with an increase in membrane potential and decrease in amplitude of excitatory and inhibitory synaptic potentials (Phillis *et al.*, 1968c). The lack of effect of histamine on spinal neurones

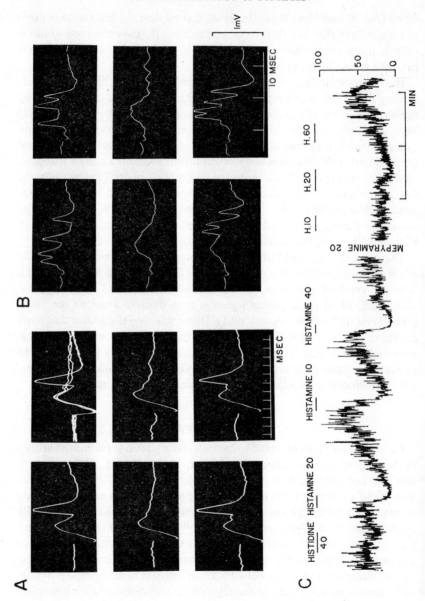

reported previously (Curtis *et al.*, 1961a) may have been due to the use of barbiturate anaesthesia.

2. *Cerebral Cortex*

Histamine depresses spontaneous, antidromic, orthodromic, L-glutamate and acetylcholine induced firing of feline cerebral cortical neurones (Fig. 8.15). Larger amounts of histamine frequently excite cortical neurones, potentiating L-glutamate firing and initiating a discharge of spikes in some neurones. Both depressant and excitant effects of histamine were observed on many neurones and the interaction of these conflicting actions frequently obscured the fact that histamine had a powerful effect on such cells (Phillis *et al.*, 1968a).

Iontophoretically applied antihistamines antagonized both the excitant and depressant actions of histamine. The application of one of these compounds to a neurone that was initially depressed by histamine, frequently resulted in the uncovering of an excitant action (Fig. 8.15c). Tripelennamine, mepyramine and chlorcyclizine were extensively tested as histamine antagonists on cortical neurones, and the specificity of their antagonism ascertained. Unfortunately, amounts of these antagonists which were sufficient to affect histamine excitation or inhibition also antagonized the depressant effects of acetylcholine, noradrenaline and 5-hydroxytryptamine on cortical neurones (Phillis *et al.*, 1968a). Strychnine also blocked the inhibitory actions of histamine.

FIG. 8.15. Histamine depression of antidromic (A), synaptic (B) and spontaneous (C) firing of three cortical neurones. (A) Pairs of consecutive records of antidromic spikes evoked by PT stimulation. At threshold stimulus intensity the spike appeared in an all-or-none manner (top records). 10 sec after the application of histamine (80 nA) antidromic invasion had failed (middle records). Recovery occurred within 12 sec (lower records). (B) A similar series of synaptic responses evoked by lateral hypothalamic stimulation. Histamine (30 nA) abolished the response. Recovery followed within 15 sec of the termination of histamine application. (C) Depression of spontaneous firing by histamine (10 nA, 20 nA and 40 nA). (+) (−) histidine (40 nA) had a weakly depressant action. After the application of mepyramine (20 nA), histamine depression was reduced and larger amounts (60 nA) now had an excitant action. Record (C) and the subsequent records in this paper were obtained with an electronic counter and ink recorder. The vertical scale on the right of each of these records indicates actual discharge rates. Drug applications are indicated by horizontal solid lines above and below the traces (Phillis, Tebēcis and York, 1968a).

Histidine, the precursor of histamine, had a depressant action on cortical neurones. 1-Methylhistamine, the major product of histamine metabolism in brain, was generally comparable to histamine in its actions, causing either excitation, inhibition or a combination of these effects. Applications with low currents frequently excited neurones that were inhibited by histamine. Imidazoleacetic acid, another catabolite of histamine which is probably not synthesized in the feline brain to a significant extent (Burkard, Gey and Pletscher, 1963; White, 1959, 1960) was an extremely potent depressant of cortical neurones.

In summary, it may be said that histamine has many of the attributes required of a transmitter in the central nervous system and interest in the neuropharmacological properties of this substance is likely to increase in the future.

D. THE INHIBITORY AMINO ACIDS

Several monocarboxylic ω-amino acids and closely related compounds with potent depressant effects on neuronal excitability are present in the central nervous system. These include γ-aminobutyric acid (GABA), β-alanine, glycine, taurine and guanidino-acetic acid (Tallan, Moore and Stein, 1954; Pisano and Udenfriend, 1958; Tallan, 1962). Of these, GABA occurs in the largest amounts and is moreover restricted in its distribution to the central nervous system (Roberts and Eidelberg, 1960). Studies on the subcellular distribution of γ-aminobutyric acid and glutamic acid have shown that they are associated with a synaptic vesicle fraction of mouse brain and that the vesicles accumulate these amino acids by a sodium dependent process (Kuriyama, Roberts and Kakefuda, 1968). The metabolism of γ-aminobutyric acid has recently been reviewed in some detail by Roberts and Kuriyama (1968).

Much of the current interest in the pharmacology of amino acids has stemmed from accounts of the effects of a brain extract, known as Factor I (Florey, 1954) on various invertebrate and vertebrate nervous preparations (McLennan, 1963). It now seems probable that most of the Factor I activity is attributable to the amino acid content of the brain extracts (Elliott, 1958; Levin, Lovell and Elliott, 1961).

Various methods have been used to administer amino acids to different portions of the central nervous system and the results obtained have been remarkably consistent. The pharmacological actions of GABA and related amino acids on neurones of the central nervous system have been comprehensively reviewed by Curtis and Watkins (1965). A comparison of the relative depressant activities of some of these compounds is shown in Table 11. The present account attempts to cover only a few of the many investigations into the actions of these compounds.

1. *Spinal Cord*

Effects on spinal reflexes have been observed with intravenously (Kuno, 1961; Muneoka, 1961; Basil, Blair and Holmes, 1964) or topically administered GABA (Honour and McLennan, 1960; Bhargava and Srivastava, 1964; Basil *et al.*, 1964). The effects varied with dose and route of administration and included both depression and potentiation of various spinal reflexes. Topically applied GABA depresses dorsal and ventral root reflexes of the isolated toad spinal cord (Curtis, Phillis and Watkins, 1961b). Associated with this is a reduction in the amplitude and duration of the underlying dorsal and ventral root potentials, a depolarization of dorsal root terminals, and on several occasions a hyperpolarization of motoneurones (Tebēcis and Phillis, 1967). Comparisons of the depressant potencies of a series of related amino acids on the toad spinal cord reveal that GABA, β-alanine, taurine and β-guanidinoproprionic acid are of comparable potency and are exceeded in depressant activity only by 3-aminopropanesulphonic acid (Curtis *et al.*, 1961b).

An extensive analysis has been made of the action of amino acids, ejected iontophoretically, upon spinal neurones (Curtis, Phillis and Watkins, 1959; Curtis and Watkins, 1960a, 1963; Curtis, Hösli, Johnston and Johnston, 1967, 1968; Curtis, Hösli and Johnston, 1967; Werman, Davidoff and Aprison, 1967, 1968). All types of spinal neurone investigated, including interneurones, motoneurones and Renshaw cells, appeared to be equally sensitive to any one amino acid. GABA was initially thought to have a non-specific depressant rather than inhibitory action on nerve cells, because although it reduced the amplitude of inhibitory and excitatory postsynaptic potentials of motoneurones and increased membrane conductance it did not produce any membrane hyperpolarization. Moreover, its action was not antagonized by strychnine, which effectively prevents the inhibitory transmitter action on motoneurones (Curtis *et al.*, 1959; Curtis and Watkins, 1965). Although recent experiments have shown that GABA depression of motoneurones is accompanied by a hyperpolarization,

TABLE 11.

STRUCTURE-ACTIVITY RELATIONSHIPS OF SOME EXCITANT AND DEPRESSANT AMINO ACIDS ON CNS NEURONES.

Inhibitory monocarboxylic and related amino acids	Structure	Relative potency	Corresponding excitatory amino acids	Structure	Potency
Glycine	$H_2N.CH_2.COOH$	—	DL-Aminomalonic acid	$HOOC.CH(NH_2).COOH$	+++
β-Alanine	$H_2N.(CH_2)_2.COOH$	—	L-Aspartic acid	$HOOC.CH_2.CH(NH_2).COOH$	++++
γ-Aminobutyric acid	$H_2N.(CH_2)_3.COOH$	—	L-Glutamic acid	$HOOC.(CH_2)_2.CH(NH_2).COOH$	++++
δ-Amino-n-valeric acid	$H_2N.(CH_2)_4.COOH$	—	DL-Aminoadipic acid	$HOOC.(CH_2)_3.CH(NH_2).COOH$	+++
ε-Amino caproic acid	$H_2N.(CH_2)_5.COOH$	—	DL-Aminopimelic acid	$HOOC.(CH_2)_4.CH(NH_2).COOH$	+++
Taurine	$H_2N.(CH_2)_2.SO_3H$	—	L-Cysteic acid	$HO_3S.CH_2.CH(NH_2).COOH$	+++
3-Aminopropane sulphonic acid	$H_2N.(CH_2)_3.SO_3H$	—	DL-Homocysteic acid	$HO_3S.(CH_2)_2.CH(NH_2).COOH$	+++
Glycocyamine	$H_2N.C(:NH).NH.CH_2.COOH$	—			
β-Guanidinopropionic acid	$H_2N.C(:NH).NH.(CH_2)_2.COOH$	—			
γ-Guanidinobutyric acid	$H_2N.C(:NH).NH.(CH_2)_3.COOH$	0			

this is not prevented by strychnine (Curtis *et al.*, 1967). It is unlikely therefore that GABA is the transmitter responsible for the hyperpolarizing, strychnine-antagonized, inhibitory postsynaptic potentials of motoneurones.

Recent evidence indicates that the related amino acid, glycine, may be the transmitter responsible for the generation of strychnine-antagonized hyperpolarizing inhibitions in the spinal cord. Studies on the distribution of glycine in the spinal cord before and after selective destruction of interneurones suggest that glycine (and aspartic acid) are located in interneurones whereas GABA and glutamic acid are not (Davidoff *et al.*, 1967b; Davidoff *et al.*, 1967a). Interneurones are interpolated in inhibitory and polysynaptic excitatory pathways from dorsal root fibres to spinal motoneurones and the association of glycine with these cells suggests that it might be an inhibitory transmitter. Glycine increased the membrane conductance of all the motoneurones tested (Fig. 8.16) and decreased the amplitude of excitatory and inhibitory postsynaptic potentials (Werman, Davidoff and Aprison, 1967, 1968). The amplitude of inhibitory postsynaptic potentials declined to minimal values as the glycine hyperpolarizations reached a maximum (Fig. 8.17), indicating that the equilibrium potentials for the inhibitory transmitter and glycine were almost identical. Injection of bromide and iodide ions into motoneurones, resulting in an inversion of inhibitory postsynaptic potentials (Ito, Kostyuk and Oshima, 1962) also caused glycine to depolarize. Depolarizing inhibitory potentials disappeared at the maximum glycine depolarization, confirming that the equilibrium potentials for the two processes are similar. Glycine hyperpolarization of motoneurones is antagonized by strychnine and other strychnine-like substances such as thebaine and bruceine (Curtis *et al.*, 1967).

This evidence suggests that glycine initiates similar permeability changes in the membrane to those induced by the inhibitory transmitter. Is glycine therefore identical with the inhibitory transmitter? The effectiveness of strychnine as an antagonist of depression by monoamines, acetylcholine and histamine on cerebral neurones (Phillis and York, 1967b) suggests that it may not be a selective antagonist of inhibitory transmission to motoneurones. The mechanisms of action of many of the substances which depress neuronal excitability may be similar and strychnine may antagonize their effects in an identical manner. If strychnine merely opposes the increase in membrane conductance resulting from receptor activation, it is not necessary that transmitter and applied drug act on the same receptor.

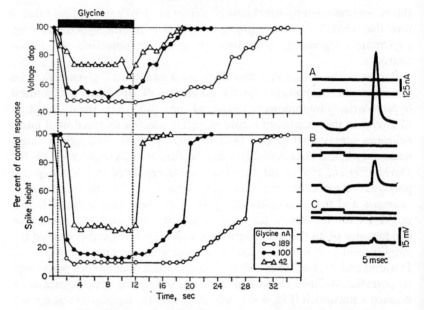

FIG. 8.16. Inhibitory action of glycine on spinal neurones in the cat. Simultaneous extracellular drug application and intracellular recording by using a fixed assembly of two micropipettes. Effect of three different amounts of glycine on membrane resistance and antidromic spike height in an L_7 motoneuron. Measurements were made at 1-sec intervals; inward current pulses of constant amplitude ($3 \cdot 5$ nA) were administered before each spike. Horizontal traces indicate glycine current. Current calibration shown is for glycine only. A. Control. B. During administration of glycine by 42 nA of iontophoretic current. Note failure of invasion of the SD membrane. C. During administration of glycine using 189 nA of current. The IS spike was greatly attenuated and the resistance decreased markedly. The upper graph shows the time course of resistance changes during and after 42, 100 and 189 nA of glycine current. The lower graph shows, on the same time base, the related changes in antidromic spike amplitude (Werman, Davidoff and Aprison, 1968).

Antagonism by strychnine may thus be reduced to the status of a necessary rather than a sufficient requirement for identification of an inhibitory transmitter. A final answer to the question posed above may therefore have to await the discovery of a truly selective blocking agent, a situation that has become almost commonplace for decisions of this nature. In the meanwhile, the claims of glycine appear to be stronger than those of the other substances.

2. Brain

GABA has been shown to act in a comparable manner to the physiological inhibitory transmitter on neurones in two regions of the brain, namely the lateral vestibular nucleus (Obata, Ito, Ochi and Sato, 1967) and cerebral cortex (Krnjević and Phillis, 1963d; Krnjević and Schwartz, 1967b).

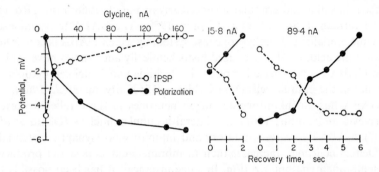

FIG. 8.17. Inhibitory action of glycine on spinal cord neurones of the cat. Simultaneous intracellular recording and extracellular drug applications. The effects of glycine on IPSP amplitude and membrane polarization. IPSP elicited in L_7 motoneuron by stimulation of L_6 dorsal root. The IPSP is seen to approach zero as the membrane potential approaches a plateau. Recovery from the effects of glycine at two different amounts of iontophoretic current are shown in the graphs on the right. There was a close parallelism in time in the increase in IPSP amplitude and the decrease in membrane polarization (Werman, Davidoff and Aprison, 1968).

(a) *Cerebellum and lateral vestibular nucleus.* Extensive correlative neuro-anatomical and neurophysiological analyses have been made of the cerebellum. These are described in a recent monograph (Eccles, Ito and Szentágothai, 1967). The overall function of the cerebellum, as indicated by these studies, appears to be entirely inhibitory, the Purkinje cells of the cerebellar cortex inhibiting Deiters neurones in the lateral vestibular nucleus and neurones in the intracerebellar nuclei monosynaptically. Basket, Stellate and Golgi cells are believed to play inhibitory roles within the cerebellum. Basket cells make numerous powerful inhibitory synapses on Purkinje cell somata; superficial stellate cells form inhibitory synapses on the dendrites of Purkinje cells and Golgi cells are thought to make inhibitory synapses on the dendrites of granule cells. The granule cells have an excitatory function, relaying afferent volleys to the Purkinje cell dendrites.

Within the cerebellar cortex GABA is present in the greatest amounts in the layer containing Purkinje cells, with progressively lower levels occurring in the molecular layer, granular layer and white matter (Hirsch and Robins, 1962; Kuriyama, Haber, Sisken and Roberts, 1966). Glutamic acid decarboxylase, the enzyme which catalyzes the formation of GABA also occurs in the greatest concentrations in the Purkinje cell layer, with lower levels in the molecular and granular layers (Kuriyama et al., 1966; Lowe, Robins and Eyerman, 1958; Albers and Brady, 1959). The GABA transaminase-succinic semialdehyde dehydrogenase system by which GABA is converted to succinic acid, can be visualized histochemically and studies have shown that GABA transaminase is present in Purkinje and Golgi cell cytoplasm but not in the granule cells (Van Gelder, 1965; Kuriyama et al., 1966).

GABA has an inhibitory action on neurones in the cerebellar cortex (Krnjević and Phillis, 1961) and lateral vestibular nucleus (Obata et al., 1967). GABA depresses excitatory and inhibitory postsynaptic potentials of Deiters neurones, increases their membrane conductance and produces a membrane hyperpolarization. In some instances, it has been possible to potentiate the monosynaptic inhibitory postsynaptic potentials evoked in Deiters neurones by cerebellar cortical stimulation with hydroxylamine, an inhibitor of GABA-transaminase. Purkinje cell and Deiters neurone inhibitions are strychnine-resistant (Andersen et al., 1963; Crawford et al., 1963; Obata et al., 1967) which might be anticipated if GABA is the inhibitory transmitter for these cells.

(b) *Cerebral cortex.* Since the discovery that topically applied solutions of GABA exert an inhibitory action on cortical activity (Hayashi and Nagai, 1956), many experiments have been performed utilizing this technique in an attempt to elucidate the mechanism of action of GABA. However, although the observations have been reproducible in several laboratories, interpretations of the data have differed. There is general agreement that topical application of GABA to the exposed surface of the cerebral cortex causes a reduction or even an inversion of the negative component of a variety of evoked responses recorded in or just below the surface (Iwama and Jasper, 1957; Purpura, Girado and Grundfest, 1957; Rech and Domino 1960; Mahnke and Ward, 1960). Different interpretations have been placed on these observations, which contrast with the finding that cerebellar potentials are merely reduced in amplitude and not inverted (Purpura et al.,

1957). Amongst other interpretations, it has been proposed that GABA is a specific inactivator of excitatory synapses of superficial dendrites (Purpura *et al.*, 1957). Iontophoretic studies on cortical neurones have shown, however, that GABA has a similar type of action on cortical neurones as has been proposed for spinal motoneurones and Deiters neurones (Krnjević and Phillis, 1963d; Krnjević and Schwartz, 1967b; Obata *et al.*, 1967).

Although the blood–brain barrier is considered to be relatively impermeable to amino acids such as GABA (van Gelder and Elliot, 1958; Purpura, Girado, Smith and Gomez, 1958; Strasberg, Krnjević, Schwartz and Elliott, 1967), intra-carotid injections of GABA have been reported to produce a considerable, though transient, depression of the surface negative component of the transcallosally evoked cortical potentials (Marrazzi, Hart and Rodriguez, 1958). This suggests that GABA can, in fact, pass across the blood–brain barrier to some extent.

Application of GABA to single cortical neurones, whilst recording their membrane potential and resistance with an intracellular electrode has revealed that its actions in the cerebral cortex are comparable to those on Deiters neurones and motoneurones (Krnjević and Schwartz, 1967b). GABA hyperpolarized cortical neurones and increased their membrane conductance. The equilibrium potentials for GABA and the inhibitory transmitter appeared to be comparable. These effects of GABA were seen only when it was applied outside the neurones. Short duration cortical inhibitions are resistant to strychnine (Andersen *et al.*, 1963; Krnjević *et al.*, 1966) as was the effect of GABA. Krnjević and his collaborators (Krnjević, 1964; Krnjević *et al.*, 1966; Krnjević and Schwartz, 1967b) have suggested that GABA is the main inhibitory transmitter in the cerebral cortex.

This suggestion has been supported by the demonstration of a release of GABA from the cortical surface which varies with the level of cortical activity (Jasper, Khan and Elliott, 1965). Several possible sources of origin of amino acids released from the cerebral cortex must, however, be considered. As well as being derived from nerve cells, the amino acids may have had their origins from cerebrospinal fluid or non-neuronal elements. As the rate of release of amino acids from the cortex is influenced by changes in blood pressure, a vascular origin for these substances may also be possible (van Harreveld and Kooiman, 1965).

It has recently been shown that relatively large anions can contribute to the membrane current of cortical neurones during inhibition (Kelly,

Krnjević, Morris and Yim, 1968). As several of these anions have a greater hydrated diameter than sodium, the membrane is unlikely to be permeable to small cations. Cortical inhibitory postsynaptic potentials may thus differ from those of motoneurones not only in their duration and sensitivity to strychnine and likely chemical transmitters, but also in the underlying permeability changes.

E. THE EXCITATORY AMINO ACIDS

The dicarboxylic amino acid, L-glutamic acid, and related amino acids, such as aspartic, cysteic and homocysteic acid, have pronounced excitant actions on nerve cells in many regions of the brain and spinal cord (Table 11).

Iontophoretic application of these substances into the immediate vicinity of nerve cells causes them to discharge repetitively, just as does a Renshaw cell responding to acetylcholine. The responses have a short latency and rapid cessation upon termination of the application (Curtis, Phillis and Watkins, 1960). The rate of firing can be controlled by varying the strength of the iontophoretic current applying the amino acid; if the rate of release is excessive, the cell fires maximally and then its responses fail, probably because of an over-depolarization. This effect is also rapidly reversible and there is no evidence that the cell is in any way damaged or desensitized by such applications. No comparable effects are produced when these substances are injected intracellularly (Coombs, Eccles and Fatt; 1955; Araki, Ito and Oscarsson, 1961) and hence it appears that their actions are on the external surface of the cell.

The excitant actions of L-glutamate are duplicated by a variety of structurally related compounds (Table 11) and the requirements for excitant activity are an amino group and two acidic groups (Curtis and Watkins, 1960a, 1963; Curtis et al., 1961b). The acidic groups may be carboxyl, sulphonic or sulphinic and the optimal separation between the α-amino and ω-acidic groups is two or three carbon atoms.

L-glutamic and L-aspartic acids have been detected in the mammalian central nervous system (Waelsch, 1957; Hayashi, 1959; Singh and Malhotra 1962). L-glutamate is widely distributed in the neuronal cytoplasm (Ryall, 1964). Nerve endings contain a substantial amount, mainly in the terminal cytoplasm (Ryall, 1964) but an appreciable quantity is also associated with the synaptic vesicles (Kuriyama et al., 1968). L-glutamate, and possibly

L-aspartate, are released from the cerebral cortex during states of cortical activity (Jasper et al., 1965; Van Harreveld and Kooiman, 1965; Jasper and Koyama, 1968). Stimulation of the reticular formation or mesial thalamus produced a 2–3-fold increase in acetylcholine output from the cerebral cortex, but a far greater increase in the output of glutamic acid (Jasper and Koyama, 1968). The absolute quantities of glutamic acid were about 10–20 times greater than of acetylcholine. Thalamic stimulation failed to produce an increase in the cortical glutamate release of *cerveau isolé* preparations, although an increased release of acetylcholine was still observed, suggesting that the glutamate release was dependent on an activation of structures below the level of transection.

Dorsal root fibres and dorsal columns of the spinal cord contain substantial amounts of L-glutamate (Aprison, Graham, Livengood and Werman, 1965; Graham, Werman and Aprison, 1965). It is not known whether the relevant nerve endings release glutamate, but there is some evidence that glutamate is released from peripheral nerve trunks during activity (Wheeler, Boyarski and Brooks, 1966). The concentrations of these amino acids in the grey matter of the spinal cord are diminished by procedures, such as asphyxiation, which cause damage to the feline spinal cord and a correlation between the aspartate concentration and the number of spinal interneurones has been postulated (Davidoff et al., 1967).

These findings suggest that L-glutamate and L-aspartate may be transmitters in the central nervous system but Curtis (Curtis and Watkins, 1960b; Curtis, 1965) has argued against identification with the synaptic transmitter agent and suggested instead that they are non-specific excitants that act at receptor sites on the subsynaptic membrane other than the sites of action of the synaptic transmitters. The original objections were based on evidence for the probable absence of enzymic destruction as a factor terminating the action of these compounds since the D- and L-isomers of these amino acids were comparable in potency and duration of action when applied iontophoretically onto spinal neurones (Curtis and Watkins, 1960a). Other evidence suggests, however, that enzymic destruction may be a factor in the removal of L-glutamate. Thiosemicarbazide, a known inhibitor of vitamin B_6-dependent enzymes such as glutamic acid decarboxylase has been shown to enhance the excitant effects of L-glutamate on neurones in the rat brain. The enhancement was partially antagonized by concomitant microelectrophoresis of the enzymic co-factor pyridoxal-5'-phosphate (Steiner and Ruf, 1966).

Enzymic destruction of L-glutamate is also suggested by the finding that topically applied D-glutamic acid is more effective than the L-isomer in the initiation of cortical spreading depression (Van Harreveld, 1959) and as an excitant of toad spinal cord neurones (Curtis et al., 1961). Alternatively, the slower rate of uptake of the D-isomer by brain tissue may account for its greater potency when applied topically (Stern, Eggleston, Hems and Krebs, 1949; Takagaki, Hirano and Nagata, 1959; Tsukada, Nagata, Hirano and Matsutani, 1963). In any case enzymic destruction need not be a feature of all transmitter systems, as diffusion would also account for removal of the transmitter from the synaptic cleft (Ogston, 1955; Eccles and Jaeger, 1958).

Further evidence for the mode of action of the acidic amino acids has been adduced from experiments which involved intracellular recording from motoneurones with extracellular drug application. By means of a coaxially arranged double microelectrode it is possible to inject amino acid extracellularly from the outer barrel and employ the inner barrel to record intracellularly (Curtis et al., 1960; Curtis, 1965). This technique has been employed to study the magnitude of the depolarization induced by L-glutamate and to compare the reversal (equilibrium) potential for amino-acid-induced depolarization with that of the depolarization induced by excitatory synaptic action. Figure 8.18 illustrates the results of such an experiment and in all cases it has been possible to demonstrate an amino acid-induced hyperpolarization at a membrane potential at or near the reversal potential for the excitatory postsynaptic potential. The arrangement of excitatory postsynaptic receptors on the motoneurone soma and dendrites may, however, introduce errors into the estimation of reversal potentials by passing current through a microelectrode inserted into the cell soma (Smith, Wuerker and Frank, 1967; Rall, 1967; Rall et al., 1967). Curtis (1965) has argued that the amino acid action in experiments of this nature is likely to have been mediated through both soma and dendritic receptors and should thus be comparable with the locus of action of the synaptically released transmitter. As the results suggest that the reversal potential for amino acid depolarization is less positive than that for synaptic activation, he postulates that it is unlikely that the two types of depolarization are produced by an identical alteration in membrane permeability. It would follow therefore that the amino acid depolarization is not a consequence of the interaction between amino acid molecules and the specific transmitter receptors of excitatory synapses. However, the experi-

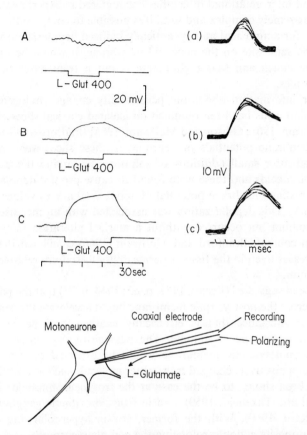

FIG. 8.18. Potentials recorded from a Flexor digitorum longus (FDL) motoneurone by means of one barrel of a double intracellular electrode in response
to the extracellular administration of L-glutamic acid (A-C) and the electrical
stimulation of the lowest threshold FDL afferent fibres (a-c). An electrophoretic
current of 400 nA was used to eject the amino acid from the outer barrel of
coaxial electrode; the time course of ejection is indicated by the lower record of
A, B and C and the amino acid induced potentials have been corrected for the
artifact introduced by the coupling resistance between inner and outer
barrels. The responses B, b were recorded at a resting potential of 58 mV;
those of A, a while depolarizing current of 30 nA was passed through the
other barrel of the intracellular electrode, those of C, c whilst a hyperpolarizing
current of 30 nA was flowing. Calibrations: 20 mV for A-C beneath A, 10 mV
for a-c beneath b; 30 sec for A-C beneath C, msec for a-c beneath c. In all
records depolarization is indicated as an upward deflection (Curtis, 1965).

mental and interpretational difficulties encountered in experiments of this type are extremely complex and until it is possible to compare the reversal potentials for amino acid and synaptically induced depolarizations generated at the same site on the neuronal membrane, it would be unwise to accept the conclusion that L-glutamate is not a transmitter for spinal motoneurones.

Further information about the permeability changes induced by the acidic amino acids has been obtained on isolated cortical slices (Hillman and McIlwain, 1961; Gibson and McIlwain, 1965; Bradford and McIlwain, 1966). Membrane potentials of neurones in these slices were measured before and after small additions of solutions containing the excitatory acidic amino acids and these were found to cause prompt depolarization from the resting membrane potential of about −60 mV to values of −30 to −45 mV. This depolarization was associated with an increased intracellular sodium but occurred without a marked alteration in the tissue potassium content. Bradford and McIlwain (1966) calculated that glutamate increases fivefold the tissue's permeability to sodium relative to that to potassium.

It has been suggested (Eccles, 1957, p. 63; 1964, p. 73) that the passage of current across the postsynaptic membrane might accelerate the removal of transmitter substance that is electrically charged, and hence indicate whether it is cationic or anionic. The passage of depolarizing current across the postsynaptic membrane would be expected to facilitate the removal of a positively charged transmitter molecule such as acetylcholine. This has been shown to be the case at the frog neuromuscular junction (Takeuchi and Takeuchi, 1959), and in frog sympathetic ganglion (Nishi and Koketsu, 1960). With the former, strong hyperpolarizing currents have the opposite action, prolonging the end plate current.

Eccles (1964) has cited the "less than predicted" increase in size and faster decay of excitatory postsynaptic potential during motoneuronal hyperpolarization as evidence that the transmitter may be an anion, such as glutamate. These findings are, however, more likely to be a result of the decrease in membrane resistance which occurs during motoneuronal hyperpolarization (Nelson and Frank, 1967). Evidence of a synaptic role for L-glutamate at invertebrate neuromuscular junctions has accumulated (Chapter 9) and this substance may well be the transmitter at such synapses. It is tempting to speculate that L-glutamate may ultimately prove to be an important synaptic transmitter in the vertebrate central nervous system.

F. PROSTAGLANDINS

The term, prostaglandin, was used by Euler (1935) to describe a pharmacologically active compound present in extracts of prostate glands and semen. Prostaglandins, of which 14 types have been identified, are widely distributed in mammalian tissues (Samuelsson, 1965; Horton, 1965). They were first isolated in a pure form by Bergström and Sjövall (1957, 1960a, b) and their structure determined by Bergström, Ryhage, Samuelsson and Sjövall (1962).

Prostaglandins appear to have a hormonal role in human reproductive physiology. They are secreted in large amounts by the seminal vesicular glands of the male (Bygdeman and Samuelsson, 1966) and are absorbed from the vagina of the female in amounts sufficient to modify the tone of reproductive smooth muscle (Horton, Main and Thompson, 1965; Eliasson and Posse, 1965; Sandberg, Ingelmann-Sundberg and Rydén, 1963). Thus prostaglandins are hormones produced by the male but acting on the reproductive tract of the female. Prostaglandin E_2 has been identified as the principal vasodepressor lipid of the rabbit renal medulla (Daniels *et al.*, 1967).

Prostaglandins have been isolated from the brains of oxen, dogs, cats, rabbits and chickens (Samuelsson, 1964; Holmes and Horton, 1967; Horton and Main, 1967; Pickles, 1967). Prostaglandins E and F are widely distributed in the brain and spinal cord (Holmes and Horton, 1968) and a release of prostaglandin-like substances from many regions of the brain and spinal cord has been described (Coceani and Wolfe, 1965; Feldberg and Meyer, 1966; Ramwell and Shaw, 1966; Ramwell, Shaw and Jessup, 1966). Subcellular fractionation has shown that prostaglandins are present in several fractions, including the nerve ending fraction (Kataoka, Ramwell and Jessup, 1967; Hopkin, Horton and Whittaker, 1967). The enzyme systems which metabolize prostaglandins have been described (Änggärd and Samuelsson, 1964b; Samuelsson, 1965) but so far these enzymes have not been looked for in the central nervous system.

Evidence that prostaglandins have actions on the central nervous system has now accumulated from work in several laboratories. Prostaglandins E_1, E_2 and E_3 produce a catatonic stupor in the cat and sedation in the chick when administered intravenously (Horton, 1964), whereas $F_{2\alpha}$ causes dorsiflexion of the neck and extension of the legs (Horton and Main, 1965). In spinal cats prostaglandin E_1, injected intravenously, increases muscle tension and potentiates crossed extensor reflexes. Topical application of E_1 to the spinal cord induces muscular contraction (Horton and Main, 1967b). In experiments on cats anaesthetized with chloralose, prostaglandin $F_{1\alpha}$ (50μg) injected close arterially to the spinal cord produced a potentiation of monosynaptic reflexes which lasted more than 4 hr. In contrast, prostaglandin E_1 (50μg) inhibited the monosynaptic reflex (Duda and McPherson, quoted by Horton, 1967).

Similar results have been observed when prostaglandins were tested on the isolated toad spinal cord (Phillis and Tebēcis, 1968). This is of some interest as prostaglandins are released from the amphibian spinal cord during hind limb stimulation (Ramwell et al., 1966). On this preparation, three prostaglandins, E_1, $F_{1\alpha}$ and $F_{2\alpha}$, produced distinct changes in reflexes and polarization levels in the dorsal and ventral roots. Simultaneous DC records from dorsal and ventral roots showed comparable changes, except that those in the dorsal root records were usually more pronounced. The prostaglandins caused a slowly developing, long-lasting depolarization of dorsal root terminals and motoneurones associated with a potentiation of polysynaptic reflexes. During its application, E_1 frequently caused a hyperpolarization in the dorsal and ventral roots which was associated with a decrease in the magnitude of dorsal and ventral root reflexes. Such hyperpolarizations rapidly reversed into depolarizations when the drug was removed from the preparation. E_1 has the most pronounced excitant actions and $F_{1\alpha}$ was generally more potent than $F_{2\alpha}$.

Iontophoretically applied prostaglandins have a selective excitatory or inhibitory action on neurones in the brain stem (Avanzino, Bradley and Wolstencroft, 1966) and cerebral cortex (Phillis and York, unpublished observations). The negative results obtained by Krnjević (1965) when testing E_1 on cortical neurones could possibly have been due to the type of anaesthetic employed. On brain stem neurones, desensitization to both excitatory and inhibitory effects was a common finding and was specific for the compound applied. An example of the effects of prostaglandins E_1, $F_{1\alpha}$ and $F_{2\alpha}$ on cerebral cortical neurones is shown in Fig. 8.19. The effects of these three compounds on a given neurone were usually of the same type although varying in magnitude.

The presence of prostaglandins in the central nervous system, their release on nerve stimulation from various regions and their actions on neurones of the spinal cord, brain stem and cerebral cortex suggests that these compounds may have some function related to transmission in the

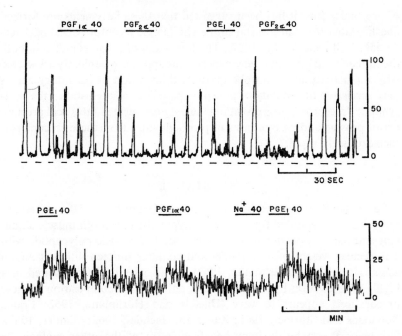

FIG. 8.19. Depressant and excitant effects of prostaglandins on cerebral cortical neurones. Upper record. L-glutamate (40 nA) evoked firing of this neurone was depressed by prostaglandins $F_{1\alpha}$, $F_{2\alpha}$ and E_1 (all applied by currents of 40 nA). Prostaglandin $F_{2\alpha}$ was the most potent depressant. Lower record. Excitant effects of prostaglandins E_1 and $F_{1\alpha}$ on a cortical neurone. Applications by currents of 40 nA. Sodium ions (40 nA) passed from another barrel as a control were without effect (Phillis and York, unpublished observations).

brain. The prolonged actions of prostaglandins may mean that these substances act as modulators of synaptic processes, influencing either the release of transmitter or the excitability of the postsynaptic membrane. Such an interpretation may explain the finding that prostaglandin E_1 is released from the phrenic nerve-diaphragm preparation during nerve stimulation both before and after block of neuromuscular transmission with d-tubocurarine (Ramwell, Shaw and Kucharski, 1965). Prostaglandin release from the rat stomach is also increased by stimulation of the cholinergic, parasympathetic nerve supply, but in this case the effect is blocked by hyoscine. However, as hyoscine does not prevent the spontaneous release of prostaglandins, it has been suggested that these fatty acids are formed and liberated from sites distal to the cholinergic receptor (Coceani, Pace-Asciak, Volta and Wolfe, 1967). The formation of prostaglandins in both the stomach and brain in *in vitro* experiments appears to be closely associated with the activity of a phospholipase A. Stimulation of excitatory nerves may accelerate the activity of phospholipase A at a site distal to the post-synaptic "receptor", thus providing the polyunsaturated fatty acid precursors of prostaglandins. Synthesis of prostaglandins from these precursors is then extremely rapid.

G. SUBSTANCE P

Substance P, discovered by von Euler and Gaddum (1931) in extracts of several tissues, is noted for its intense hypotensive, smooth muscle stimulant and pain-producing actions. Substance P is a basic polypeptide with a molecular weight of about 1600 and contains thirteen different amino acids (Haefely and Hürlimann, 1962). It has recently been isolated in a highly purified form by several groups, although the composition of these preparations appears to vary (Haefely and Hürlimann, 1962; Franz, Boissonas and Stürmer, 1961; Zuber and Jacques, 1962; Winder, 1967). Substance P can be distinguished from most of the other biologically active peptides. It has, however, many similarities in structure and pharmacological activity to the polypeptide, eledoisin (Pisano, 1968).

Substance P is present in the brains of mammals, birds, reptiles and fish and is localized especially in the cell-rich, phylogenetically oldest, parts of the brain, with high values in the hypothalamus, thalamus and basal nuclei (Pernow, 1953; Haefely and Hürlimann, 1962; Lembeck and Zetler, 1962). It is present in high concentrations in the dorsal columns and dorsal roots of the spinal cord. Studies on the subcellular distribution of substance P have shown that it is present in the ultracentrifuge fraction containing synaptic vesicles (Inouye and Kataoka, 1962; Ryall, 1964; Whittaker, 1964).

The numerous publications on the central nervous effects of substance P can be placed into one of two categories describing either "a general tranquillizing effect" or the postulated role of substance P as a neurotransmitter in the primary sensory pathway.

A sedative effect of substance P extracts on the spontaneous activity of mice (Zetler, 1959), hares (Stern and Milin, 1959) and the Japanese fighting fish, *Betta splendens* (Stern and Huković, 1958) has been described. Whilst Kissel and Domino (1959) found that substance P was without effect on mono and polysynaptic spinal cord reflexes, Stern, Dobrić and Mitrović-Kocić (1957) have described an inhibition of the homolateral flexor reflex and the contralateral extensor reflex but no effect on the knee jerk response. Caspers and Stern (1961) applied substance P topically on to the cerebral cortex and recorded an increased negative component of the direct cortical response together with a positive Dc potential shift. This they attributed to a hyperpolarization of neurones in the superficial layers of the cortex, which might have been due to a transmitter function of substance P at inhibitory synapses. An enhancement of the surface negative, recruiting component of the cortical potential evoked by mid-line thalamic stimulation has also been described (Schneiderman, Monnier and Lembeck, 1965).

Lembeck (1953) has suggested that the high concentration of substance P in dorsal roots may indicate a connection with primary sensory synaptic transmission. Direct evidence in support of this suggestion has, however, not been forthcoming. Umrath (1961) is of the opinion that substance P is the precursor of the primary sensory synaptic transmitter.

Many of the studies described above were carried out with very impure preparations of substance P, which has only recently been obtained in a purified form. The presence of other biologically active substances in these extracts may have led to false conclusions concerning the effects of substance P. Experiments with a highly purified extract of substance P have yielded results which are in conflict with those of many earlier investigations and have led to the conclusion that most of the reported effects on the nervous system ascribed to Substance P were in fact due to impurities in the preparations (Vogler *et al.*, 1963).

It is likely therefore, that a definite conclusion concerning the physiological significance of substance P in the central nervous system will not be reached until synthetic substance P becomes available.

CONCLUSIONS

1. Catecholamines depress or excite neurones in many areas of the central nervous system. In conjunction with the fluorescent histochemical results, these findings indicate that catecholamines may be extensively involved as synaptic transmitters in the central nervous system.

2. Inhibitory effects of noradrenaline are the most frequently observed,

although a high proportion of particular groups of neurones, such as those in the floccular lobe of the cerebellum or thalamocortical and geniculo-cortical relay cells are excited. A combination of inhibitory and excitatory effects are sometimes observed on the same neurone. The excitatory actions of noradrenaline are liable to desensitization during repeated applications.

Dopamine has pronounced inhibitory actions on neurons in many areas of the brain. Excitation with this compound has been consistently observed only in the basal ganglia.

3. The α- and β-adrenergic antagonists frequently have comparable actions to the catecholamines on the excitability of neurones, suggesting that they have agonist properties. Once cell excitability has recovered, the depressant effects of the catecholamines are often reduced or abolished by applications of their antagonists. This antagonism does not always appear to be specific as the depressant effects of other monoamines and acetylcholine are also reduced.

4. The convulsants, picrotoxin and strychnine antagonize the depressant actions of noradrenaline, as well as those of the other monoamines and acetylcholine. Figures 8.4 and 8.5 present examples of picrotoxin and strychnine antagonism of noradrenergic and synaptic inhibitions in the thalamus and medial geniculate nucleus.

5. Noradrenaline, 5-hydroxytryptamine and histamine hyperpolarize motoneurones in the spinal cord, inhibiting both orthodromic and antidromic activation of these neurones.

6. 5-hydroxytryptamine depresses many cells in the brain and spinal cord. Relatively few neurones are excited, and desensitization of the excitatory response occurs with repeated applications. The evidence strongly suggests that 5-hydroxytryptamine is a transmitter in various areas of the central nervous system. 5-Hydroxytryptamine inhibits many cortical neurones and excites others. Its excitant actions are antagonized by lysergic acid diethylamide and the inhibitory effects by strychnine and other monoaminergic antagonists.

7. Histamine may also be a transmitter in the cerebral cortex as it has comparable actions to 5-hydroxytryptamine and noradrenaline. Histamine antagonists, which block both the excitant and depressant actions of histamine, also antagonize the actions of other monoamines and acetylcholine.

8. Glycine and γ-aminobutyric acid have been proposed as inhibitory neurotransmitters in the spinal cord and brain respectively. The actions of

glycine, but not of γ-aminobutyric acid are antagonized by strychnine. Recent experiments have shown that amino acids of this type affect the permeability of the postsynaptic membrane in an identical manner to the inhibitory transmitters.

9. Glutamic acid and related amino acids have pronounced excitatory actions on nerve cells and may be important excitatory transmitters in the central nervous system. Glutamic and aspartic acids have also been proposed as excitatory transmitters in the spinal cord and cerebral cortex on the basis of studies on their distribution and release.

10. The actions of various prostaglandins and substance P on nerve cells are described. The significance of the prostaglandins in both central and peripheral nervous systems is not yet apparent. Recent studies with substance P indicate that many of the actions attributed to this compound were in fact due to impurities in the preparations.

CHAPTER 9

NEUROMUSCULAR TRANSMISSION IN INVERTEBRATES

SKELETAL muscle fibres of many invertebrates differ from those of the more advanced vertebrates in that they receive both excitatory and inhibitory inputs. Extensive research has revealed that muscle fibres of Crustacea and Insecta share many anatomical and physiological features. Skeletal muscle fibres in both are innervated multiterminally and frequently also polyneuronally. Both usually exhibit graded responses to stimulation of their excitatory axons, which may be either "fast" or "slow" in type. The existence of peripheral postsynaptic inhibition is well documented in both Crustacea and Insecta. In Crustacea, this is supplemented by presynaptic inhibition. A detailed account of the anatomy and physiology of the neuromuscular systems of invertebrates can be found in the extensive monographs by Bullock and Horridge (1965).

A. GAMMA-AMINOBUTYRIC ACID

1. *Inhibition in Crustacea*

Peripheral inhibition of contraction in crustacean muscles has been a well-established phenomenon for several years. At present, two actions of the inhibitory transmitter agent are distinguished. One is a direct effect on the muscle membrane resulting in increased conductance of chloride ions and a shift of membrane potential towards the chloride equilibrium potential (Boistel and Fatt, 1958). The other is an effect which is considered to occur in the presynaptic motor axon terminals, causing a reduction in the amount of excitatory transmitter released (Dudel and Kuffler, 1961), and thus a reduction in the excitatory junctional potential. According to Dudel (1965a) the effect is mediated through reduction of the spread of the excitatory nerve impulse into the axon terminals.

Crustacean leg muscles often receive two motor axons, termed "fast" and "slow" on the basis of the differences in speed of the contractions they evoke. In muscles of this type, the fast contraction is invariably less influenced by stimulation of the inhibitory axon than is the slow. For example, the fast contraction of the closer muscle of the shore crab, *Pachygrapsus crassipes* Randall, is hardly affected by inhibition, whereas the slow contraction is efficiently suppressed. Atwood, Parnas and Wiersma (1967) have shown that the fast contraction of this muscle is attributable to a group of specialized phasic fibres which respond almost exclusively to fast axons. Many of these fibres lack both a slow exciter axon and an inhibitory input, explaining the insensitivity of the fast contraction to inhibition. Phasic muscle fibres in the crab leg that have been found to be relatively insensitive to inhibitory stimulation are also insensitive to the inhibitory effects of γ-aminobutyric acid (Atwood, 1965), suggesting that the amino acid acts only on fibres which receive an inhibitory innervation.

Presynaptic inhibitory effects, such as those seen in the crayfish leg opener (Dudel and Kuffler, 1961) may be restricted in their occurrence. The inhibitions in the slow abdominal flexor muscles of the crayfish (*Procambarus clarkii*) and lobster (*Homarus americanus*) (Kennedy and Evoy, 1966) and deep abdominal extensors of the same species of crayfish and the rock lobster (*Panulirus interruptus*) (Atwood *et al.*, 1967) appear to be entirely postsynaptic.

The postulate that γ-aminobutyric acid is an inhibitory transmitter at the crustacean neuromuscular junction is based on several lines of experimental evidence. *Gamma*-aminobutyric acid mimics the actions of the inhibitory transmitter at neuromuscular junctions of several species of Crustacea (Kuffler and Edwards, 1958; Hagiwara, Kusano and Saito, 1960; Takeuchi and Takeuchi, 1965, 1966a, b). It is present in high concentrations in the cell bodies and axons of inhibitory nerves of the lobster, *Homarus americanus* (Kravitz, Kuffler and Potter, 1963; Otsuka, Kravitz and Potter, 1967). The concentration of γ-aminobutyric acid in inhibitory fibres is about $0 \cdot 1$ M if it is freely dissolved in the axoplasm, representing about 100 times the concentration found in excitatory axons. The activity of glutamic decarboxylase, the enzyme that synthesizes γ-aminobutyric acid from glutamate, is ten times as high in inhibitory, as in excitatory nerves (Kravitz, Mollinoff and Hall, 1965). *Gamma*-aminobutyric acid transaminase, the enzyme for the breakdown of GABA, is present in lobster nervous tissue (Hall and Kravitz, 1967). *Gamma*-aminobutyric acid is released by inhibitory nerves during their activation (Otsuka, Iversen, Hall and Kravitz, 1966).

The effects of γ-aminobutyric acid on pre- and postjunctional membranes of neuromuscular junctions of the abductor muscle of the dactylopodite of the first or second walking legs of the crayfish *Cambarus clarkii* have been described by Takeuchi and Takeuchi (1965, 1966a, b). The drug was applied iontophoretically and the resulting potential changes recorded with intra- and extracellular microelectrodes. Only certain circumscribed regions of the muscle responded to γ-aminobutyric acid and these coincided with the foci at which inhibitory junctional potentials could be recorded. Both γ-aminobutyric acid and inhibitory nerve stimulation produced small transient depolarizations; the reversal potentials of the inhibitory nerve and amino-acid-induced depolarizations coincided within half a millivolt of each other (Fig. 9.1). Injection of γ-aminobutyric acid into the interior of muscle fibres was without effect. The average size of both L-glutamate-induced depolarizations and excitatory junctional potentials were reduced by the application of γ-aminobutyric acid. The effect of γ-aminobutyric acid on glutamate-induced potentials is shown in Fig. 9.2.

These results indicate that γ-aminobutyric acid has a specific action on the inhibitory neuromuscular junction and that the γ-aminobutyric acid potential is produced by the same ionic mechanisms as the inhibitory junctional potential, namely by an increase in the membrane permeability to chloride ions (Boistel and Fatt, 1958).

It had previously been shown that stimulation of the inhibitory nerve reduces the number of quanta of excitatory transmitter released at crustacean nerve-muscle junctions by stimulation of the motor nerve, although the quantum size remains unchanged (Dudel and Kuffler, 1961). A decrease in the amplitude of the presynaptic nerve spike during inhibitory nerve stimulation has also been observed at the crayfish neuromuscular junction (Dudel, 1963), and this presumably accounts for the reduction in the amount of transmitter released. Investigations by Takeuchi and Takeuchi (1966a, b) have now confirmed that γ-aminobutyric acid has a similar action on presynaptic terminals at the crustacean neuromuscular junction, causing a reduction in the size of the presynaptic spike in the motor nerve and a reduction in the number of quanta of excitatory transmitter released. No change in amplitude of the inhibitory nerve spike was observed.

A similar pre- and postsynaptic combination of actions have been shown for β-alanine and γ-aminobutyric acid (Dudel, 1965b). On the other hand,

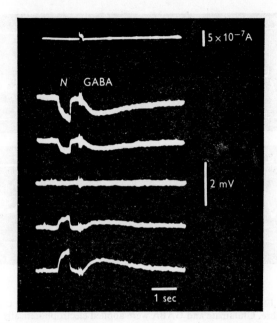

Fig. 9.1. Actions of γ-aminobutyric acid (GABA) on a crustacean muscle fibre. A comparison of the reversal potentials of inhibitory junctional potentials (i.j.p.s.) and GABA potential. N, i.j.p.s. produced by stimulating the inhibitory nerve at 30 sec; GABA, potentials produced by iontophoretic injection of GABA on the sensitive area of the same muscle fibre. Upper trace, monitored injection current. Bottom trace was obtained at the resting potential (−70 mV), and the muscle fibre was depolarized in 2 mV steps. The reversal potential, in this case, was about −66 mV. Potassium propionate—filled electrode used for intracellular recording (Takeuchi and Takeuchi, 1965).

β-guanidinopropionic acid and various other compounds have the presynaptic actions, but do not affect the postjunctional membrane. There is, therefore, a clear difference in the pharmacological specificity of the pre- and postjunctional receptors. The pre- and postjunctional effects of both the synaptically released inhibitory transmitter, and γ-aminobutyric acid are blocked by picrotoxin (Robbins, 1959). When chloride ion in the perfusion fluid is replaced by various large anions, such as propionate or acetate, stimulation of the inhibitory nerve or an application of γ-amino-butyric acid fails to reduce the quantum content of excitatory junctional

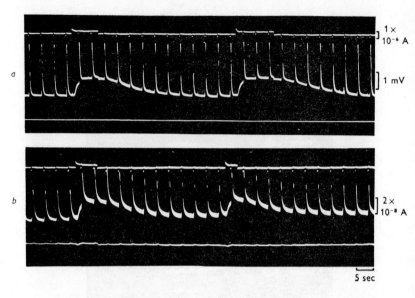

FIG. 9.2. Effect of GABA on the glutamate-induced potential of a crustacean muscle fibre. Glutamate and GABA were applied electrophoretically through separate pipettes to a junctional area. Upper traces are monitored injection current, upward deflexion, GABA injection; downward deflexion, L-glutamate injection. *a*, Intracellularly recorded glutamate—(brief depolarization) and GABA—potentials (slow depolarization). *b*. The clamping current for the L-glutamate injection (brief deflexions) and for the GABA injection (slow deflexions) when the membrane potential was clamped at the resting level. Lower trace; the clamped membrane potential (Takeuchi and Takeuchi, 1966a).

potentials. It appears therefore, that the action of the inhibitory transmitter on the presynaptic nerve terminals is a result of an increase in chloride permeability, as in the postsynaptic membrane.

The possibility that γ-aminobutyric acid might exert direct inhibitory effects on crustacean muscle fibres by competing with the excitatory transmitter has been considered (Fatt and Katz, 1953). However, Takeuchi and Takeuchi (1966a) have since shown that there is no appreciable competition for postsynaptic receptors between γ-aminobutyric acid and L-glutamic acid, the postulated excitatory transmitter.

A note of caution has been sounded by Florey (1965) about the acceptance of γ-aminobutyric acid as the inhibitory transmitter at crustacean neuromuscular synapses. Experiments in Florey's laboratory have shown that crustacean nerve extracts contain a labile inhibitory factor which has about 20 times the potency of γ-aminobutyric acid (Florey and Chapman, 1961). Florey (1965) has used the data presented by Kravitz and his colleagues (Kravitz, Kuffler, Potter and Van Gelder, 1963) to show that the γ-aminobutyric acid content of lobster muscle is considerably higher than can be accounted for by the amino acid content of the nerve terminals and suggests that it is also present in the muscle fibres.

2. Inhibition in Insects

Gamma-aminobutyric acid, which occurs in insect nervous systems (Frontali, 1964; Ray, 1964), has recently been implicated as an inhibitory transmitter at insect nerve–muscle junctions. Experiments by Usherwood and Grundfest (1965) have established that inhibitory postsynaptic potentials can be recorded from muscles of the locust (Schistocerca gregaria) and grasshopper (Romalea microptera). Only those fibres of the extensor tibiae muscle which were innervated by the slow exciter axon received an inhibitory innervation. These numbered about 20% of all fibres of the grasshopper and about 10% in the locust. The hyperpolarizing inhibitory postsynaptic potentials were the result of an increase in chloride permeability, as substitution of the chloride of the medium with an impermeable anion caused a reversal of the postsynaptic potential. Applications of γ-aminobutyric acid caused an increase in membrane conductance and a hyperpolarization of those muscle fibres which were innervated by the slow exciter and inhibitory axons. Stimulation of the inhibitory nerve and applications of γ-aminobutyric acid reduced the mechanical response of the muscle to stimulation of the slow exciter axon but did not affect the responses to the fast exciter axon, indicating that γ-aminobutyric acid acts only on those muscle fibres which receive an inhibitory innervation. Picrotoxin blocked the effects of inhibitory nerve stimulation and γ-aminobutyric acid. The potentiating effect of picrotoxin on the responses of locust muscles to stimulation of the slow nerve fibres suggests that γ-aminobutyric acid may also act presynaptically on slow fibre endings in Insecta, as well as in crustaceans.

Gamma-aminobutyric acid inhibits glutamic acid-evoked contractions of the dorsal and ventral longitudinal body muscles of the centipede (Pachymerinus millepunctatus) (Florey and Florey, 1965) and leg muscles of the cockroach, *Periplaneta americana* (Kerkut, Shapira and Walker, 1965). It does not affect the contractions of the cockroach leg evoked by acetylcholine. The amplitude and frequency of miniature endplate potentials of cockroach leg muscle decreased when γ-aminobutyric acid was allowed to diffuse from micropipettes on to the muscle fibres (Kerkut and Walker, 1966). Although it was not determined whether these effects were due to pre- or postsynaptic actions of γ-aminobutyric acid, the results suggest that this amino acid should be given consideration as an inhibitory transmitter at the cockroach nerve–muscle junction.

In contrast to its actions on muscles of crustaceans and insects, (both members of the phylum *Arthropoda*), γ-aminobutyric acid has no effect on the dorsal and ventral longitudinal body muscles of a species of annelid, *Abarenicola pacifaca* (Florey and Florey, 1965). These authors used pharmacology as a tool to explore the evolutionary relationships of the Onychophoran, *Opisthopatus costesi*, which has been regarded as a transition stage between annelids and arthropods. Muscles of *Opisthopatus* proved to be cholinoceptive, like those of the annelids and did not respond to either glutamic acid or γ-aminobutyric acid.

B. GLUTAMIC ACID

1. *Crustacea*

Glutamic acid is present in comparable amounts in excitatory and inhibitory fibres of the legs of the lobster, *Homarus americanus* (Kravitz *et al.*, 1965; Otsuka *et al.*, 1967). Relatively low concentrations of glutamate produce contraction and depolarization of various crustacean muscles (Robbins, 1959; Van Harreveld and Mendelson, 1959; Takeuchi and Takeuchi, 1964). Glutamate is released from perfused legs of the crab, *Carcinus maenas* during limb nerve stimulation (Kerkut *et al.*, 1965) and Baker (1964) has observed that the isolated nerve trunk of the crab, *Maia*, releases glutamate and aspartate during stimulation.

Takeuchi and Takeuchi (1964) applied glutamate iontophoretically to the surface of the abductor muscle of the dactylopodite of the crayfish *Cambarus clarkii*. The regions which depolarized when glutamate was applied were sharply localized (Fig. 9.3) and coincided exactly with the points from which junctional potentials could be recorded with an extracellularly located electrode. Injection of glutamate into the interior of the

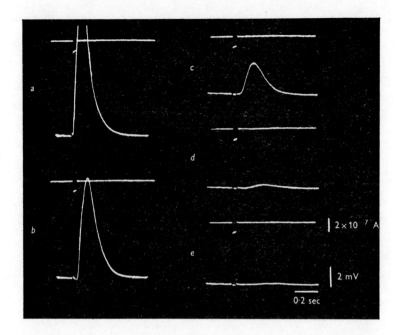

FIG. 9.3. L-glutamate depolarization at a junctional area of a crustacean muscle fibre recorded with an intracellular electrode. Lower traces, L-glutamate induced depolarizations. Upper traces, monitored injection current. *a*, L-glutamate filled pipette was located near a nerve-muscle junction. The amplitude of the depolarization was about 16 mV in a record at a lower gain. From *a* to *e* the L-glutamate pipette was moved along muscle fibre in 8 μ steps (Takeuchi and Takeuchi, 1964).

muscle fibres produced no appreciable depolarization. When the changes in sensitivity of the receptor during and after a conditioning dose of L-glutamate were investigated, it became apparent that a small conditioning dose caused a transient increase in the test responses, and that as the conditioning dose increased, desensitization of the receptor occurred (Fig. 9.4). During the administration of L-glutamate, the size of excitatory junctional potentials was decreased. This interaction between applied L-glutamate and the excitatory transmitter suggests that they share a common receptor. D-glutamate had no depolarizing action on crustacean muscle (Fig. 9.5).

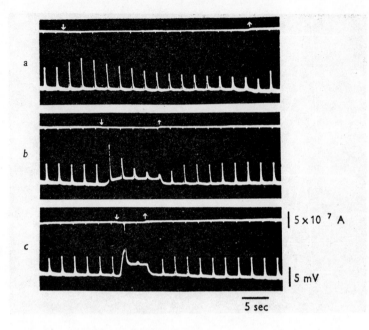

5×10^{7} A

5 mV

5 sec

FIG. 9.4. Action of L-glutamate on crustacean muscle fibres. Lower traces, L-glutamate induced depolarizations. Desensitization and potentiation of glutamate potential by conditioning doses of L-glutamate. Brief test responses were recorded and during the period indicated by arrows a steady conditioning dose was injected through another pipette. From *a* to *e* the strength of conditioning dose was increased. Upper trace. Monitored injection current (Takeuchi and Takeuchi, 1964).

Thus, L-glutamate or a related amino acid may be an excitatory transmitter at crustacean neuromuscular synapses. The possibility that another substance may be involved in neuromuscular transmission in the crayfish is suggested by the work of Van der Kloot (1960). He found a substance in the crayfish, *Cambarus clarkii*, which stimulated the closer muscle of the claw. This substance, called factor S, was detected in perfusates from stimulated, but not unstimulated claws. Van der Kloot extracted factor S by the aluminium hydroxide precipitation of Von Euler (1948) and he noted that it had several properties in common with an unidentified catechol-4 isolated by Ostlund (1954) from various invertebrate species.

Cook (1967) has employed the Von Euler extraction procedure on several species of arthropods, including crayfish, cockroaches, a grasshopper and a fly. A factor S-like substance was found in all the extracts, and the distribution of biological activity indicated that it was concentrated in nervous tissue. Factor S elicited an excitatory response from motor neurones in the cockroach and potentiated muscular contractions in this species. Factor S, which may be an amine, must therefore be considered as a potential neurotransmitter in arthropods.

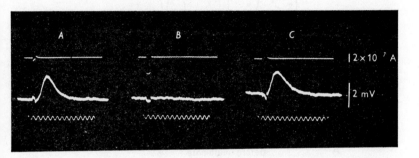

FIG. 9.5. Comparison of effects of L- and D-glutamate on crustacean muscle fibres. A. Depolarization produced by L-glutamate injection from one barrel of a double-barrelled pipette. B. D-glutamate was injected at the same spot from another barrel. C. L- and D-glutamate of the same doses with those in A and B were applied simultaneously to the same spot. Upper traces, monitored injection currents. Middle traces, intracellular potential changes. Time scale, 25 c/s (Takeuchi and Takeuchi, 1964).

2. *Insects*

Glutamic acid occurs in the nervous systems of various insects (Frontali, 1964; Ray, 1964) and its release from the legs of the cockroach, *Periplaneta*, during nerve stimulation has been demonstrated (Kerkut *et al.*, 1966). Glutamic acid decarboxylase activity has been demonstrated in insect brain tissue by Frontali (1964) and from the work of McAllan and Chefurka (1961) it appears that the muscle of *Periplaneta* is capable of transaminating glutamate.

Glutamate (10^{-5} g/ml) causes an increase in the frequency and amplitude of the contractions of the cockroach leg (Kerkut and Walker, 1966). The frequency of miniature junctional potentials of insect muscle fibres is

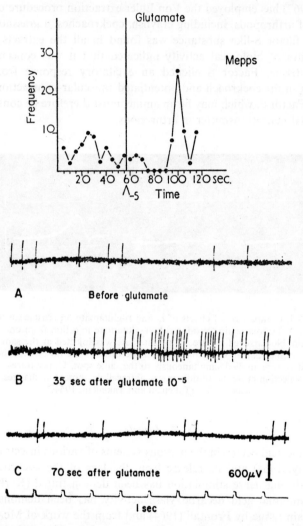

FIG. 9.6. Action of L-glutamate on miniature endplate potentials (mepps) recorded from cockroach leg muscle fibres. Glutamate applied by diffusion from a coarse, 50 μ tip, microelectrode filled with 10^{-5} M glutamate, which was brought into close proximity with the recording microelectrode at the muscle surface. Graph shows increase in frequency of mepps brought about by the addition of glutamate. A, B and C are series of pen recordings showing the mepps before and after the addition of glutamate (Kerkut and Walker, 1966).

increased by glutamic acid (Fig. 9.6) (Kerkut and Walker, 1966; Usherwood and Machili, 1966), suggesting that the amino acid is facilitating the release of transmitter from the excitatory presynaptic nerve terminals. This could be the result of a glutamate-induced depolarization of the terminals. Usherwood and Machili (1966) treated a locust muscle preparation with glutamic acid decarboxylase and demonstrated a decrease in nerve-evoked muscle contractions, which was reversed by washing. The decarboxylase inhibitor, phenylhydrazine, potentiated the response of the muscle to nerve stimulation. Both of these observations favour the hypothesis that L-glutamate may be an excitatory transmitter in this muscle.

3. *Mollusca*

Glutamate (10^{-7} g/ml) contracts the pharyngeal retractor muscle of the snail *Helix aspersa* and it appears in the muscle perfusate when the nerves are stimulated, the amount increasing according to the number of stimuli (Kerkut *et al.*, 1965). The significance of these results has yet to be evaluated.

C. ACETYLCHOLINE

1. *Annelids*

The presence of cholinergic nerves innervating the body-wall musculature of the leech was suggested by Bacq and Coppee (1937). Intracellular records from the body-wall musculature of *Hirudo medicinalis* have shown that iontophoretically applied acetylcholine produces depolarizations, similar in their characteristics to the muscle action potentials (Walker, Woodruff and Kerkut, 1968). Acetylcholine, may, therefore, be an excitatory transmitter at synapses on these muscles, but further comparisons of the pharmacology of the synaptically released transmitter and acetylcholine will be essential before this hypothesis can be confirmed.

2. *Crustacea*

Acetylcholine is unlikely to have a transmitter function at the crustacean neuromuscular junction. Motor fibres in crustacea do not contain detectable amounts of acetylcholine (Florey and Biaderman, 1960). Moreover, acetylcholine, anticholinesterases and acetylcholine antagonists are without effect on crustacean muscle (Bullock and Horridge, 1965).

The hearts of many crustaceans are excited by low concentrations of acetylcholine (Krijgsman, 1952). Eserine potentiates the effect of acetyl-choline (Bullock and Horridge, 1965). The action resembles that observed when the excitatory nerve fibres are stimulated. However, although the action of applied acetylcholine is blocked by atropine, the effects of nerve stimulation are not. Florey (1960) has concluded that acetylcholine is not the transmitter released by the cardio-accelerator axons.

3. *Insects*

The identity of the chemical agent responsible for impulse transmission across the insect neuromuscular junction is still unknown. Evidence derived from a number of studies with topically applied drugs has indicated that the mechanism is not a cholinergic one. The ineffectiveness of applied acetylcholine in modifying the transmission process (Harlow, 1958), the absence of potentiating effects of anticholinesterases (Usherwood, 1961), the failure of curare to act as a neuromuscular blocking agent (Ellis, Thienes and Wiersma, 1942; Roeder and Weiant, 1950) and the failure to show the presence of cholinesterase at the neuromuscular junction (Iyatomi and Kaneshina, 1958) have been interpreted as evidence to support the contention that acetylcholine is not the effective agent in insects.

When injected into the abdominal cavity of the fly, *Sarcophaga bullata*, acetylcholine, eserine and curare had pronounced effects on the electrical activity of single dorsal longitudinal flight-muscle fibres, even though they were without effect when applied topically (McCann, 1966; McCann and Reece, 1967). After an intra-abdominal injection of curare, stimulation of the central thoracic ganglion failed to elicit action potentials from the flight muscles, indicating that the drug had blocked neuromuscular trans-mission. When injected into the abdomen, acetylcholine depolarized flight muscles, and small irregular potentials, similar in appearance to miniature endplate potentials, appeared. An injection of eserine into the abdominal cavity evoked sporadic repetitive firing of muscle fibres. McCann and Reece interpret their results as evidence for a cholinergic mechanism of neuromuscular transmission and suggest that topically applied drugs may fail to reach the target areas. The concept of barriers to drug diffusion in insects has also been discussed by Twarog and Roeder (1956) and Treherne (1966). However, after injection into the abdominal cavity drugs would be widely distributed through the insect and the effects of acetylcholine and curare observed by McCann and Reece may have been due to actions on elements of the nervous system. Until the pharmacology of neuromuscular transmission in *Sarcophaga* is studied with drugs applied iontophoretically directly on to the muscle fibres, it will not be possible to evaluate the significance of these findings.

Acetylcholine stimulates the cockroach heart (Metcalf, Winton and Fukuto, 1964). Anticholinesterases were also found to accelerate the heart, their actions being prevented by atropine. The authors suggest that the neurogenic pacemaker system has cholinergic properties.

4. *Molluscs*

Neuromuscular transmission in molluscs, unlike that in the arthropods, appears to be mediated by acetylcholine.

The anterior byssus retractor muscles of the mussel, *Mytilus edulis*, has provided a model for the study of neuromuscular transmission in pelecypod molluscs. Acetylcholine, which is present in the muscle, produces a depolarization and prolonged contraction (Twarog, 1954). Electrically induced phasic contractions of this muscle are blocked by acetylcholine antagonists, including methantheline (Banthine) (Twarog, 1959, 1960). Cambridge, Holgate and Sharp (1959) have confirmed the acetylcholine blocking action of methantheline and offered evidence that the closely related agent, propantheline (Pro-Banthine), also blocks responses to stimulation of the excitatory nerves. The acetylcholine antagonists did not relax sustained contractions, which could, however, be abolished by 5-hydroxytryptamine. Anticholinesterases potentiated the effects of excitatory nerve stimulation. Methantheline (10^{-4}M) has also been shown to cause a progressive reduction in the amplitude of intracellularly recorded junctional potentials in *Mytilus* muscle (Twarog, 1967a).

The pharyngeal retractor muscles (PRM) of two gastropods, *Helix aspersa* (Kerkut and Leake, 1966) and *Euhadra hesperia* (Ozeki, 1962) differ in their responses to acetylcholine. At concentrations of up to 10^{-5} g/ml, acetylcholine had no effect on the PRM of *Euhadra* but in higher concentrations it depressed the responses of the muscle to electrical stimulation. Low concentrations ($10^{-9} - 10^{-4}$ g/ml) of acetylcholine inhibited the contractions of *Helix* PRM's evoked by brain stimulation. At higher concentrations it increased the contractions of the muscle. Curare ($10^{-5} - 10^{-4}$ g/ml) depressed and abolished the excitant effects of brain stimulation.

Dual effects of acetylcholine on other molluscan muscle tissues have been recorded and the effects of curare suggest that acetylcholine may be an excitatory transmitter for the *Helix* PRM. However, the PRM is a complex preparation containing smooth muscle fibres, nerve cells and axons, sensory nerve endings and secretory cells. Thus, acetylcholine and curare may exert their effects on various components of the muscle mass other than at the neuromuscular junction itself.

There is some evidence that acetylcholine could be the transmitter at other molluscan nerve–muscle preparations. Jaeger (1962) showed that the penis retractor muscle of *Strophocheilos oblongus* was stimulated to contract by acetylcholine at 10^{-7} g/ml and that the contraction was blocked by benzoquinonium and curare. Duncan (1964) showed that acetylcholine excited the penis retractor muscle of *Limnaea stagnalis*. Similarly, acetylcholine stimulates the radula muscle of *Buccinum undatum* (Fange and Mattisson, 1958) and the radular protractor muscle of *Busycon canaliculatum* (Hill, 1958).

The most obvious effect of acetylcholine on the hearts of gastropod and lamellibranch molluscs is an inhibition (S.-Rozsa and Pecsi, 1967; Greenberg, 1965). However, the hearts from many of these species also show an excitatory response, manifest as an increase in tone or amplitude of beat, to very high or very low doses of acetylcholine, or in the presence of benzoquinonium. With a few species such as *Strophocheilos oblongus* and *Mytilus galloprovincialis* the excitatory effect predominates (Jaeger, 1961; Greenberg, 1965).

The actions of acetylcholine on the hearts of two members of the family of *Veneridae*, *Mercenaria mercenaria* and *Tapes watlingi*, have been related to nervously mediated inhibition (Prosser, 1940; Welsh and Slocombe, 1952; Welsh, 1961; Phillis, 1966). Acetylcholine inhibits the contractions of both hearts at concentrations of $10^{-10} - 10^{-9}$ g/ml and its actions, as well as those of stimulation of the cardio-inhibitory nerves, are blocked by benzoquinonium (Mytolon) (Fig. 9.7). After the application of benzoquinonium, stimulation of the cardio-regulator nerves excites the hearts of both species and this excitant effect can be abolished by the 5-hydroxytryptamine antagonist, methysergide (Fig. 9.7c). Higher concentrations of acetylcholine excite the *Tapes* heart, especially after pretreatment with benzoquinonium. The acetylcholine-induced excitation is resistant to both methysergide and higher concentrations of benzoquinonium. The possibility therefore arises that the methysergide-sensitive nervous transmission

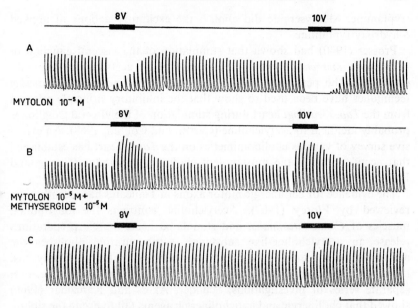

FIG. 9.7. The effects of stimulation of the cardio-regulator nerves on ventricular contractions of the *Tapes watlingi* heart. Trace A illustrates the inhibitory effects of nervous stimulation, applied during the period indicated on the marker trace. on ventricular activity. B. Was recorded after the ventricle had been soaked in mytolon (benzoquinonium) (10^{-5} M) for 20 min and C after a further 20 min period of application of mytolon and methysergide (10^{-5} M). Time calibration: 1 min (Phillis, 1966a).

of excitation occurs at a ganglionic synapse and that the postganglionic fibres are cholinergic but benzoquinonium resistant. However, this suggestion has been refuted by the demonstration that the drug, mytelase, abolishes the excitant actions of acetylcholine but not the action of the cardio-excitor nerves.

Pécsi (1968) has studied the innervation of the heart of the freshwater mussel, *Anodonta cygnea*. Electrical stimulation of the visceral ganglion of this species results in both excitatory and inhibitory effects on the heart, with the inhibitory effect dominating. After pretreatment with benzoquinonium the inhibitory effect is blocked and only excitation can be observed. However, unlike its actions on the two marine molluscs discussed above, methysergide failed to antagonize the cardio-excitor substance of *Anodonta*, which is therefore unlikely to be related to 5-hydroxytryptamine. Methysergide did abolish the excitatory actions of applied 5-hydroxytryptamine.

Prosser (1940) had shown that stimulation of the visceral ganglion of *Mercenaria mercenaria* evokes the release of an acetylcholine-like substance into the perfusion fluid. Chromatographic and parallel-bioassay techniques have been used to show that the inhibitory principle released from the *Tapes watlingi* heart during stimulation of the visceral ganglion is probably identical to acetylcholine (Carroll and Cobbin, 1968). An extensive survey of various cholinomimetics on the *Tapes* heart has established that acetylcholine is the most potent cholinergic inhibitor (Chong and Phillis, 1965; Phillis, 1966).

The evidence for cholinergic motor axons in Tunicates has recently been reviewed by Florey (1967). Acetylcholine contracts the longitudinal muscles of *Ciona intestinalis*, and stimulated nerve-muscle preparations release an acetylcholine-like substance. D-tubocurarine abolishes the actions of both acetylcholine and motor nerve stimulation. Florey has, therefore, concluded that the motor nerves in *Ciona* are cholinergic. In a separate series of investigations, Scudder, Akers and Karczmar (1966) showed that cholinergic and anticholinergic agents fail to excite the siphon muscles of *Ciona* or alter the response of the siphon to electrical stimulation. These authors suggested that the motor systems controlling the siphon are not cholinergically mediated. However, intact animals were used in these experiments, with the drugs added to the surrounding sea-water, and the negative results may therefore be a reflection of the impermeability of the outer body wall of *Ciona* to the drugs used.

D. 5-HYDROXYTRYPTAMINE

The history of the discovery of 5-hydroxytryptamine as a naturally occurring substance involves several invertebrates. Enteramine, now known to be identical with 5-hydroxytryptamine, was found in the alimentary tract of two ascidians, *Tethium plicatum* and *Ciona intestinalis* (Erspamer, 1946). Enteramine-like activity was also noted in extracts of the posterior salivary glands of *Octopus vulgaris* and *Eledone moschata* (Erspamer, 1948).

1. Cellular Localization

The histochemical localization of 5-hydroxytryptamine in the nerve cells of invertebrates has now been investigated with the fluorescent technique.

Both 5-hydroxytryptamine- and dopamine-containing neurones were found in the cerebral, visceral and pedal ganglia of *Anodonta piscinalis, Helix pomatia* and *Buccinum undatum* (Dahl *et al.*, 1966). Small fluorescent granules, arranged in rows, and suggesting the presence of nerve fibres with varicosities were observed in the neuropile of the ganglia. These were thought to be nerve terminals similar to those of the adrenergic system of vertebrates.

In *Astacus astacus*, a decapod crustacean, neurones containing 5-hydroxytryptamine were found in small numbers in the protocerebrum, medulla externa and ventral nerve cord (Elofsson, Kauri, Nielsen and Stromberg, 1966). Catecholamine-containing neurones were more abundant. In the polychaete, *Nephthys caeca*, Clark (1966) found neurones containing 5-hydroxytryptamine in the cerebral ganglion and ventral nerve cord of the central nervous system, in the segmental nerves and in the intestinal wall. Longitudinal fibres in the ventral nerve cord had but few varicosities. Clark suggests that in the annelids these 5-hydroxytryptamine-containing axons are motor in function but the longitudinal fibres may also be association fibres running between ganglia. Catecholamine-containing neurones were concentrated in the supraoesophageal ganglia. As catecholamine-containing cells were widely distributed, Clark suggests that they may have a sensory function.

At least one tenth of the motor and interneuronal population of a typical ganglion of the ventral nerve cord of the earthworm, *Lumbricus terrestris*, contains either 5-hydroxytryptamine or a catecholamine (Rude, 1967). Both Rude (1967) and Myhrberg (1967) have suggested that 5-hydroxytryptamine containing neurones in *Lumbricus* may have a motor function. 5-Hydroxytryptamine has been found in the cytoplasm of the two segmental giant neurones (Retzius cells) of the ganglia of the leech, *Hirudo medicinalis* (Kerkut, Sedden and Walker, 1967a). These cells send axons down the segmental nerves to innervate the body wall musculature. As 5-hydroxytryptamine depressed the amplitude of excitatory junctional potentials in the body wall musculature, it may be an inhibitory transmitter (Walker, Woodruff and Kerkut, 1968).

2. *Crustacea and Annelids*

The occurrence and role of 5-hydroxytryptamine in phyla other than the Mollusca is incompletely known. Studies on the hearts of decapod

Crustacea have shown that 5-hydroxytryptamine causes an acceleration and increase in stroke volume (Florey, 1965). 5-hydroxytryptamine appears to act directly on the neurones of the cardiac ganglion, driving the burst frequency to a higher rate and increasing the duration of the bursts (Cooke, 1966).

A facilitatory effect of 5-hydroxytryptamine on crayfish neuromuscular transmission has been shown by Grundfest, Reuben and Rickles (1959) and Dudel (1965a). Excitatory postjunctional potentials become larger due to an increase in the number of quanta released per stimulus.

5-Hydroxytryptamine has a relaxing action on annelid muscles (Schain, 1961; Walker et al., 1968).

3. Molluscs

Whereas 5-hydroxytryptamine excites the smooth muscle of molluscan hearts, it relaxes prolonged contractions in certain molluscan non-cardiac smooth muscles, including the anterior byssus retractor muscle of *Mytilus* (Twarog, 1954, 1960) and muscles of the gastropod radula apparatus (Hill, 1958; Fänge and Mattisson, 1958). Nerve fibres specifically inducing relaxation of prolonged contractions probably exist in molluscs, as it has been demonstrated that direct stimulation of the byssus retractor muscle with brief repetitive electrical pulses, or stimulation of the pedal ganglion, can lead to relaxation of prolonged contractions. In the byssus retractor muscle, the relaxing effect of 5-hydroxytryptamine, (which occurs naturally in *Mytilus* ganglia) supports the hypothesis that 5-hydroxytryptamine may be involved as a transmitter in neurally-induced relaxation.

The byssus retractor muscle of *Mytilus* remains contracted for long periods after stimulation by acetylcholine or cathodal current. Washing does not relax this sustained tension but 5-hydroxytryptamine (10^{-9} — 10^{-7} M) causes or produces an immediate relaxation (Fig. 9.8). In the presence of relaxing concentrations of 5-hydroxytryptamine, tension development in response to acetylcholine and direct cathodal current is not blocked (Fig. 9.8) but somewhat increased, while the phase of sustained tension following stimulation is abolished. Since neither muscle action potentials nor prolonged depolarization are found during sustained contractions, and as relaxation by 5-hydroxytryptamine causes essentially no change in membrane polarization, it has been concluded that prolonged tension does not involve continued activation of the muscle membrane (Twarog, 1960).

On this assumption, 5-hydroxytryptamine-induced relaxation would involve a direct action on the muscle fibres, in such a way as not to alter membrane polarization, or on the excitation-contraction coupling mechanism or the contractile mechanism itself. Twarog (1967b) has speculated that actomyosin in *Mytilus* muscle is activated by a calcium releasing mechanism. The maintenance of a sustained tension or "catch" would depend on sustained high levels of free intracellular calcium. If 5-hydroxytryptamine, in proportion to its concentration, increases the binding of intracellular calcium to a "relaxing" system, the reduction of intracellular free calcium could explain the apparent paradox that "catch" is released while the excitability of the membrane is increased. Woolley and Campbell

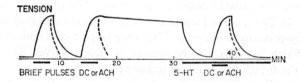

FIG. 9.8. Diagram of contractile responses of a small bundle from the anterior byssus retractor muscle of *Mytilus*. In response to repetitive brief pulses (0·5–10 msec duration), a brief tetanus is seen. Prolonged cathodal direct current pulses (DC) or acetylocholine (ACH) produce a contraction which persists after stimulation has ceased: catch. In the presence of 5-hydroxytryptamine (5-HT), contraction no longer persists after stimulation; catch is abolished. Solid line, tension; interrupted line, active state (Tarwog, 1967b).

(1960) have provided evidence that 5-hydroxytryptamine increases calcium binding to lipid fractions.

One of the earliest suggestions concerning the role of 5-hydroxytryptamine in invertebrates was that it is a cardio-excitatory transmitter in molluscs (Welsh, 1953). 5-Hydroxytryptamine is widely distributed in the nervous systems of invertebrates (Welsh and Moorhead, 1960) and homogenates of molluscan nerve tissue have been shown to have considerable 5-hydroxytryptophan decarboxylase activity (Welsh and Moorhead, 1959). Excitation of the hearts of various lamellibranch molluscs following stimulation of the visceral ganglion or its connectives can be blocked by 5-hydroxytryptamine antagonists such as methysergide (Fig. 9.7) and bromolysergic acid (Loveland, 1963; S.-Rozsa and Graul, 1964; Phillis, 1966). Release of 5-hydroxytryptamine from molluscan hearts has been detected during stimulation of the cardio-regulator nerves (S.-Rozsa and Perényi, 1966). S.-Rozsa and Perényi also detected a second cardio-excitatory factor in the perfusate of stimulated *Helix pomatia* hearts, thought to be a derivative of arginine. An unidentified cardio-excitatory substance is also released from the heart of another gastropod, *Strophocheilos*, during stimulation (Jaeger, 1966).

A cardio-excitatory substance has been isolated from *Mercenaria* ganglia. This substance, called substance X, can be distinguished from 5-hydroxytryptamine both chromatographically and by the use of specific 5-hydroxytryptamine antagonists (Cottrell, 1966). Further analysis of substance X on Sephadex columns has established that it contains four factors which are excitatory on *Mercenaria* hearts treated with acetylcholine and 5-hydroxytryptamine antagonists (Frontali, Williams and Welsh, 1967). Three of the factors appear to be peptides as they are readily attacked by proteolytic enzymes. They may be part of the neurosecretory material which has shown to be present in cardiac nerves. The chemical nature of the fourth factor is still unknown.

Density gradient centrifugation of homogenates of *Mercenaria* ganglia has been used to separate the particles binding acetylcholine, 5-hydroxytryptamine and substance X. From the results of an electron microscopic study of different homogenate fractions of *Anadonta*, Zs-Nagy and his colleagues concluded that 5-hydroxytryptamine in molluscan nervous tissue is associated with endoplasmic reticulum vesicles (Zs-Nagy *et al.*, 1965) though this has been disputed by Cottrell and Maser (1967).

Fluorescence microscopy of the heart of *Limnaea stagnalis* has revealed the presence of catecholamine-containing cells and axons in the auricles. 5-Hydroxytryptamine appeared to be restricted to small vesicles in the muscle cells themselves (S.-Rozsa and Zs-Nagy, 1967). As a result of these findings, it has been postulated that stimulation of the cardio-excitatory nerves may release an unidentified transmitter on to the catecholamine-containing "postganglionic" neurones. These release a catecholamine at their junctions with muscle cells which subsequently liberates 5-hydroxytryptamine within the muscle fibres. The metabolic effects of 5-hydroxytryptamine precipitate a contraction.

In support of their hypothesis, S-Roza and Zs-Nagy have shown that dopamine, adrenaline, noradrenaline and 5-hydroxytryptamine excite the *Limnaea* heart in concentrations of $10^{-10} - 10^{-9}$M. Acetylcholine (10^{-12}M) inhibits the heart.

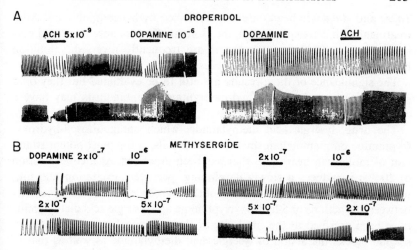

FIG. 9.9. Records from heart of the bivalve mollusc, *Tapes watlingi*. A. Dopamine (10^{-6} g/ml) inhibited one of these hearts and excited the other. Acetylcholine (ACH, $5\text{--}10^{-9}$ g/ml) inhibited both. After perfusing both hearts with droperidol (5×10^{7} g/ml) for 20 min, the inhibitory actions of dopamine and acetylcholine were reduced or abolished, but the excitant action of dopamine was unaffected. B. Two *Tapes* hearts, the actions of dopamine on which were either blocked or reversed by methysergide (2×10^{-5} g/ml), a 5-hydroxytryptamine antagonist. This record illustrates the complexity of some drug-receptor interactions on this preparation (Phillis, unpublished observations).

The involvement of 5-hydroxytryptamine in nervously-induced cardio-excitation of molluscs appears to have been established, even though the precise role it plays is still uncertain. With the fluorescence histochemical technique, further studies of the distribution of monoamines in the hearts of different species may clarify some of the confusion. The autofluorescence of molluscan tissues is, however, a serious obstacle to the interpretation of such experiments. Much of the evidence in support of a transmitter role for 5-hydroxytryptamine in the molluscan heart is derived from experiments with antagonists such as methysergide and bromolysergic acid. It is disturbing, therefore, that recent experiments in the author's laboratory on *Tapes* hearts and by S.-Rozsa and Pécsi on *Anodonta* hearts have shown that these agents also antagonize the effects of catecholamines. Methysergide depresses both the excitant and depressant actions of dopamine on the *Tapes* heart (Fig. 9.9). The depressant actions of dopamine on both

Tapes and *Anodonta* hearts are also abolished by benzoquinonium. After treatment with benzoquinonium, the excitant effects of adrenaline and noradrenaline on *Helix pomatia* hearts are frequently reversed, inhibition becoming apparent (S.-Rozsa and Pécsi, 1967).

The significance of these results has still to be evaluated but they offer some indications that the 5-hydroxytryptamine antagonists may have a complex action on molluscan hearts.

The drug, lysergic acid diethylamide, which antagonizes 5-hydroxytryptamine on mammalian smooth muscle cells, is the most potent stimulant of molluscan heart cells that has been described. At a concentration of 10^{-16}M it induces a slowly developing, persistent excitation and ultimately causes maximal contractions of the *Mercenaria* heart. The similarity between the actions of 5-hydroxytryptamine and lysergic acid diethylamide have been ascribed to the similarity of their chemical structures. Methysergide blocks the action of lysergic acid diethylamide as well as that of 5-hydroxytryptamine (Wright, Moorhead and Welsh, 1962; Chong and Phillis, 1965).

E. CATECHOLAMINES

Catecholamines are widely distributed in the invertebrate nervous system. Dopamine, noradrenaline and adrenaline have all been found (Cottrell and Laverack, 1968). Fluorescent histochemical studies have demonstrated the presence of catecholamine-containing neurones in coelenterates (Dahl, Falck, Mecklenburg and Myhrberg, 1963), annelids (Clark, 1966; Rude, 1967; Kerkut *et al.*, 1967a), molluscs (Dahl *et al.*, 1966; S-Rozsa and Zs-Nagy, 1967) and insects (Frontali and Norberg, 1966). The catecholamine-type fluorescence in molluscs may be largely due to dopamine as Sweeney (1963) has demonstrated large amounts of this amine in molluscan ganglia.

On histochemical grounds it appears that at least some of the catecholamine-containing neurones in annelids and molluscs are sensory in nature. With the exception of the catecholamine-containing cells in the *Lymnaea* heart (S.-Rozsa and Zs-Nagy, 1967), no histochemical evidence of a motor function has been reported.

In contrast to the molluscan nervous system, on which the actions of the catecholamines have been extensively investigated, there have been few recent publications on their actions on invertebrate neuromuscular transmission. The literature concerning the actions of catecholamines on invertebrate hearts is difficult to evaluate as the type of heart and experimental conditions have varied greatly. Although some differences exist in the literature, the general conclusion is that adrenaline excites arthropod hearts (Crescitelli and Geissman, 1962).

Diverse effects of adrenaline and noradrenaline on molluscan hearts, including excitation, inhibition or both, have been reported (Krijgsman and Divaris, 1955). Dopamine was the most potent catecholamine tested on the heart of the lamellibranch mollusc, *Tapes watlingi*, having a threshold concentration of about 10^{-7}M (Chong and Phillis, 1965). The effects of dopamine varied considerably, as it excited some hearts and depressed others. The depressant actions of dopamine were reduced by droperidol (Fig. 9.9A) (Droleptan), mytolon and methysergide (Fig. 9.9B), and the excitant actions by methysergide (Fig. 9.9B). Droperidol also antagonized the inhibitory actions of acetylcholine, and the effects of both this substance and benzoquinonium can be explained if it is assumed that dopamine releases acetylcholine from cholinergic terminals, either by a direct action on the terminals or by exciting cholinergic neurones in the heart. It is more difficult to postulate an explanation for the actions of methysergide, which blocked both excitant and depressant actions of dopamine, frequently reversing the initial effect.

Elimination of the excitant effects of the catecholamines on *Helix pomatia* hearts and elimination or reversal of their inhibitory effects on *Anodonta cygnea* hearts by mytolon and bromolysergic acid have also been described (S-Rozsa and Pécsi, 1967).

The effects of noradrenaline and adrenaline on the *Tapes* heart were invariably weaker than those of dopamine (Chong and Phillis, 1965). On *Helix* and *Anodonta* hearts, the effects of noradrenaline and adrenaline did not differ appreciably from those of dopamine as regards threshold concentrations or the maximum effect produced.

Neuronal excitation of the light organ of the firefly, *Photinus pyralis* may afford an example of adrenergic transmission in insects (Smalley, 1965). Noradrenaline, adrenaline and amphetamine induce glowing of the organ *in situ*. Pretreatment with reserpine or denervation blocks the response to amphetamine but not to noradrenaline and adrenaline. Electrical stimulation of the light organ results in two flashes, a fast response followed by a slower one. Only the slow response was thought to be under direct neuronal control as it was selectively blocked by yohimbine and amphetamine.

CONCLUSIONS

1. Gamma-aminobutyric acid has been identified as an inhibitory transmitter at crustacean neuromuscular junctions and may also be implicated as an inhibitory transmitter at insect nerve–muscle junctions. There is some evidence that other inhibitory substances are present in inhibitory motor nerves in crustacea.

2. Glutamic acid may be an excitatory transmitter at nerve–muscle junctions in crustacea, insects and molluscs. The action of glutamic acid on crustacean muscles closely parallels those of the synaptically released transmitter. In insects, a depolarizing action of glutamic acid on nerve terminals has also been demonstrated. Extracts from several arthropod species contain a substance, called factor S, which has also been proposed as a muscle excitant.

3. Acetylcholine has been identified as an excitatory transmitter at nerve–muscle synapses in mollusca and as an inhibitory transmitter in molluscan hearts. It does not appear to be involved in neuromuscular transmission in insects and crustacea.

4. 5-Hydroxytryptamine excites the smooth muscle of molluscan hearts and relaxes prolonged contractions in certain molluscan non-cardiac smooth muscles. In both instances it is thought to act as a transmitter.

5. There is as yet no convincing evidence that catecholamines are involved as neural transmitters at invertebrate nerve–muscle junctions.

6. Fluorescent histochemical studies have revealed the presence of 5-hydroxytryptamine and catecholamines in the nervous systems of coelenterates, annelids, molluscs, insects and crustacea. The actions of these monoamines on molluscan neurones will be described in Chapter 10.

CHAPTER 10

DRUGS, TRANSMISSION
AND MOLLUSCAN NEURONES

A. STRUCTURE

The development of interest in neural transmission in molluscan central nervous systems reflects the ease with which their nerve cells can be impaled by microelectrodes and the fact that many of these cells can be recognized by their colour, location or physiological properties.

In a typical molluscan ganglion, a central core of fibrous matter, or neuropil, is surrounded by an outer covering of cell bodies. The nerve cells are mostly unipolar with no somatic dendrites and usually one axonic process which often divides into collaterals. Bipolar and occasional multipolar neurones are found along the course of nerves and connectives or in the centre of the ganglia in the neuropil. Some of the cells in gastropods have diameters of several hundreds of microns, one of the largest being the giant cell of the abdominal ganglion of the sea hare, *Aplysia*, which may have a diameter of nearly 1 mm. Each of the giant cells usually has a specific place in the ganglion and can be identified in different individuals. The ganglion cells frequently contain an intracellular pigment, which may be brown, red or yellow and this also aids in the identification of different cells. An axonal process leaves the cell body at the axon hillock and may divide into collaterals at different distances from the soma.

All known synaptic junctions in Mollusca are axo-axonic (Tauc, 1966, 1967). Light and electron microscopic studies have failed to find any evidence of nerve fibre endings on the cell body or the base of the axon (Bullock, 1961; Gerschenfeld, 1963). The ultrastructure of synapses in gastropods has been analyzed by Gerschenfeld (1963). Synaptic contacts are formed in the neuropil between complex presynaptic endings and thin branches of the postsynaptic axons. Synaptic areas are revealed by well defined synaptic clefts, bordered by areas of dense membrane. The

267

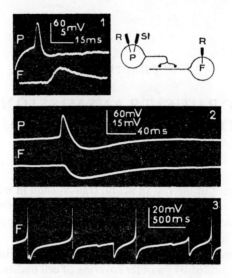

FIG. 10.1. Postsynaptic potentials in *Aplysia* neurons. In (1) and (2), simultaneous recordings from internuncial (P) and follower (F) neurons are shown. The spike in (1) is produced by direct stimulation (St) of P; in (2), the spike is spontaneous. In (1) P is an excitatory neuron whose activity is followed, in F, by an excitatory postsynaptic potentials; in (2), P is an inhibitory interneuron giving, in F, inhibitory postsynaptic potentials (IPSP's). In (3), spontaneous activity of spike is altered by IPSP's as a result of spontaneous activity of an inhibitory internuncial neuron (Tauc, 1966).

structure and properties of the molluscan nervous system have been described in detail by Tauc (1966, 1967).

B. SYNAPTIC TRANSMISSION IN GASTROPODS

Ganglion cells in the gastropods are integrative neurones, each receiving multiple excitatory and inhibitory connections from other neurones or receptors. Both excitatory and inhibitory postsynaptic potentials are therefore observed in ganglion cells (Fig. 10.1). Excitatory postsynaptic potentials originating from the activation of one presynaptic fibre have a duration of 50–400 msec in direct relation to the diameter of the cell body. In relatively small cells of 70μ diameter, the duration of the excitatory postsynaptic potential is many times greater than that of a passive electrotonic decay, suggesting a prolonged action of the transmitter. In larger cells, the long falling phase of the excitatory potential has been attributed to the slow decay of the potential induced by the initial part of the excitatory postsynaptic potential (Tauc, 1966).

Initiation of an action potential by an excitatory postsynaptic potential occurs at some distance from the cell soma in an axonal region with an excitability surpassing that of the surrounding membranes (Fig. 10.2).

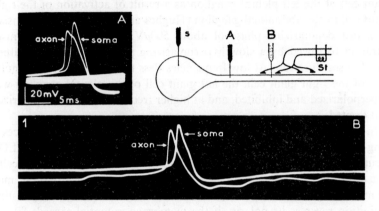

Fig. 10.2. Simultaneous intracellular recordings from the soma and axon of the giant cell of *Aplysia*, stimulated orthodromically at *St* (the stimulus artifacts are outside the records). The distance of the axonal microelectrode is 350 μ in (A), 2 mm in (B). (A) and (B) were taken from different neurons. Excitatory postsynaptic potentials can be seen on the record taken from the axonal region in (B) (Tauc, 1966).

Between the trigger zone and the soma there is a region of transitional excitability, where conduction of the spike towards the soma may fail. The soma is then excited by the electrotonic spread of the axonic spike potential.

The inhibitory postsynaptic potentials observed in many cells are a result of spontaneous discharges of inhibitory presynaptic neurones. More rarely, the inhibitory postsynaptic potential can be induced by stimulation of preganglionic nerves. The form and duration of inhibitory potentials are similar to the excitatory potentials, but with reversed polarity. The amplitude and polarity of the inhibitory potentials are closely related to the membrane potential. If the latter is increased, the inhibitory postsynaptic potential first decreases in amplitude, falling to zero at about −60mV. With increasing polarity the inhibitory potential reappears, but as a depolarizing potential with excitatory properties. Both chloride and potassium ions appear to be involved in the inhibitory process at cholinergic inhibitory synapses in gastropods, whilst at the non-cholinergic inhibitory synapses in snails potassium only has been implicated (Gerschenfeld and Chiarandini, 1965).

In *Aplysia* a biphasic postsynaptic potential has been observed in the left giant cell of the left pleural ganglion as a result of activation of the right giant cell in the abdominal ganglion (Hughes and Tauc, 1965). It consists of a fast depolarizing phase of about $500\mu V$ amplitude and 200 msec duration followed by a slow hyperpolarizing phase of $500\mu V$ amplitude and 1–3 sec duration. At low frequencies (less than 3 per sec) of stimulation of the right giant cell, the left giant cell of the pleural ganglion was hyperpolarized and inhibited, and at higher frequencies it was depolarized and excited.

In *Aplysia* and some snail neurones, synaptic stimulation produces a long-lasting hyperpolarizing potential, the "long-lasting inhibition" (ILD). Neurones showing long duration inhibitions are known as CILDA cells. The duration of these inhibitions is usually 20–60 sec (Fig. 10.3) but may be much longer, attaining 30 min in some cells (Tauc, 1966). Long lasting inhibition reverses its polarity if the membrane potential exceeds 80mV, which indicates that an ionic process is involved but excludes the possibility that repetition of the normal short duration inhibition is a cause as the reversal potential for the latter is −60mV. During the long duration inhibitions the postsynaptic membrane conductance increases considerably.

A prolonged depolarizing effect of synaptic stimulation with a duration of up to several minutes has been observed in some other molluscan neurones (Fig. 10.3) (Tauc, 1966). Although the possibility that this effect is due to repetitive short duration excitatory postsynaptic potentials has not yet been excluded, it may represent a phenomenon opposite to long duration inhibitions.

1. *Pharmacological Characterization of Neurones in Gastropod Ganglia*

Several pharmacological cell-types have been described in various gastropods, including *Aplysia*, *Helix* and *Cryptomphallus*. These are described briefly below.

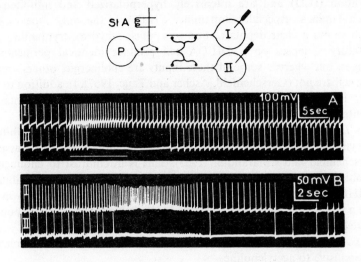

FIG. 10.3. Residual effects observed in spontaneously firing ganglion cells of *Aplysia*. Simultaneous intracellular records. In A, a brief repetitive orthodromic stimulation (horizontal line) of an excitatory afferent pathway, including interneuron, P, accelerates for a long period cell I, whereas cell II is first accelerated, then inhibited, giving after recovery a frequency greater than the resting level (inhibition of long duration). In B, an increase of frequency of excitatory synaptic potentials (EPSP's) due to a common internuncial neuron accelerates cell I and inhibits cell II (Tauc, 1966).

(a) *D and H cells*. These cells receive cholinergic excitatory and inhibitory synapses respectively. Application of acetylcholine depolarizes and excites D cells and hyperpolarizes and inhibits H cells. Threshold effects are seen with acetylcholine concentrations as low as 10^{-10} g/ml. In both D and H cells, acetylcholine causes a fall in membrane resistance. The action of acetylcholine on cells of both types is abolished by *d*-tubocurarine. Hexamethonium blocks the action of acetylcholine on D cells.

The excitatory input to H cells is not affected by curarizing drugs and is therefore unlikely to be cholinergic. Moreover, the H cells are excited by catecholamines, especially dopamine (Gerschenfeld and Tauc, 1964). 5-hydroxytryptamine is completely without effect.

(b) *CILDA cells*. These cells are depolarized (DILDA type) or hyperpolarized (HILDA type) by acetylcholine. Both types show long lasting inhibition (ILD) and are intensively hyperpolarized and inhibited by catecholamines, especially dopamine. CILDA is the only type of cell which shows a clear depolarization to applied 5-hydroxytryptamine. All excitatory synapses on a DILDA cell produce identical permeability changes, but whereas some of these inputs are cholinergic, others on the same cell are not (Gerschenfeld, Ascher and Tauc, 1967). In addition to the ILD, HILDA cells have classical cholinergic inhibitory postsynaptic potentials.

(c) *DINHI cells.* Cells of this type show non-cholinergic inhibitory postsynaptic potentials resulting from a permeability change to potassium (Gerschenfeld and Chiarandini, 1965). This is in contrast to cholinergic inhibitions which are the result of an increase in chloride permeability. DINHI cells are depolarized by acetylcholine and have been shown to have a cholinergic excitatory input and to give hyperpolarizing responses to catecholamines, especially to dopamine.

(d) *Acetylcholine-insensitive cells.* A small group of cells are completely unresponsive to acetylcholine.

2. Cholinergic Mechanisms in Molluscan Ganglia

Acetylcholine is the only drug which has been firmly established as a transmitter substance at ganglionic synapses in gastropods. Studies have been carried out on *Aplysia depilans* and *californica, Cryptomphallus aspersa, Helix pomatia, Helix aspersa* and *Onchidium.*

The application of acetylcholine by perfusion or local injection, produces one of two types of response from neurones in gastropod ganglia. Cells of one type, conventionally designated as D neurones, are depolarized and excited (Fig. 10.4) and cells of another type, H neurones, are hyper-polarized and inhibited (Fig. 10.5). Threshold effects are observed with acetylcholine concentrations of less than 10^{-10} g/ml. D neurones show only excitatory synaptic inputs, whereas H neurones have both excitatory and inhibitory inputs. In both D and H cells acetylcholine decreases the membrane resistance to a low level. The reversal potential level of the acetylcholine action is identical to that of the excitatory postsynaptic potentials in D cells and to that of the inhibitory postsynaptic potential in H cells (Fig. 10.5).

In the presence of atropine or *d*-tubocurarine, the effects of acetylcholine on both types of cell are diminished or abolished (Fig. 10.6) and at the same

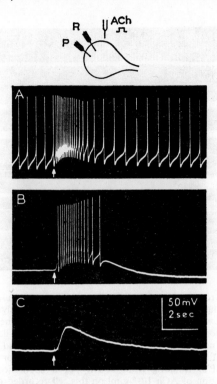

FIG. 10.4. Effects of brief (200 msec) electrophoretic application of acetylcholine (at arrows) on somatic membrane potential of a D cell of a ganglion of the opisthobranch (Gastropoda) *Aplysia depilans*. Above the records is a diagram of the set-up, showing the recording microelectrode (R), and the polarizing microelectrode (P) inserted in the cell body, and the acetylcholine-filled micropipet (ACh) applied to the outside of the cell. In A, the cell shows rhythmic activity, accelerated by ACh action. In B, the cell was slightly hyperpolarized to avoid spontaneous firing; ACh depolarizes transiently and induces spikes. In C, the cell was hyperpolarized further; the depolarizing wave produced by ACh action does not reach the firing level (Tauc and Gerschenfeld, 1962).

time excitatory and inhibitory postsynaptic potentials in D and H cells respectively, are reduced or abolished (Fig. 10.7). A notable difference between the specificity of the D and H cholinergic receptors is evident in the presence of hexamethonium, which depresses the excitatory postsynaptic potentials and depolarization by acetylcholine of D cells (Fig.

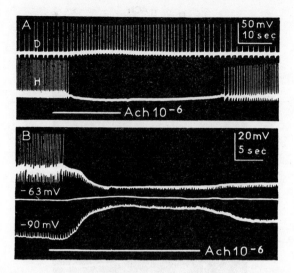

Fig. 10.5. Records from *Aplysia* ganglion cells. A. Simultaneous intracellular recordings from two contiguous and spontaneously firing D and H cells perfused with ACh 10^{-6} g/ml (white line below) showing their different patterns of response. While the D neuron (upper record) is depolarized and excited, the H neuron (lower record) is hyperpolarized and inhibited. B. Spontaneously firing H cell presenting elementary inhibitory postsynaptic potentials (IPSP's) resulting from activity of a spontaneous inhibitory interneuron. Action of ACh 10^{-6} g/ml on this cell recorded during normal conditions (upper record), hyperpolarization to −63 mV (middle record) and to −90 mV (lower record). Influence of membrane potential level is similar in amplitude and polarity for both IPSP's and for ACh action. Note that for the IPSP's inversion potential (−63 mV) no overt action of ACh is observed (Tauc and Gershenfeld, 1962).

10.6) whereas inhibitory postsynaptic potentials and the hyperpolarizing action of acetylcholine on H cells are not affected.

The suggestion by Tauc and Gerschenfeld (1961) that synaptic endings of the same interneurone in *Aplysia* ganglia might have a cholinergic excitatory action on some D cells and a cholinergic inhibitory one on some H cells has been confirmed by Kandel, Frazier, Waziri and Coggeshall (1967). Different specified neurones in the abdominal ganglion of *Aplysia californica* were impaled and recordings made simultaneously from two or more such cells. Synchronous postsynaptic potentials of opposite

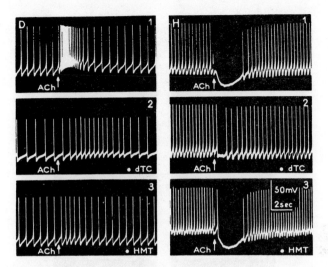

FIG. 10.6. (1) Effect of brief electrophoretic injections of acetylcholine (arrows) on the somatic membrane of a D cell (left column) and an H cell (right column) of *Aplysia* ganglion, firing spontaneously. The drug depolarizes the D cell and accelerates its firing, while it hyperpolarizes the H cell and inhibits firing. (2) The same amount of acetylcholine as in (1) is injected into the D cell (left) and into the H cell (right), but in the presence of the bathing fluid of 10^{-4} g/ml of d-tubocurarine, which clearly inactivates both D and H cell membranes to the action of acetylcholine. (3) The same electrophoretic injection of acetylcholine on D and H cells as in (1), but in the presence of 10^{-4} g/ml of hexamethonium bromide. This drug inactivates the D cell membrane to the action of acetylcholine (left) but has no effect on the response of the II cell membrane to acetylcholine (Tauc and Gerschenfeld, 1961).

polarity were seen between certain combinations of cells, suggesting that the opposite synaptic actions were mediated by the same interneurone. By searching among the identified cells of the ganglion Kandel *et al.* (1967) found an interneurone (L10) which produces hyperpolarizing synaptic potentials in neurones of the left rostral quarter ganglion and depolarizing potentials in neurones in the right quarter ganglion.

Figure 10.8A is a simultaneous high sweep speed record from three cells, showing an action potential in the L10 interneurone and postsynaptic potentials of opposite polarity in the two follower cells. When both follower cells were hyperpolarized about 10–15mV (Fig. 10.8B) the excitatory potential remained almost unaltered whilst the inhibitory potential

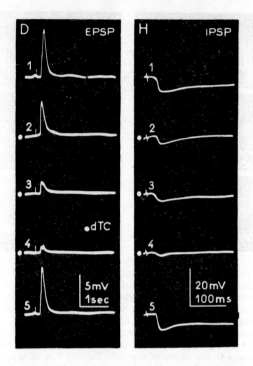

FIG. 10.7. Effects of d-tubocurarine in 10^{-4} g/ml concentration (white dots, 2–4) on the evoked excitatory postsynaptic potential (EPSP) in a D cell (left column) and on the inhibitory postsynaptic potential (IPSP) in an H cell (right column) of *Aplysia*. The synaptic potential in the D cell is composed of two unitary excitatory synaptic potentials. In both cells the drug inactivates the postsynaptic membrane to natural excitatory and inhibitory transmitters, respectively, as indicated by the gradual diminution (2–4) of the postsynaptic potentials. The removal of the curare restores the initial amplitude of the synaptic potentials (5) (Tauc and Gerschenfeld, 1961).

was reversed to a depolarizing potential as would be expected of an inhibitory postsynaptic potential.

Iontophoretically applied acetylcholine depolarized and excited the follower cell which was excited by L10 interneurone and hyperpolarized and inhibited the other follower cell. D-tubocurarine abolished the excitant and inhibitory effects of both the L10 interneurone and acetylcholine on the two follower cells. Hexamethonium blocked only the excitant responses.

This finding provides corroboration of "Dale's principle", which is simply that the same transmitter is liberated at all the synaptic terminals of a neurone. The differentiation in this case being in the specific properties of the acetylcholine receptors on the postsynaptic membrane. "Double action" neurones appear not to be limited to molluscs. Recently a double-action neurone was discovered in the third abdominal ganglion of the

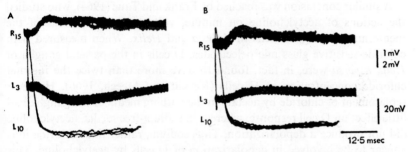

FIG. 10.8. Demonstration of different equilibrium potentials for the two types of PSP's mediated by L10 interneurone of *Aplysia* ganglion. Intracellular recordings from the interneuron (lowermost trace), and two bursting follower neurons, R15 (uppermost trace) and L3 (middle trace). The interneuron was stimulated intracellularly and its action potential was used to trigger the oscilloscope. Several sweeps were superimposed. In A the membrane potential of the follower cells is at the resting level. In B the membrane potential of the follower cells was hyperpolarized causing the hyperpolarizing PSP in L3 to be inverted to a depolarizing PSP (Kandel, Frazier, Waziri and Coggeshall, 1967).

lobster by Otsuka, Kravitz and Potter (1967). In this ganglion, the inhibitory neurones to muscle are electrically coupled with the symmetrical inhibitory neurones of the other side. These cells mediate chemical inhibition to muscle (by the release of γ-aminobutyric acid) and electrical excitation to the contralateral inhibitory interneurone.

Studies on the ionic mechanisms underlying the excitatory and inhibitory actions of acetylcholine have yielded somewhat contradictory results. However, a recent paper by Chiarandini, Stefani and Gerschenfeld (1967), which demonstrates the presence of two different mechanisms of acetylcholine depolarization in ganglia of the land snail *Cryptomphallus aspersa*, suggests that some of the contradictions may have been a result of the type of neurone tested.

Oomura, Ooyama and Sawada (1965) found that the hyperpolarizing and depolarizing actions of acetylcholine on neurones in *Onchidium* were due to an increase in chloride permeability. A difference between the internal chloride concentrations of D and H cells was postulated to account for this finding. Hyperpolarization or depolarization occurs according to whether the equilibrium potential for chloride ions is above or below the membrane potential.

A similar conclusion was reached by Frank and Tauc (1964), who studied the actions of acetylcholine on minute, voltage clamped, areas of the membrane of ganglion cells in *Aplysia* and *Helix*. When measured with chloride-sensitive glass microelectrodes, D cells in the parietal ganglia of *Helix aspersa* were, in fact, found to have more than twice the internal chloride concentration of H cells (Kerkut and Meech, 1966). However replacement of chloride by acetate in the bathing media of the ganglia had little effect on D cell response, whereas in sodium-free media, acetylcholine did not produce a depolarization. Thus sodium, rather than chloride ions appear to be involved in depolarization of D cells by acetylcholine. This contrasts with the inhibitory postsynaptic potential and acetylcholine-induced hyperpolarization of H cells in *Helix aspersa* where chloride is the major, if not the only, ion responsible for changes in membrane potentials (Kerkut and Thomas, 1964).

The ionic permeability changes during acetylcholine-induced responses in D and H cells of *Aplysia californica* have been investigated by Sato, Austin, Yai and Maruhashi (1968). The results were comparable to those obtained by Kerkut and Meech (1966) in *Helix*, as the acetylcholine-induced depolarization of D cells was markedly decreased when the external sodium was reduced. Acetylcholine depolarization was slightly depressed in chloride-free media. If an increased chloride ion permeability had been involved in the action of acetylcholine the depolarization should have been greatly enhanced. Acetylcholine-induced hyperpolarization of H cells decreased almost linearly as the external chloride was reduced until it reversed into a depolarization in chloride-free media. These results strongly suggest that inhibition in the abdominal ganglion cells of *Aplysia* is due to an increase in chloride permeability.

The ionic mechanism of cholinergic inhibition of neurones in the perioesophageal ganglia of the land snail, *Cryptomphallus aspersa*, is similar to those in *Aplysia* and *Onchidium*, namely due to an increase in the permeability of the subsynaptic membrane to chloride ions (Chiarandini and Gerschenfeld, 1967). The presence of an outward pump of chloride ions has been postulated to account for the required electrochemical gradient. On the other hand, Kerkut and Thomas (1964) have suggested that potassium, as well as chloride, permeability changes may be involved in synaptic inhibition of neurones in *Helix aspersa*.

Acetylcholine appears to be an excitatory transmitter at synapses on two different types of nerve cell in *Cryptomphallus aspersa* (Chiarandini, Stefani and Gerschenfeld, 1967). In D-type neurones, acetylcholine increases chloride permeability and through a net efflux of this ion depolarizes the cell. Reductions in the chloride content of the perfusing fluid increase the amplitude of acetylcholine-induced depolarizations (Fig. 10.9) whereas a reduction in the extracellular sodium has little effect. On neurones which exhibit long duration inhibitions (CILDA), acetylcholine depolarization is dependent on extracellular sodium (Fig. 10.10) and is not altered by removal of chloride ion. An increase in sodium permeability is definitely implicated in the acetylcholine depolarization of CILDA neurones and potassium may also be involved.

A further complication has been the discovery of an identified interneurone in the abdominal ganglion of *Aplysia californica* which mediates both direct excitation and inhibition of the same follower cell (Wachtel and Kandel, 1967). At low firing rates the interneurone produces excitatory postsynaptic potentials. However, at higher firing rates these gradually diminish in size and eventually invert to inhibitory postsynaptic potentials. Electrophysiological and pharmacological evidence indicates that the connection between these cells is monosynaptic and that a single transmitter, acetylcholine, mediates both actions. These opposite synaptic responses appear to result from the transmitter acting on two types of postsynaptic receptor having different thresholds for activation and different susceptibilities for desensitization. The excitatory receptor has the lower threshold but is quickly desensitized. Both receptors are blocked by *d*-tubocurarine.

Kehoe (1967) has described a cell in the pleural ganglion of *Aplysia* in which short and long duration inhibitions can be evoked by single or repetitive drops of sea water falling on a tentacle. The reversal potentials for the two inhibitory processes are separated by about 20mV and both can be reproduced by acetylcholine. However, whilst the short duration

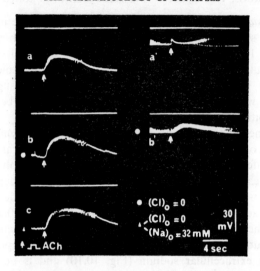

FIG. 10.9. Effect of changes in the ionic composition of the bathing solution on the acetylcholine (ACh) response of a D-neuron of the land snail *Cryptomphallus aspersa*. The recordings were displayed in a double-beam cathoderay oscilloscope. The upper trace corresponds to the zero potential level, and the lower trace displays the intracellular recording. Acetylcholine was applied iontophoretically (arrows) by passing currents of 100 nA during 300 msec. (a) The ACh-potential recorded when the neuron was artificially hyperpolarized from -44 to -60 mV; control saline solution. (b) The neuron was immersed in a Cl^- free solution. Notice the increase in the amplitude of the ACh-potential. (c) The Na^+ content of the Cl^--free Ringer was lowered to 32 mmole/liter (25% of the normal content). Notice that the depolarizations in (b) and (c) are similar. (a') The neuron was artificially depolarized to -20 mV. Application of ACh produced a hyperpolarizing response. (b') The E_m is maintained at -20 mV, and the neuron is bathed in a Cl-free Ringer solution. Application of ACh produces a depolarization (Chiarandini, Stefani and Gerschenfeld, 1967).

inhibition is blocked by curare, the long duration effect is resistant to acetylcholine antagonists. An iontophoretic application of dopamine on these cells caused a single, phased hyperpolarization, which like the second phase of the acetylcholine potential reversed at -80 mV.

3. *Catecholamines*

The effects of catecholamines have been studied on neurones in the ganglia of *Helix aspersa* (Kerkut and Walker, 1961, 1962; Walker *et al.*,

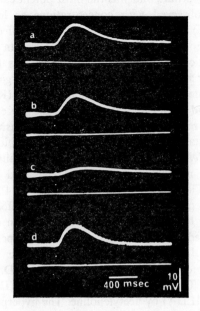

FIG. 10.10. Effect of changes in the ionic composition of the bathing solution on the ACh response of a CILDA neuron of *Cryptomphallus aspersa*. Recording displaying in a double beam cathode-ray oscilloscope. Upper trace corresponds to intracellular recording. Lower trace monitors the ACh injecting current. (a) The E_m equals -58 mV. The bathing solution is normal saline. (b) Cl-free Ringer. (c) Cl-free Ringer containing only 25% of the normal Na^+ content (32 mM). Notice the lack of effect of changes of Cl^- and the decrease of ACh response when Na^+ is lowered. (d) The ACh-potential recovers its initial amplitude after the neuron has been washed with normal saline (Chiarandini, Stefani and Gerschenfeld, 1967).

1968), *Cryptomphallus aspersa* (Gerschenfeld, 1964; Gerschenfeld and Chiarandini, 1965) and *Aplysia depilans* (Gerschenfeld and Tauc, 1961).

Individual neurones of *Helix aspersa* responded to comparatively low concentrations of the catecholamines in the perfusion fluid. Generally, adrenaline increased the firing rate of neurones at concentrations of 10^{-7} g/ml or above, while noradrenaline decreased the rate of firing of most neurones studied although it excited some. Dopamine decreased the rate of firing of most neurones and was the most potent catecholamine tested, inhibition being observed with concentrations as low as 10^{-11} g/ml. Walker *et al.* (1968) have shown that the inhibitory effects of dopamine on specific cells in the suboesophageal mass of *Helix* can be antagonized by several α-adrenergic antagonists but not by various β-antagonists. The dopamine receptor appears to resemble the α-adrenergic receptor of vertebrates. As dopamine is synthesized in the *Helix* brain (Kerkut, Sedden and Walker, 1966) and is located within neurones (Kerkut, Sedden and Walker, 1967b), it may be involved in inhibitory transmission. The effects of α-adrenergic antagonists on neurally evoked inhibitions of dopamine-sensitive cells in *Helix* ganglia have still to be ascertained.

Adrenaline and noradrenaline excite H cells and inhibit D cells in *Aplysia depilans* (Gerschenfeld and Tauc, 1961, 1964). Noradrenaline is considerably more potent than adrenaline and the effects of both amines are approximately ten times greater on D cells than on H cells. Iontophoretically applied dopamine depolarizes or hyperpolarizes various identified cells in *Aplysia* (Ascher, Kehoe and Tauc, 1967). The hyperpolarizing effects occur in the two groups of CILDA cells defined by Gerschenfeld and Tauc (1964); those depolarized (DILDA) and those hyperpolarized (HILDA) by acetylcholine. The hyperpolarizing action of dopamine can be reversed by artificially hyperpolarizing the neurone. The inversion potential depends on the external potassium concentrations and does not alter when external chloride is replaced by methylsulphate (Ascher, 1968). In all HILDA cells the synaptic "inhibition of long duration" (ILD) can be inverted and appears also to be due to a selective increase in potassium permeability.

4. 5-*Hydroxytryptamine*

5-Hydroxytryptamine excites neurones in the ganglia of various molluscs (Kerkut and Walker, 1961, 1962; Gerschenfeld and Tauc, 1964). When applied iontophoretically on to cells in *Cryptomphallus aspersa*, 5-hydroxytryptamine excited only CILDA neurones (Gerschenfeld and Stefani, 1966). Repeated applications of 5-hydroxytryptamine produced desensitization which lasted for about 40 sec. Membrane conductance was increased by 5-hydroxytryptamine. The receptors were blocked by lysergic acid diethylamide and its derivatives. Atropine blocked the excitant actions of both acetylcholine and 5-hydroxytryptamine; the 5-hydroxytryptamine receptors being blocked to a greater extent. It is unlikely, however, that the two drugs act on a common receptor as there was no evidence of a crossed desensitization between acetylcholine and 5-hydroxytryptamine. Bromolysergic acid 148 has been observed to block the excitatory postsynaptic potentials of some CILDA neurones, which may indicate that 5-hydroxytryptamine is a transmitter in gastropod ganglia.

5. *Histamine*

The effects of histamine and other naturally occurring imidazoles on neurones of *Helix aspersa* have been studied by Kerkut, Walker and Woodruff (1968). Drugs were applied iontophoretically or by perfusion. Histamine excited 45 percent of the cells tested and inhibited 16%. Both the excitatory and inhibitory actions of histamine were blocked by low concentrations of mepyramine. L-Histidine, 1.4-methylhistamine and N-methylhistamine had no effect on histamine-sensitive neurones. As histamine and the enzymes which metabolize it are present in the snail brain, it may function as a synaptic transmitter.

6. *Gamma-aminobutyric and Glutamic acids*

The specific effects of γ-aminobutyric acid on molluscan neurones have been demonstrated by Kerkut and Walker (1961). The overall effect of γ-aminobutyric acid on neurones in whole ganglia of *Helix aspersa* was excitation, although it did cause inhibition of some neurones. Glutamic acid appeared to accelerate the firing of some neurones and to inhibit others. The excitatory action was only noticeable about 1 min after application although inhibition occurred within 5–10 sec.

Gerschenfeld and Lasansky (1964) showed several different effects of γ-aminobutyric acid and glutamic acid, applied topically or iontophoretically, on neurones in *Cryptomphallus aspersa* and *Helix pomatia*. (Fig. 10.11 and 12). Some cells were excited by glutamate and inhibited by γ-aminobutyric acid, whereas others were also excited by the latter. Others were excited by glutamate and unaffected by γ-aminobutyric acid and yet others were inhibited by both γ-aminobutyric acid and glutamate. The excitant, but not the inhibitory actions of the amino acids, were subject to desensitization with repeated applications. The possible functions of these amino acids is not yet clear.

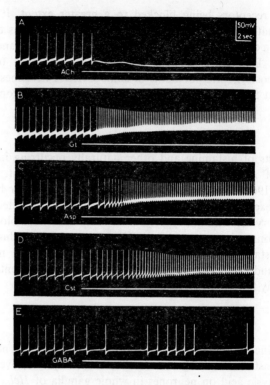

FIG. 10.11. Comparison of the actions of A: acetylcholine (ACh); B: glutamic acid (Gt); C: aspartic acid (Asp); D: cysteic acid (Cst) and E: γ-aminobutyric acid (all 10^{-3}M) on an H-type land snail neuron (Gerschenfeld and Lasansky, 1964).

CONCLUSIONS

1. The synaptic relationships between molluscan neurones are unusual in that all known synaptic junctions are axo-axonic. The cell soma and axon hillock do not appear to form junctions with terminals.

2. Excitatory and inhibitory junctional potentials in molluscan neurones may be of either short (50–400 msec) or long (20–60 sec or longer) duration. Short and long duration inhibitions reverse their polarity at different levels of membrane polarization, indicating that different ionic processes are involved.

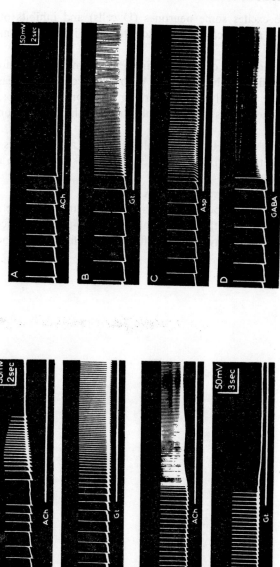

FIG. 10.12. Left hand records: effect of sodium glutamate (Gt) 10^{-3}M applied by perfusion on two different neighbouring cells of the same snail ganglion: A' shows a depolarizing effect and B', an hyperpolarizing effect. Notice in A and B that both neurons show the same response to acetylcholine (ACh). In all the figures the white streaks indicate the application of the drug by perfusion. Right hand records: comparative action of different amino-acids on a snail neuron hyperpolarized by ACh (A). All the drugs were perfused with 10^{-3}M drug solutions. In B: with glutamic acid. In C: with aspartic acid; in D: with γ-aminobutyric acid. Notice the similarity of effect between mono- and dicarboxylic acids (Gerschenfeld and Lasansky, 1964).

3. Acetylcholine excites some neurones (D cells) and inhibits others (H cells). These cells receive cholinergic excitatory and inhibitory synaptic inputs respectively.

4. The depolarizing action of acetylcholine on some molluscan neurones is the result of an efflux of chloride ions. With other cells, an increase in sodium permeability is involved. An increase in chloride, and possibly potassium, ion permeabilities is responsible for the inhibitory actions of acetylcholine.

5. Catecholamines excite H cells and inhibit D cells and neurones with long duration inhibitions (CILDA cells). Dopamine is usually the most potent catecholamine.

6. 5-Hydroxytryptamine excites CILDA cells.

7. Histamine has been reported to excite some neurones in the snail *Helix aspersa* and to inhibit others. Glutamic acid and γ-aminobutyric acid have also been reported to have variable effects on molluscan neurones.

CHAPTER 11

CONCLUSIONS

THE preceding chapters of this book have been devoted to an account of the actions of various substances on a variety of structures in both vertebrates and invertebrates. Wherever possible, the evidence has been related to the seven criteria for acceptance of transmitter action discussed in Chapter 1. As the reader will now appreciate, it has frequently been impossible to conclude otherwise than that "the criteria for this substance at a given synaptic structure" are only partially satisfied. In many instances, satisfaction of the criteria of identical action (6) and pharmacological identification (7) remains as the greatest obstacle to acceptance of a substance as a transmitter. The technical difficulties of intracellular recording in the central nervous system may preclude a detailed analysis of the actions of potential transmitters on many of the small nerve cells in the brain and spinal cord and every effort should be made to develop potent, specific antagonists for the various compounds which are postulated as transmitters.

The availability of cholinergic antagonists, such as atropine and dihydro-β-erythroidine, has contributed extensively to the establishment of cholinergic transmission in several areas of the brain and spinal cord (see Chapter 7). Until it becomes possible to selectively antagonize the actions of the various monoamines, it will be difficult to establish, beyond doubt, their involvement as synaptic transmitters in the central nervous system. The same comment can be applied to amino acids such as glycine, γ-aminobutyric acid and glutamic acid.

The substances that have been considered in this book are those that the author considers to have a reasonable claim to be synaptic transmitters. Other compounds, such as ergothionine and adenosine triphosphate, have been omitted in the belief that the available evidence does not justify their inclusion. It would be surprising if the future did not reveal new promising candidates for the role of synaptic transmitters. Many indeed are the reports of biological activity in brain extracts, which are difficult to adequately explain on the basis of known substances. With improvements in the techniques for extraction and identification, a whole plethora of biologically active compounds may yet emerge from the vaults of the brain.

Of particular importance to the neuropharmacologist must be the re-emergence of the electrical hypothesis of synaptic transmission. It has been claimed that recent data on monosynaptic transmission from dorsal root afferents to spinal cord motoneurones is consistent with either electrical or chemical models of transmission (Rall *et al.*, 1967). The difficulties inherent in evaluating the results obtained from cells in which the excitatory synaptic input is largely restricted to the dendritic tree have been stressed in Chapter 7. A particularly significant paper on the distribution of excitatory and inhibitory synapses on the lateral dendrites of Mauthner cells in goldfish has recently been published by Diamond (1968). The large size of these dendrites makes them particularly suitable for intracellular recording. Evidence was adduced for the presence of both excitatory and inhibitory receptors on both the proximal and distal parts of the lateral dendrites. The distally-located inhibitory endings were the cause of *dendritic remote inhibition*, which was not detectable by an electrode in the cell soma. Excitatory junctional potentials generated out on the dendrites were most affected by this inhibition, whereas those produced in the cell body and axon hillock were least affected. *Gamma*-aminobutyric acid had a similar action to the inhibitory transmitter and also appeared to act presynaptically, reducing the output of excitatory transmitter. These findings raise some doubts concerning the assumption that depolarization of the presynaptic terminals is solely responsible for the phenomenon of presynaptic inhibition in the vertebrate spinal cord (Eccles, 1964). Generation of remote dendritic inhibition could also account for the observed phenomena and it is conceivable that the release of a substance such as γ-aminobutyric acid from inhibitory synapses on the motoneurone dendrites would cause a depolarization of adjacent afferent fibre terminals at the same time as a postsynaptic inhibition. A depolarizing action of γ-aminobutyric acid on dorsal root terminals and simultaneous hyperpolarization of motoneurones has been reported in the toad spinal cord (Tebēcis and Phillis, 1967). Presynaptic inhibition in the vertebrate spinal cord is blocked by picrotoxin (Eccles, 1964), which also antagonized the actions of γ-aminobutyric acid at ganglionic and crustacean neuromuscular junctions (De Groat, 1966; Robbins, 1959).

The observation that artificially applied transmitters will react with the synapse-free cell soma of molluscan neurones in a comparable manner to their action on the axonal synaptic receptors has important implications. The possibility that diffusion of these agents to axonal receptors is responsible for the permeability changes has been excluded by the experiments of Frank and Tauc (1964), who studied the actions of acetylcholine on minute, voltage clamped areas of the membrane of ganglion cells in *Helix* and *Aplysia*. The presence of receptors for various transmitters may thus constitute a basic property of neuronal membranes. In this instance, a synapse would be constituted when a developing presynaptic terminal "recognized" the correct receptor for its particular transmitter and formed a morphologically distinct junction. A hypothesis along these lines might account for the high proportion of nerve cells which respond to the various potential transmitters. For example, although dopamine, noradrenaline and adrenaline depress the excitability of many cells in the neocerebellar cortex (Phillis, 1965; Yamamoto, 1967), histochemistry reveals only a limited noradrenergic innervation of the cerebellar cortex (Andén, Fuxe and Ungerstedt, 1967).

This hypothesis derives support from the studies of the distribution of acetylcholine receptors on skeletal muscles described in Chapter 4. These clearly demonstrate that the ability to produce acetylcholine-receptor sites is an inherent property of the muscle membrane (Miledi, 1960a). It is the process of innervation which results in a contraction of the area of receptive membrane to the junctional region.

The response of a cell to a particular substance may therefore indicate the presence of potential synaptic receptors rather than of actual junctional synapses.

REFERENCES

ABRAHAMS, V. C. and EDERY, H. (1964) Brain stem electrical activity and the release of acetylcholine. *Progr. Brain Res.* **6**, 26–35.

ADAM, H. M. (1961) Histamine in the central nervous system and hypophysis of the dog. In: *Regional Neurochemistry*, pp. 293–305. Ed. S. S. Kety and J. Elkes. Oxford: Pergamon Press.

ADAM, H. M. and HYE, H. K. A. (1964) Effect of drugs on the concentration of histamine in the hypophysis and proximate parts of the brain. *J. Physiol. (Lond.)* **171**, 37–38P.

ADAM, H. M. and HYE, H. K. A. (1966) Concentration of histamine in different parts of brain and hypophysis of cat and its modification by drugs. *Br. J. Pharmac. Chemother.* **28**, 137–152.

ADRIAN, E. D. (1941) Afferent discharges to the cerebral cortex from peripheral sense organs. *J. Physiol. (Lond.)* **100**, 159–191.

AGHAJANIAN, G. K. and BLOOM, F. E. (1967a) Electron-microscopic localization of tritiated norepinephrine in rat brain: Effect of drugs. *J. Pharmac. exp. Ther.* **156**, 407–416.

AGHAJANIAN, G. K. and BLOOM, F. E. (1967b) Localization of tritiated serotonin in rat brain by electron-microscopic autoradiography. *J. Pharmac. exp. Ther.* **156**, 23–30.

AGHAJANIAN, G. K., ROSECRANS, J. A. and SHEARD, M. H. (1967) Serotonin: Release in the forebrain by stimulation of midbrain raphé. *Science, N.Y.* **156**, 402–403.

AHLQUIST, R. P. (1948) A study of adrenotropic receptors. *Am. J. Physiol.* **153**, 586–600.

AHLQUIST, R. P. and LEVY, B. (1959) Adrenergic receptive mechanism of the canine ileum. *J. Pharmac. exp. Ther.* **127**, 146–156.

ALBE-FESSARD, D. and HESSE, O. (1953) Le facteur de pression artérielle dans l'accroissement adrénalinique de l'activité corticale chez le lapin. *J. Physiol. (Paris)* **45**, 16–20.

ALBERS, R. W. and BRADY, R. O. (1959) Distribution of glutamic decarboxylase in the nervous system of the Rhesus monkey. *J. biol. Chem.* **234**, 926–928.

ALDRIDGE, W. N. and JOHNSON, M. K. (1959) Cholinesterase, succinic dehydrogenase, nucleic acids, esterase and glutathione reductase in sub-cellular fractions from rat brain. *Biochem. J.* **73**, 270–276.

AMBACHE, N. (1946) Interaction of drugs and the effect of cooling on the isolated mammalian intestine. *J. Physiol. (Lond.)* **104**, 266–287.

AMBACHE, N. (1951) Unmasking after cholinergic paralysis by botulinum toxin, of a reversed action of nicotine on the mammalian intestine, revealing the probable presence of local inhibitory ganglion cells in the enteric plexuses. *Br. J. Pharmac. Chemother.* **6**, 51–67.

AMBACHE, N. (1955) The use and limitations of atropine for pharmacological studies on autonomic effectors. *Pharmac. Rev.* **7**, 467–494.

AMBACHE, N. (1957a) Properties of irin, a physiological constituent of the rabbit's iris. *J. Physiol. (Lond.)* **135**, 114–132.

AMBACHE, N. (1957b) A rapid purification of irin and the use of the hamster colon for its assay. *J. Physiol. (Lond.)* **138**, 6–7P.

AMBACHE, N., BRUMMER, H. C., ROSE, J. G. and WHITING, J. (1966) Thin layer chromatography of spasmogenic unsaturated hydroxy-acids from various tissues. *J. Physiol.* (*Lond.*) **185**, 77–78P.

AMBACHE, N., KAVANAGH, L. and WHITING, J. (1965) Effect of mechanical stimulation on rabbits' eyes: Release of active substance in anterior chamber perfusates. *J. Physiol.* (*Lond.*) **176**, 378–408.

AMBACHE, N., PERRY, W. L. M. and ROBERSTON, P. A. (1956) The effects of muscarine on perfused superior cervical ganglia of cats. *Br. J. Pharmac. Chemother.* **11**, 442–448.

AMIN, A. H., CRAWFORD, T. B. B. and GADDUM, J. H. (1954) The distribution of substance P and 5-hydroxytryptamine in the central nervous system of the dog. *J. Physiol.* (*Lond.*) **126**, 596–618.

ANDÉN, N.-E. (1964) On the mechanism of noradrenaline depletion by α-methylmetatyrosine and metaraminol. *Acta pharmac. tox.* **21**, 260–271.

ANDÉN, N.-E. (1965) Distribution of monoamines and dihydroxyphenylalanine decarboxylase activity in the spinal cord. *Acta physiol. scand.* **64**, 197–203.

ANDÉN, N.-E., CARLSSON, A., DAHLSTRÖM, A., FUXE, K., HILLARP, N.-Å and LARSSON, K. (1964) Demonstrating and mapping out of nigro-neostriatal dopamine neurones. *Life Sci.* (*Oxford*) **3**, 523–530.

ANDÉN, N.-E., CARLSSON, A. HILLARP, N.-Å. and MAGNUSSON, T. (1964) 5-hydroxytryptamine release by nerve stimulation of the spinal cord. *Life Sci.* (*Oxford*) **3**, 473–478.

ANDÉN, N.-E., CARLSSON, A., HILLARP, N.-Å. and MAGNUSSON, T. (1965) Noradrenaline release by nerve stimulation of the spinal cord. *Life Sci.* (*Oxford*) **4**, 129–132.

ANDÉN, N.-E., DAHLSTRÖM, A., FUXE, K. and LARSSON, K. (1965) Further evidence for the presence of nigro-neostriatal dopamine neurones in the rat. *Am. J. Anat.* **116**, 329–334.

ANDÉN, N.-E., DAHLSTRÖM, A., FUXE, K., LARSSON, K., OLSON, L. and UNGERSTEDT, U. (1966) Ascending monoamine neurons to the telencephalon and diencephalon. *Acta physiol. scand.* **67**, 313–326.

ANDÉN, N.-E., FUXE, K., HAMBERGER, B. and HÖKFELT, T. (1966) A quantitative study on the nigro-neostriatal dopamine neuron system in the rat. *Acta physiol. scand.* **67**, 306–312.

ANDÉN, N.-E., FUXE, K. and UNGERSTEDT, U. (1967) Monoamine pathways to the cerebellum and cerebral cortex. *Experientia* **23**, 838–839.

ANDÉN, N.-E., HÄGGENDAL, J., MAGNUSSON, T. and ROSENGREN, E. (1964) The time-course of the disappearance of noradrenaline and 5-hydroxytryptamine in the spinal cord after transection. *Acta physiol. scand.* **62**, 115–118.

ANDÉN, N.-E., JUKES, M. G. M. and LUNDBERG, A. (1964) Spinal reflexes and monoamine liberation. *Nature* (*Lond.*) **202**, 1222–1223.

ANDÉN, N.-E., JUKES, M. G. M. and LUNDBERG, A. (1966) The effect of DOPA on the spinal cord. 2. A pharmacological analysis. *Acta physiol. scand.* **67**, 387–397.

ANDÉN, N.-E., JUKES, M. G. M., LUNDBERG, A. and VYKLICKY, L. (1966a) The effect of DOPA on the spinal cord. 1. Influence on transmission from primary afferents. *Acta physiol. scand.* **67**, 373–386.

ANDÉN, N.-E., JUKEŠ, M. G. M., LUNDBERG, A. and VYKLICKY, L. (1966b) The effect of DOPA on the spinal cord. 3. Depolarisation evoked in the central terminals of ipsilateral Ia afferents by volleys in the flexor reflex afferents. *Acta physiol. scand.* **68**, 322–336.

ANDERSEN, P. and CURTIS, D. R. (1964a) The excitation of thalamic neurones by acetylcholine. *Acta physiol. scand.* **61**, 85–99.

ANDERSEN, P. and CURTIS, D. R. (1964b) The pharmacology of the synaptic and acetylcholine-induced excitation of ventrobasal thalamic neurones. *Acta physiol. scand.* **61**, 100–120.

ANDERSEN, P., ECCLES, J. C., LØYNING, Y. and VOORHOEVE, P. E. (1963) Strychnine-resistant inhibition in the brain. *Nature (Lond.)* **200**, 843–845.

ANDERSON, E. G. and CUDIA, J. (1962) The anatomical localisation of norepinephrine and 5-hydroxytryptamine in cat spinal cord. *Am. Soc. exp. Biol.* **21**, 341.

ANDERSON, E. G. and HOLGERSON, L. O. (1966) The distribution of 5-hydroxytryptamine and norepinephrine in cat spinal cord. *J. Neurochem.* **13**, 479–485.

ANDERSON, E. G. and SHIBUYA, T. (1966) The effects of 5-hydroxytryptophan and L-tryptophan on spinal synaptic activity. *J. Pharmac. exp. Ther.* **153**, 352–360.

ANGELUCCI, L. (1956) Experiments with perfused frog's spinal cord. *Br. J. Pharmac. Chemother.* **11**, 161–170.

ÄNGGÅRD, E. and SAMUELSSON, B. (1964a) Smooth muscle stimulating lipids in sheep iris. The identification of prostaglandin F2α. *Biochem. Pharmacol.* **13**, 281–283.

ÄNGGÅRD, E. and SAMUELSSON, B. (1964b) Metabolism of prostaglandin E_1 in guinea pig lung: the structure of two metabolites. *J. biol. Chem.* **239**, 4097–4102.

ANTON, A. H. and SAYRE, D. F. (1964) The distribution of dopamine and dopa in various animals and a method for their determination in diverse biological material. *J. Pharmac. exp. Ther.* **145**, 326–336.

APRISON, M. H., GRAHAM, L. T., LIVENGOOD, D. R. and WERMAN, R. (1965) Distribution of glutamic acid in the cat spinal cord and roots. *Fed. Proc.* **24**, 462.

ARAKI, T., ITO, M. and OSCARSSON, O. (1961) Anion permeability of the synaptic and non-synaptic motoneurone membrane. *J. Physiol. (Lond.)* **159**, 410–435.

ARIËNS, E. J. and SIMONIS, A. M. (1962) Drug-receptor interaction. *Acta physiol. pharmac. Neerl.* **11**, 151–172.

ARNAIZ, R. G. DE L. and DE ROBERTIS, E. D. P. (1962) Cholinergic and non-cholinergic nerve endings in the rat brain. II. Subcellular localization of monoamine oxidase and succinate dehydrogenase. *J. Neurochem.* **9**, 503–508.

ARNAIZ, R. G. DE L. and DE ROBERTIS, E. D. P. (1964) 5-Hydroxytryptophan decarboxylase activity in nerve endings of the rat brain. *J. Neurochem.* **11**, 213–219.

ASCHER, P. (1968) Electrophoretic injections of dopamine in *Aplysia* neurones. *J. Physiol. (Lond.)*

ASCHER, P., KEHOE, J. S. and TAUC, L. (1967) Effets d'injections électrophorétiques de dopamine sur les neurones d'Aplysie. *J. Physiol. (Paris)* **59**, 331–332P.

ATWOOD, H. L. (1965) Excitation and inhibition in crab muscle fibres. *Comp. Biochem. Physiol.* **16**, 409–426.

ATWOOD, H. L., PARNAS, I. and WIERSMA, C. A. G. (1967) Inhibition in crustacean phasic neuromuscular systems. *Comp. Biochem. Physiol.* **20**, 163–177.

AUGUSTINSSON, K.-B. and NACHMANSOHN, D. (1949) Distinction between acetylcholinesterase and other choline ester-splitting enzymes. *Science, N.Y.* **110**, 98–99.

AUSTIN, L. and PHILLIS, J. W. (1965) The distribution of cerebellar cholinesterases in several species. *J. Neurochem.* **12**, 709–717.

AVANZINO, G. L., BRADLEY, P. B. and WOLSTENCROFT, J. H. (1966) Actions of prostaglandins E_1, E_2, and F2α on brain stem neurones. *Br. J. Pharmac. Chemother.* **27**, 157–163.

AXELROD, J. (1962) Purification and properties of phenylethanolamine-N-methyltransferase. *J. biol. Chem.* **237**, 1657–1660.

AXELROD, J. (1968) The fate of norepinephrine and the effect of drugs. *Physiologist* **11**, 63–73.

AXELROD, J., ALBERS, W. and CLEMENTE, C. D. (1959) Distribution of catechol-O-methyltransferase in the nervous system and other tissues. *J. Neurochem.* **5**, 68–72.

AXELROD, J., MACLEAN, P. D., ALBERS, R. W. and WEISSBACH, H. (1961) Regional distribution of methyltransferase enzymes in the nervous system and glandular tissues. In: *Regional Neurochemistry*, pp. 307–311. Ed. S. S. Kety and J. Elkes, Oxford: Pergamon Press.

AXELROD, J. and WEISSBACH, H. (1960) Enzymatic O-methylation of N-acetylserotonin to melatonin. *Science, N.Y.* **131**, 1312.

AXELROD, J. and WEISSBACH, H. (1961) Purification and properties of hydroxyindole-O-methyltransferase. *J. biol. Chem.* **236**, 211–213.

AXELSSON, J. and THESLEFF, S. (1958) The "desensitizing" effect of acetylcholine on the mammalian motor endplate. *Acta physiol. scand.* **43**, 15–26.

AXELSSON, J. and THESLEFF, S. (1959) A study of supersentivity in denervated mammalian skeletal muscle. *J. Physiol. (Lond.)* **147**, 178–193.

BACQ, Z. M. and BROWN, G. L. (1937) Pharmacological experiments on mammalian voluntary muscle in relation to the theory of chemical transmission. *J. Physiol. (Lond.)* **89**, 45–60.

BACQ, Z. M. and COPPEE, G. (1937) Réaction des vers et des mollusques a l'éserine. Existence de nerfs cholinergiques chez les vers. *Arch. int. Physiol.* **45**, 310–324.

BACQ, Z. M. and GOFFART, M. (1939) L'Acetylcholine libre du sang veineux du tube digestif chez le chien. *Arch. int. Physiol.* **49**, 179–188.

BACQ, Z. M. and MONNIER, A. M. (1935) Recherches sur la physiologie et la pharmacologie du système nerveux autonome. XV. Variations de la polarisation des muscles lisses sous l'influence du système nerveux autonome et de ses mimétiques. *Arch. int. Physiol.* **40**, 467–484.

BAGCHI, S. P. and McGEER, P. L. (1964) Some properties of tyrosine hydroxylase from the caudate nucleus. *Life Sci. (Oxford)* **3**, 1195–1200.

BAKER, P. F. (1964) An efflux of ninhydrin-positive material associated with the operation of the Na+ pump in intact crab nerve immersed in Na+ free solutions. *Biochem. Biophys. Acta* **88**, 458–460.

BALDESSARINI, R. J. and KOPIN, I. J. (1966) S-Adenosylmethionine in brain and other tissues. *J. Neurochem.* **13**, 769–777.

BALZER, H., HOLTZ, P. and PALM, D. (1961) Reserpine and γ-aminobutyric acid content of the brain. *Experientia* **17**, 38–40.

BARLOW, R. B. (1955) *Introduction to Chemical Pharmacology*. London: Methuen.

BARRNETT, R. J. (1962) The fine structural localization of acetylcholinesterase at the myoneural junction. *J. cell. Biol.* **12**, 247–262.

BARRON, D. H. and MATTHEWS, B. H. C. (1938) The interpretation of potential changes in the spinal cord. *J. Physiol. (Lond.)* **92**, 276–321.

BARSTAD, J. A. B. (1962) Presynaptic effect of the neuromuscular transmitter. *Experientia* **18**, 579–580.

BASIL, B., BLAIR, A. M. J. N. and HOLMES, S. W. (1964) The action of sodium 4-hydroxybutyrate on spinal reflexes. *Br. J. Pharmac. Chemother.* **22**, 318–328.

BAUST, W. and KATZ, P. (1961) Untersuchungen zur Tonisierung einzelner Neurone in hinteren Hypothalamus. *Pflügers Arch. ges. Physiol.* **272**, 575–590.

BAUST, W. and NIEMCZYK, H. (1963) Studies on the adrenaline-sensitive component of the mesencephalic reticular formation. *J. Neurophysiol.* **26**, 692–704.

BAUST, W., NIEMCZYK, H. and VIETH, J. (1963) The action of blood pressure on the ascending reticular activating system with special reference to adrenaline-induced EEG arousal. *Electroen. Neurophysiol.* **15**, 63–72.

BELESLIN, D., RADMANOVIĆ, B. and VARAGIĆ, V. (1960) The effect of substance P on the superior cervical ganglion of the cat. *Br. J. Pharmac. Chemother.* **15**, 10–13.

BENNETT, M. V. L., ALJURE, E., NAKAJIMA, Y. and PAPPAS, G. D. (1963) Electrotonic junctions between teleost spinal neurones: electrophysiology and ultrastructure. *Science. N.Y.* **141**, 262–264.

BENTLEY, G. A. and SMITH, G. (1967) Effects of alpha-adrenergic receptor blocking drugs on the response of vas deferens and arterial muscle to sympathetic drugs and stimulation. *Circulation Res.* **21**, Suppl. III, 101–110.

BERGER, W. (1963) Die Doppelsaccharosetrennwandtechnik. Eine Methode zur Untersuchung des Membranpotentials und der Membraneigenschaften glatter Muskelzellen. *Pflügers Arch. ges. Physiol.* **277**, 570–576.

BERGSTRÖM, S., ELIASSON, R., EULER, U. S. VON and SJÖVALL, J. (1959) Some biological effects of two crystalline prostaglandin factors. *Acta physiol. scand.* **45**, 133–144.

BERGSTRÖM, S., RYHAGE, R., SAMUELSSON, B. and SJÖVALL, J. (1962) The structure of prostaglandin E, F_1 and F_2. *Acta chem. scand.* **16**, 501–502.

BERGSTRÖM, S. and SJÖVALL, J. (1957) The isolation of prostaglandin. *Acta. chem. scand.* **11**, 1086.

BERGSTRÖM, S. and SJÖVALL, J. (1960a) The isolation of prostaglandin F from sheep prostate glands. *Acta chem. scand.* **14**, 1693–1700.

BERGSTRÖM, S. and SJÖVALL, J. (1960b) The isolation of prostaglandin E from sheep prostate glands. *Acta chem. scand.* **14**, 1701–1705.

BERNHARD, C. G. and SKOGLUND, C. R. (1963) Potential changes in spinal cord following intra-arterial administration of adrenaline and noradrenaline as compared with acetylcholine effects. *Acta physiol. scand.* **29**, Suppl. 106, 435–454.

BERNHARD, C. G., SKOGLUND, C. R. and THERMAN, P. O. (1947) Studies of the potential level in the ventral root under varying conditions. *Acta physiol. scand.* **14**, Suppl. 47, 8.

BERTLER, Å. (1961) Occurrence and localization of catecholamines in the human brain. *Acta physiol. scand.* **51**, 97–107.

BERTLER, Å., FALCK, B., GOTTFRIES, C. G., LJUNGGREN, L. and ROSENGREN, E. (1964) Some observations on adrenergic connections between mesencephalon and cerebral hemispheres. *Acta pharmac. tox.* **21**, 283–289.

BERTLER, Å., HILLARP, N. Å. and ROSENGREN, E. (1960) "Bound" and "free" catecholamines in the brain. *Acta physiol. scand.* **50**, 113–118.

BERTLER, Å. and ROSENGREN, E. (1959) Occurrence and distribution of catecholamines in brain. *Acta physiol. scand.* **47**, 350–361.

BEVAN, J. A. and SU, M. S. C. (1964) The sympathetic mechanism in the isolated pulmonary artery of the rabbit. *Br. J. Pharmac. Chemother.* **22**, 176–182.

BEYCHOCK, S. (1965) On the problem of isolation of the specific acetylcholine receptor. *Biochem. Pharmacol.* **14**, 1249–1255.

BHARGAVA, K. P. and SRIVASTAVA, R. K. (1964) Nonspecific depressant action of γ-aminobutyric acid on somatic reflexes. *Br. J. Pharmac. Chemother.* **23**, 391–398.

BIRKS, R. I. (1963) The role of sodium ions in the metabolism of acetylcholine. *Can. J. Biochem. Physiol.* **41**, 2573–2597.

BIRKS, R. I. and COHEN, M. W. (1965) Effects of sodium on transmitter release from frog motor nerve terminals. In: *Muscle, Proceedings of Symposium at University of Alberta*, pp. 403–420. London: Pergamon Press.

BIRKS, R. I., HUXLEY, H. E. and KATZ, B. (1960) The fine structure of the neuromuscular junction of the frog. *J. Physiol. (Lond.)* **150**, 134–144.

BIRKS, R. I. KATZ, B. and MILEDI, R. (1960) Physiological and structural changes at the amphibian myoneural junction, in the course of nerve degeneration. *J. Physiol. (Lond.)* **150**, 145–168.

BIRKS, R. I. and MACINTOSH, F. C. (1957) Acetylcholine metabolism at nerve endings. *Br. med. Bull.* **13**, 157–161.

BIRKS, R. I. and MacINTOSH, F. C. (1961) Acetylcholine metabolism of a sympathetic ganglion. *Can. J. Biochem. Physiol.* **39**, 787–827.

BISCOE, T. J. and CURTIS, D. R. (1966) Noradrenaline and inhibition of Renshaw cells. *Science, N.Y.* **151**, 1230–1231.

BISCOE, T. J., CURTIS, D. R. and RYALL, R. W. (1966) An investigation of catecholamine receptors of spinal interneurones. *Int. J. Neuropharmac.* **5**, 429–434.

BISCOE, T. J. and STRAUGHAN, D. W. (1966) Micro-electrophoretic studies of neurones in the cat hippocampus. *J. Physiol. (Lond.)* **183**, 341–359.

BISHOP, P. O., BURKE, W., DAVIS, R. and HAYHOW, W. R. (1960) Drugs as tools in visual physiology with particular reference to (a) the effects of prolonged disuse, and (b) the origin of the electroencephalogram. *Trans. ophthal. Soc. Aust.* **20**, 50–65.

BISHOP, P. O., BURKE, W. and HAYHOW, W. R. (1959) Lysergic acid diethylamide block of lateral geniculate synapses and relief by repetitive stimulation. *Expl. Neurol.* **1**, 556–568.

BISHOP, P. O., FIELD, G., HENNESSY, B. L. and SMITH, J. R. (1958) Action of D-lysergic acid diethylamide on lateral geniculate synapses. *J. Neurophysiol.* **21**, 529–549.

BLABER, L. C. (1967) Personal communication. Quoted by Karczmar, A. G. in *Neuromuscular Pharmacology. A. Rev. Pharmac.* **7**, 241–276.

BLABER, L. C. and BOWMAN, W. C. (1963) The effects of some drugs on the repetitive discharges produced in nerve and muscle by anticholinesterases. *Int. J. Neuropharmac.* **2**, 1–16.

BLACKMAN, J. G., GINSBORG, B. L. and RAY, C. (1963) Synaptic transmission in the sympathetic ganglion of the frog. *J. Physiol. (Lond.)* **167**, 355–373.

BLASCHKO, H. and LEVINE, W. G. (1966) Metabolism of indolealkylamines. *Handbk. exp. Pharmak.* **14**, 212–244.

BLOOM, F. E., COSTA, E. and SALMOIRAGHI, G. C. (1965) Anaesthesia and the responsiveness of individual neurones of the caudate nucleus of the cat to acetylcholine, norepinephrine and dopamine administered by microelectrophoresis. *J. Pharmac. exp. Ther.* **150**, 244–252.

BLOOM, F. E. and GIARMAN, N. J. (1968) Physiologic and pharmacologic considerations of biogenic amines in the nervous system. *A. Rev. Pharmac.* **8**, 229–258.

BLOOM, F. E., OLIVER, A. P. and SALMOIRAGHI, G. C. (1963) The responsiveness of individual hypothalamic neurones to microelectrophoretically administered endogeneous amines. *Int. J. Neuropharmac.* **2**, 181–193.

BOGDANSKI, D. F., WEISSBACH, H. and UDENFRIEND, S. (1957) The distribution of serotonin, 5-hydroxytryptamine decarboxylase and monoamine oxidase in brain. *J. Neurochem.* **1**, 272–278.

BOISTEL, J. and FATT, P. (1968) Membrane permeability change during inhibitory transmitter action in crustacean muscle. *J. Physiol. (Lond.)* **144**, 176–191.

BONVALLET, M., DELL, P. and HIEBEL, G. (1954) Tonus sympathique et activité électrique corticale. *Electroen. Neurophysiol.* **6**, 119–144.

BONVALLET, M., HUGELIN, A. and DELL, P. (1956) Milieu intérieur et activité automatique des cellules réticulaires mésencéphaliques. *J. Physiol. (Paris)* **48**, 403–406.

BORN, G. V. R. and BÜLBRING, E. (1956) The movement of potassium between smooth muscle and the surrounding fluid. *J. Physiol. (Lond.)* **131**, 690–703.

BORTOFF, A. (1961) Electrical activity of intestine recorded with pressure electrode. *Am. J. Physiol.* **201**, 209–212.

BOVET-NITTI, F., KOHN, R., MAROTTA, M., SCOGNAMIGLIO, W. P. and SILVESTRINI, B. (1964) Histamine induced modification of neuromuscular blockade by lepto- and pachycurares. *Archs. int. Pharmacodyn.* **149**, 308–317.

BOWMAN, W. C., GOLDBERG, A. A. J. and RAPER, C. (1962) A comparison between the effects of a tetanus and the effects of sympathomimetic amines on fast- and slow-contracting mammalian muscles. *Br. J. Pharmac. Chemother.* **19**, 464–484.

BOWMAN, W. C. and HEMSWORTH, B. A. (1965) Effects of triethylcholine on the output of acetylcholine from the isolated diaphragm of the rat. *Br. J. Pharmac. Chemother.* **24**, 110–118.

BOWMAN, W. C., HEMSWORTH, B. A. and RAND, M. J. (1962) Triethylcholine compared with other substances affecting neuromuscular transmission. *Br. J. Pharmac. Chemother.* **19**, 198–218.

BOWMAN, W. C. and RAND, M. J. (1961) Actions of triethylcholine on neuromuscular transmission. *Br. J. Pharmac. Chemother.* **17**, 176–195.

BOWMAN, W. C. and RAPER, C. (1964) The effects of adrenaline and other drugs affecting carbohydrate metabolism on contractions of the rat diaphragm. *Br. J. Pharmac. Chemother.* **23**, 184–200.

BOWMAN, W. C. and RAPER, C. (1965) The effects of sympathomimetic amines on chronically denervated skeletal muscles. *Br. J. Pharmac. Chemother.* **24**, 98–109.

BOWMAN, W. C. and RAPER, C. (1966) Effects of sympathomimetic amines on neuro-muscular transmission. *Br. J. Pharmac. Chemother.* **27**, 313–331.

BOYD, I. A. and MARTIN, A. R. (1956) The end-plate potential in mammalian muscle. *J. Physiol. (Lond.)* **132**, 74–91.

BOZLER, E. (1940) An analysis of the excitatory and inhibitory effects of sympathetic nerve impulses and adrenaline on visceral smooth muscle. *Am. J. Physiol.* **130**, 627–634.

BOZLER, E. (1948) Conduction, automaticity and tonus of visceral muscles. *Experientia* **4**, 213–218.

BRADFORD, H. F., and McILWAIN, H. (1966) Ionic basis for the depolarization of cere-bral tissues by excitatory acidic amino acids. *J. Neurochem.* **13**, 1163–1177.

BRADLEY, P. B. (1960) Electrophysiological evidence relating to the role of adrenaline in the central nervous system. Ciba Symp. *Adrenergic Mechanisms*, pp. 410–420. J. and A. Churchill Ltd. London.

BRADLEY, P. B., DHAWAN, B. N. and WOLSTENCROFT, J. H. (1966) Pharmacological properties of cholinoceptive neurones in the medulla and pons of the cat. *J. Phsyiol. (Lond.)* **183**, 658–674.

BRADLEY, P. B. and MOLLICA, A. (1958) The effect of adrenaline and acetylcholine on single unit activity in the reticular formation of the decerebrate cat. *Archs. ital. Biol.* **96**, 168–186.

BRADLEY, P. B. and WOLSTENCROFT, J. H. (1962) Excitation and inhibition of brain stem neurones by noradrenaline and acetylcholine. *Nature (Lond.)* **196**, 840, 873.

BRADLEY, P. B. and WOLSTENCROFT, J. H. (1965) Actions of drugs on single neurones in the brain stem. *Br. med. Bull.* **21**, 15–18.

BRADLEY, P. B., WOLSTENCROFT, J. H., HÖSLI, L. and AVANZINO, G. L. (1966) Neuronal basis for the central action of chlorpromazine. *Nature (Lond.)* **212**, 1425–1427.

BRANCH, C. L. and MARTIN, A. R. (1958) Inhibition of Betz cell activity by thalamic and cortical stimulation. *J. Neurophysiol.* **21**, 380–390.

BRODIE, B. B., COMER, M. S., COSTA, E. and DLABAC, A. (1966) The role of brain serotonin in the mechanism of the central action of reserpine. *J. Pharmac. exp. Ther.* **152**, 340–349.

BRODIE, B. B., FINGER, K. F., ORLANS, F. B., QUINN, G. P. and SULSER, F. (1960) Evidence that tranquilizing action of reserpine is associated with change in brain serotonin and not in brain norepinephrine. *J. Pharmac. exp. Ther.* **129**, 250–256.

BRODIE, B. B. and SHORE, P. A. (1957) A concept for a role of serotonin and norepine-phrine as chemical mediators in the brain. *Ann. N.Y. Acad. Sci.* **66**, 631–642.

BRODY, T. M. and DIAMOND, J. (1966) Blockade of the biochemical correlates of contraction and relaxation in uterine and intestinal smooth muscle. *Ann. N.Y. Acad. Sci.* **139**, 772–780.

BROOKS, V. B. (1954) The action of botulinum toxin on motor nerve filaments. *J. Physiol. (Lond.)* **123**, 501–515.

BROOKS, V. B. (1956) An intracellular study of the action of repetitive nerve volleys and of botulinum toxin on miniature endplate potentials. *J. Physiol. (Lond.)* **134**, 264–277.

BROOKS, V. B. and ASANUMA, H. (1965) Pharmacological studies of recurrent cortical inhibition and facilitation. *Am. J. Physiol.* **208**, 674–681.

BROOKS, V. B. and MEYERS, D. K. (1952) Cholinesterase content of normal and denervated skeletal muscle in the guinea-pig. *J. Physiol. (Lond.)* **116**, 158–167.

BROWN, D. A. (1966) Depolarization of normal and preganglionically denervated superior cervical ganglia by stimulant drugs. *Br. J. Pharmac. Chemother.* **26**, 511–520.

BROWN, D. D., TOMCHICK, R. and AXELROD, J. (1959) The distribution and properties of a histamine-methylating enzyme. *J. biol. Chem.* **234**, 2948–2950.

BROWN, G. L., DALE, H. H. and FELDBERG, W. (1936) Reactions of the normal mammalian muscle to acetylcholine and to eserine. *J. Physiol. (Lond.)* **87**, 394–424.

BROWN, G. L. and FELDBERG, W. (1936) The action of potassium on the superior cervical ganglion of the cat. *J. Physiol. (Lond.)* **86**, 290–305.

BROWN, G. L., GOFFART, M. and DIAS, M. V. (1950) The effects of adrenaline and of sympathetic stimulation on the demarcation potential of mammalian skeletal muscle. *J. Physiol. (Lond.)* **111**, 184–194.

BROWNLEE, G. and JOHNSON, E. S. (1963) The site of the 5-hydroxytryptamine receptor on the intramural nervous plexus of the guinea pig isolated ileum. *Br. J. Pharmac. Chemother.* **21**, 306–322.

BROWNLEE, G. and JOHNSON, E. S. (1965) The release of acetylcholine from the isolated ileum of the guinea pig induced by 5-hydroxytryptamine and dimethylphenyl-piperazinium. *Br. J. Pharmac. Chemother.* **24**, 689–700.

BRÜCKE, F. Th. v. (1937) Cholinesterase in sympathetic ganglia. *J. Physiol. (Lond.)* **89**, 429–437.

BRÜCKE, F., GOGOLÁK, G. and STUMPF, CH. (1961) Die wirkung von LSD auf die Makro- und Mikrotätigkeit des Hippocampus. Naunyn-Schmiedeberg's *Arch. exp. Path. Pharmak.* **240**, 461–468.

BRZIN, M. and ZAJICEK, J. (1958) Quantitative determination of cholinesterase activity in individual endplates of normal and denervated gastrocnemius muscle. *Nature (Lond.)* **181**, 626.

BUCKLEY, G., CONSOLO, S., GIACOBINI, E. and SJÖQVIST, F. (1967) Cholinacetylase in innervated and denervated sympathetic ganglia and ganglion cells of the cat. *Acta physiol. scand.* **71**, 348–356.

BUEDING, E., BÜLBRING, E., GERCKEN, G., HAWKINS, J. T. and KURIYAMA, H. (1967) The effect of adrenaline on the adenosinetriphosphate and creatine phosphate content of intestinal smooth muscle. *J. Physiol. (Lond.)* **193**, 187–212.

BULAT, M. and SUPEK, Z. (1967) The penetration of 5-hydroxytryptamine through the blood-brain barrier. *J. Neurochem.* **14**, 265–271.

BÜLBRING, E. (1944) The action of adrenaline on transmission in the superior cervical ganglion. *J. Physiol. (Lond.)* **103**, 55–67.

BÜLBRING, E. (1954) Membrane potentials of smooth muscle fibres of the taenia coli of the guinea pig. *J. Physiol. (Lond.)* **125**, 302–315.

BÜLBRING, E. (1957) Changes in configuration of spontaneously discharged spike potentials from smooth muscle of the guinea-pig's taenia coli. The effect of electronic currents and of adrenaline, acetylcholine and histamine. *J. Physiol. (Lond.)* **135,** 412–425.

BÜLBRING, E. and BURN, J. H. (1941) Observations bearing on synaptic transmission by acetylcholine in the spinal cord. *J. Physiol. (Lond.)* **100,** 337–368.

BÜLBRING, E. and BURN, J. H. (1942a) The interrelation of prostigmine, adrenaline and ephedrine in skeletal muscle. *J. Physiol. (Lond.)* **101,** 224–235.

BÜLBRING, E. and BURN, J. H. (1942b) An action of adrenaline on transmission in sympathetic ganglia, which may play a part in shock. *J. Physiol. (Lond.)* **101,** 289–303.

BÜLBRING, E. and BURNSTOCK, G. (1960) Membrane potential changes associated with tachyphylaxis and potentiation of the response to stimulating drugs in smooth muscle. *Br. J. Pharmac. Chemother.* **15,** 611–624.

BÜLBRING, E., GOODFORD, P. J. and SETEKLIEV, J. (1966) The action of adrenaline on the ionic content and on sodium and potassium movements in the smooth muscle of the guinea-pig taenia coli. *Br. J. Pharmac. Chemother.* **28,** 296–307.

BÜLBRING, E. and KURIYAMA, H. (1963) Effects of changes in ionic environment on the action of acetylcholine and adrenaline on the smooth muscle cells of guinea-pig taenia coli. *J. Physiol. (Lond.)* **166,** 59–74.

BÜLBRING, E. and LIN, R. C. Y. (1958) The effect of intraluminal application of 5-hydroxytryptamine and 5-hydroxytryptophan on peristalsis; the local production of 5-HT and its release in relation to intraluminal pressure and propulsive activity. *J. Physiol (Lond.)* **140,** 381–407.

BÜLBRING, E. and LÜLLMAN, H. (1957) The effect of metabolic inhibitors on the electrical and mechanical activity of the smooth muscle of the guinea-pig's taenia coli. *J. Physiol. (Lond.)* **136,** 310–323.

BÜLBRING, E. and TOMITA, T. (1968) The effect of catecholamines on the membrane resistance and spike generation in the smooth muscle of guinea-pig taenia coli. *J. Physiol. (Lond.)* **194,** 74–76P.

BULL, G., FEINSTEIN, A. and MORRIS, D. (1964) Sedimentation behaviour and molecular weight of choline acetyltransferase. *Nature (Lond.)* **201,** 1326.

BULL, G. and HEMSWORTH, B. A. (1963) Inhibition of biological synthesis of acetylcholine by triethylcholine. *Nature (Lond.)* **199,** 487–488.

BULLOCK, T. H. (1961) On the anatomy of the giant neurones of the visceral ganglion of *Aplysia.* In: *Nervous Inhibition,* pp. 233–240. Ed. E. Florey, London: Pergamon Press.

BULLOCK, T. H. and HORRIDGE, G. A. (1965) *Structure and Function in the Nervous Systems of Invertebrates.* London: W. H. Freeman.

BURGEN, A. S. V. and CHIPMAN, L. M. (1951) Cholinesterase and succinic dehydrogenase in the central nervous system of the dog. *J. Physiol. (Lond.)* **114,** 296–305.

BURGEN, A. S. V., DICKENS, F. and ZATMAN, L. J. (1949) The action of botulinum toxin on the neuromuscular junction. *J. Physiol. (Lond.)* **109,** 10–24.

BURKARD, W. P., GEY, K. F. and PLETSCHER, A. (1963) Diamine oxidase in the brain of vertebrates. *J. Neurochem.* **10,** 183–186.

BURKARD, W. P., GEY, K. F. and PLETSCHER, A. (1964) Inhibition of the hydroxylation of tryptophan and phenylalanine by α-methyldopa and similar compounds. *Life Sci. (Oxford)* **3,** 27–33.

BURKE, R. E. (1967) Composite nature of the monosynaptic excitatory postsynaptic potential. *J. Neurophysiol.* **30,** 1114–1137.

BURN, J. H. and DALE, H. H. (1915) The action of certain quarternary ammonium bases. *J. Pharmac. exp. Ther.* **6,** 417–438.

BURN, J. H. and RAND, M. J. (1965) Acetylcholine in adrenergic transmission. *A. Rev. Pharmac.* **5**, 163–182.

BURNSTOCK, G. (1958) The action of adrenaline on excitability and membrane potential in the taenia coli of the guinea pig and the effect of DNP on this action and on the action of acetylcholine. *J. Physiol. (Lond.)* **143**, 183–194.

BURNSTOCK, G. (1960) Membrane potential changes associated with stimulation of smooth muscle by adrenalin. *Nature (Lond.)* **186**, 727–728.

BURNSTOCK, G., CAMPBELL, G., BENNETT, M. and HOLMAN, M. E. (1964) Innervation of the guinea-pig taenia coli: Are there intrinsic inhibitory nerves which are distinot from sympathetic nerves? *Int. J. Neuropharmac.* **3**, 163–166.

BURNSTOCK, G. and HOLMAN, M. E. (1961) The transmission of excitation from autonomic nerve to smooth muscle. *J. Physiol. (Lond.)* **155**, 115–133.

BURNSTOCK, G. and HOLMAN, M. E. (1962) The effect of denervation and of reserpine treatment on transmission at sympathetic nerve endings. *J. Physiol. (Lond.)* **160**, 461–469.

BURNSTOCK, G. and HOLMAN, M. E. (1964) An electrophysiological investigation of the actions of some autonomic blocking drugs on transmission in the guinea-pig vas deferens. *Br. J. Pharmac. Chemother.* **23**, 600–612.

BURNSTOCK, G. and HOLMAN, M. E. (1966a) Effect of drugs on smooth muscle. *A. Rev. Pharmac.* **6**, 129–156.

BURNSTOCK, G. and HOLMAN, M. E. (1966b) Junctional potentials at adrenergic synapses. *Pharmac. Rev.* **18**, 481–493.

BURNSTOCK, G., HOLMAN, M. E. and PROSSER, C. L. (1963) Electrophysiology of smooth muscle. *Physiol. Rev.* **43**, 482–527.

BYGDEMAN, M., KWON, S., WIQVIST, N. (1967) The effect of prostaglandin E_1 on human pregnant myometrium *in vivo*. In *Nobel Symposium 2: Prostaglandins*. Ed. S. Bergström and B. Samuelsson. Stockholm: Almqvist & Wiksell.

BYGDEMAN, M. and SAMUELSSON, B. (1966) Analyses of prostaglandins in human semen. *Clin. chim. Acta* **13**, 465–474.

CALMA, I. and WRIGHT, S. (1944) Action of acetylcholine, atropine and eserine on the central nervous system of the decerebrate cat. *J. Physiol. (Lond.)* **103**, 93–102.

CAMBRIDGE, G. W., HOLGATE, J. A. and SHARP, J. A. (1959) A pharmacological analysis of the contractile mechanism of *Mytilus* muscle. *J. Physiol. (Lond.)* **148**, 451–464.

CANNON, W. B. and BACQ, Z. M. (1931) Studies on the conditions of activity in endocrine organs. XXVI. A hormone produced by sympathetic action on smooth muscle. *Am. J. Physiol.* **96**, 392–412.

CAPON, A. (1958) Analyse de l'effet d'éveil exercé par l'adrénaline et la noradrénaline sur électrocorticogramme du lapin non narcotisé. *J. Physiol. (Paris)* **50**, 201–204.

CAPON, A. (1960) Analyse de l'effet d'éveil exercé par l'adrénaline et d'autres amines sympathomimétiques sur l'electrocorticogramme du lapin non narcotisé. *Archs. int. Pharmacodyn. Thér.* **127**, 141–162.

CARELS, G. (1962) Depression par la sérotonine de la transmission monosynaptique dans la moelle isolée de la grenouille. *Archs. int. Pharmacodyn. Thér.* **138**. 326–328.

CARLINI, E. A. and GREEN, J. P. (1963a) Acetylcholine activity in the sciatic nerve, *Biochem. Pharmacol.* **12**, 1367–1376.

CARLINI, E. A. and GREEN, J. P. (1963b) The subcellular distribution of histamine, slow reacting substance and 5-hydroxytryptamine in the brain of the rat. *Br. J. Pharmac. Chemother.* **20**, 264–277.

CARLINI, E. A. and GREEN, J. P. (1963c) The measurement of histamine in brain and its distribution. *Biochem. Pharmacol.* **12**, 1448–1449.

CARLSSON, A. (1959) The occurrence, distribution and physiological role of catecholamines in the nervous system. *Pharmacol. Rev.* **11**, 490–493.

CARLSSON, A. (1964) Functional significance of drug-induced changes in brain monoamine levels. *Progr. Brain Res.* **8**, 9–27.

CARLSSON, A. (1966) Drugs which block the storage of 5-hydroxytryptamine and related amines. *Handb. exp. Pharmak.* **19**, 529–592.

CARLSSON, A., CORRODI, H. and WALDECK, B. (1963) [Inhibition of catechol-O-methyltransferase (COMT) and of enzymic hydroxylation of aromatic amino acids by α-substituted dopacetamides. Substances affecting catecholamine metabolism.] *Helv. chim. Acta* **46**, 2271–2285.

CARLSSON, A., DAHLSTRÖM, A., FUXE, K. and HILLARP, N. Å. (1965) Failure of reserpine to deplete noradrenaline neurons of α-methyl-noradrenaline formed from α-methyldopa. *Acta pharmac. tox.* **22**, 270–276.

CARLSSON, A., FALCK, B., FUXE, K. and HILLARP, N. Å. (1964) Cellular localisation of monoamines in the spinal cord. *Acta physiol. scand.* **60**, 112–119.

CARLSSON, A., FALCK, B. and HILLARP, N. Å. (1962) Cellular localisation of brain monoamines. *Acta physiol. scand.* **56**, Suppl. 196. 1–28.

CARLSSON, A., FALCK, B., HILLARP, N. Å. and TORP, A. (1962) Histochemical localization at the cellular level of hypothalamic noradrenaline. *Acta physiol scand.* **54**, 385–386.

CARLSSON, A. and HILLARP, N. Å. (1962) Formation of phenolic acids in brain after administration of 3,4-dihydroxy-phenylalanine. *Acta physiol. scand.* **55**, 95–100.

CARLSSON, A., LINDQVIST, M., MAGNUSSON, T. and WALDECK, B. (1958) On the presence of 3-hydroxytyramine in brain. *Science* **127**, 471.

CARLSSON, A., MAGNUSSON, T. and ROSENGREN, E. (1963) 5-Hydroxytryptamine in spinal cord, normally and after transection. *Experientia* **19**, 359.

CARLSSON, A. and WALDECK, B. (1964) A method for the fluorimetric determination of 3-methoxytyramine in tissues and the occurrence of this amine in brain. *Scand. J. clin. Lab. Inv.* **16**, 133–138.

CARROLL, P. R. and COBBIN, L. B. (1968) Acetylcholine and nervous transmission in *Tapes watlingi*. *Aust. J. exp. Biol. med. Sci.* **46**, 23P.

CASPERS, H. and STERN, P. (1961) Die Wirkung von Substanz P auf das Dendritenpotential und die Gleichspannungs-komponente des Neocortex. *Pflügers Arch. ges. Physiol.* **273**, 94–110.

CELESIA, G. G. and JASPER, H. H. (1966) Acetylcholine released from the cerebral cortex in relation to state of activation. *Neurology (Minneap.)* **16**, 1053–1063.

CERLETTI, A. and ROTHLIN, E. (1955) Role of 5-hydroxytryptamine in mental diseases and its antagonism to lysergic acid derivatives. *Nature (Lond.)* **176**, 675–686.

CHAGAS, C., PENNA-FRANCA, E., NISHIE, K., CROCKER, C. and MIRANDA, M. (1956) The fixation of triiodoethylate of radioactive gallamine on electroplates of *Electrophorus electricus*. *C.R. Acad. Sci.* **242**, 2671–2674.

CHANG, H-T., (1953) Similarity in action between curare and strychnine on cortical neurones. *J. Neurophysiol.* **16**, 221–233.

CHANG, H. C. and GADDUM, J. H. (1963) Choline esters in tissue extracts. *J. Physiol. (Lond.)* **79**, 255–285.

CHANG, V. and RAND, M. J. (1960) Transmission failure in sympathetic nerves produced by hemicholinium. *Br. J. Pharmac. Chemother.* **15**, 588–600.

CHAPMAN, J. B. and McCANCE, I. (1967) Acetylcholine-sensitive cells in the intracerebellar nuclei of the cat. *Brain Res.* **5**, 535–538.

CHASE, T. N. and KOPIN, I. J. (1968) Stimulus-induced release of substances from olfactory bulb using the push-pull cannula. *Nature (Lond.)* **217**, 466–467.

CHATFIELD, P. O. and LORD, J. T. (1955) Effects of atropine, prostigmine and acetylcholine on evoked cortical potentials. *Electroen. Neurophysiol.* **7**, 553–556.

CHATFIELD, P. O. and PURPURA, D. P. (1954) Augmentation of evoked cortical potentials by topical application of prostigmine and acetylcholine after atropinisation of cortex. *Electroen. Neurophysiol.* **6**, 287–298.

CHE SU, M. S. and BEVAN, J. A. (1967) Release of [³H] noradrenaline from vasoconstrictor nerves. *J. Pharm. Pharmac.* **19**, 625–626

CHE SU, M. S., BEVAN, J. A. and URSILLO, R. C. (1964) Electrical quiescence of pulmonary artery smooth muscle during sympathomimetic stimulation. *Circulation Res.* **15**, 26–27.

CHIARANDINI, D. J. and GERSCHENFELD, H. M. (1967) Ionic mechanism of cholinergic inhibition in molluscan neurones. *Science, N.Y.* **156**, 1595–1596.

CHIARANDINI, D. J., STEFANI, E., and GERSCHENFELD, H. M. (1967) Ionic mechanisms of cholinergic excitation in molluscan neurones. *Science, N.Y.* **156**, 1597–1599.

CHIRIGOS, M. A., GREENGARD, P. and UDENFRIEND, S. (1960) Uptake of tyrosine by rat brain *in vivo. J. biol. Chem.* **235**, 2075–2079.

CHONG, G. C. and PHILLIS, J. W. (1965) Pharmacological studies on the heart of *Tapes watlingi*, a mollusc of the family Veneridae. *Br. J. Pharmac. Chemother.* **25**, 481–496.

CHUJYO, N. (1952) Acetylcholine production in passively extended wall of the intestine. *Am. J. Physiol.* **170**, 668–672.

CLARK, W. G. (1959) Studies on inhibition of L-dopa decarboxylase *in vitro* and *in vivo. Pharmacol. Rev.* **11**, 330–349.

CLARK, M. E. (1966) Histochemical localization of monoamines in the nervous system of the polychaete *Nephtys. Proc. R. Soc. B* **165**, 308–325.

CLITHEROW, J. W., MITCHARD, M. and HARPER, N. J. (1963) The possible biological function of pseudocholinesterase. *Nature (Lond.)* **199**, 1000–1001.

CLOUET, D. H. and WAELSCH, H. (1961) Amino acid and protein metabolism of the brain. VII. The penetration of cholinesterase inhibitors into the nervous system of the frog. *J. Neurochem.* **8**, 189–200.

COBBIN, L. B., LEEDER, S. and POLLARD, J. (1965) Smooth muscle stimulants in extracts of optic nerves, optic tracts and lateral geniculate bodies of sheep. *Br. J. Pharmac. Chemother.* **25**, 295–306.

COCEANI, F., PACE-ASCIAK, C., VOLTA, F. and WOLFE, L. S. (1967) Effect of nerve stimulation on prostaglandin formation and release from the rat stomach. *Am. J. Physiol.* **213**, 1056–1064.

COCEANI, F. and WOLFE, L. S. (1965) Prostaglandins in brain and the release of prostaglandin-like compounds from the cat cerebellar cortex. *Can. J. Physiol. Pharmac.* **43**, 445–450.

COCEANI, F. and WOLFE, L. S. (1966) On the action of prostaglandin E₁ and prostaglandins from brain on the isolated rat stomach. *Can. J. Physiol. Pharmac.* **44**, 933–950.

COERS, C. (1953) La détetion histochemique de la cholinéstérase au niveau de la jonction neuro-musculaire. *Rev. belge. Path. et méd. expér.* **22**, 306–315.

COERS, C. (1955) Aspects histologiques de la régénération neuromusculaire au cours de diverse affections du neurone moteur périphérique (regeneration collatérale chez l'homme). *Acta neurol. et psychiat. belg.* **55**, 23–30.

COHEN, M. (1956) Concentration of choline acetylase in conducting tissue. *Arch. Biochem.* **60**, 284–296.

COLE, W. V. (1957) Structural variations of nerve endings in the striated muscles of the rat. *J. comp. Neurol.* **108**, 445–463.

COLLIER, B. and MURRAY-BROWN, N. (1968) Validity of a method measuring transmitter release from the central nervous system. *Nature (Lond.)* **218**, 434–435.

COLLINS, R. J. and SIMONTON, V. R. (1967) Inhibition of evoked potentials by caudate stimulation and its antagonism by centrally acting drugs. *Int. J. Neuropharmac.* **6**, 349–356.

COLOMO, F., RAHAMIMOFF, R. and STEFANI, E. (1968) An action of 5-hydroxytryptamine on the frog motor end-plate. *Europ. J. Pharmac.* **3**, 272–274.

COMIS, S. D. and WHITFIELD, I. C. (1966) The effect of acetylcholine on neurones of the cochlear nucleus. *J. Physiol. (Lond.)* **183**, 22–23P.

COOK, B. J. (1967) An investigation of Factor S, a neuromuscular excitatory substance from insects and crustacea. *Biol. Bull. mar. biol. Lab. Woods Hole* **133**, 526–538.

COOKE, I. M. (1966) The sites of action of pericardial organ extract and 5-hydroxytryptamine in the decapod crustacean heart. *Am. Zool.* **6**, 107–121.

COOMBS, J. S., ECCLES, J. C., and FATT, P. (1955) The specific ionic conductances and the ionic movements across the motoneuronal membrane that produce the inhibitory post-synaptic potential. *J. Physiol. (Lond.)* **130**, 326–373.

CORDEAU, J. P., MOREAU, A., BEAULNES, A. and LAURIN, C. (1963) EEG and behavioural changes following microinjections of acetylcholine in the brain stem of cats. *Archs. ital. Biol.* **101**, 30–47.

COSTA, E. (1960) The role of serotonin in neurobiology. *Int. Rev. Neurobiol.* **2**, 175–227.

COSTA, E. and APRISON, M. (1958) Distribution of intracarotidly injected serotonin in the brain. *Am. J. Physiol.* **192**, 95–100.

COSTA, E., PSCHEIDT, G. R., van MEETER, W. G. and HIMWICH, H. E. (1960) Brain concentrations of biogenic amines and e.e.g. patterns of rabbits. *J. Pharmac. exp. Ther.* **130**, 81–88.

COSTA, E., REVZIN, A. M., KUNTZMAN, R., SPECTOR, S., and BRODIE, B. B. (1961) Role for ganglionic norepinephrine in sympathetic synaptic transmission. *Science, N.Y.* **133**, 1822–1823.

COSTA, E. and RINALDI, F. (1958) Biochemical and electroencephalographic changes in the brain of rabbits injected with 5-hydroxytryptophan (influence of chlorpromazine premedication). *Am. J. Physiol.* **194**, 214–220.

COTTRELL, G. A. (1966) Separation and properties of subcellular particles associated with 5-hydroxytryptamine, with acetylcholine and with an unidentified cardioexcitatory substance from *Mercenaria* nervous tissue. *Comp. Biochem. Physiol.* **17**, 891–907.

COTTRELL, G. A. and LAVERACK, M. S. (1968) Invertebrate pharmacology. *A. Rev. Pharmac.* **8**, 273–298.

COTTRELL, G. A. and MASER, M. (1967) Subcellular localization of 5-hydroxytryptamine and Substance X in molluscan ganglia. *Comp. Biochem. Physiol.* **20**, 901–906.

COUTEAUX, R. (1953) Particularités histochimiques des zones d'insertion du muscle strié. *C.R. Soc. Biol., Paris* **147**, 1974–1976.

COUTEAUX, R. (1958) Morphological and cytochemical observations on the postsynaptic membrane at motor endplates and ganglionic synapses. *Exp. Cell. Res. Suppl.* **5**, 294–322.

COUTEAUX, R. and TAXI, J. (1952) Recherches histochimiques sur la distribution des activités cholinestéraisiques au niveau de la synapse myoneurale. *Arch. Anat. micr. Morph. exp.* **41**, 352–393.

CRAWFORD, J. M. and CURTIS, D. R. (1964) The excitation and depression of mammalian cortical neurones by amino acids. *Br. J. Pharmac. Chemother.* **23**, 313–329.

CRAWFORD, J. M. and CURTIS, D. R. (1966) Pharmacological studies on feline Betz cells. *J. Physiol. (Lond.)* **186**, 121–138.

CRAWFORD, J. M., CURTIS, D. R., VOORHOEVE, P. E. and WILSON, V. J. (1963) Strychnine and cortical inhibition. *Nature* (*Lond.*) **200**, 845–846.

CRAWFORD, J. M., CURTIS, D. R., VOORHOEVE, P. E. and WILSON, V. J. (1966) Acetylcholine sensitivity of cerebellar neurones in the cat. *J. Physiol.* (*Lond.*) **186**, 139–165.

CREESE, R. and TAYLOR, D. B. (1965) The effect of atropine on the uptake of labelled carbachol by rat brain slices. *Life Sci.* (*Oxford*) **4**, 1545–1547.

CRESCITELLI, F. and GEISSMAN, T. A. (1962) Invertebrate pharmacology: Selected topics. *A. Rev. Pharmac.* **2**, 143–192.

CREVELING, C. R., DALY, J. W., WITKOP, B. and UDENFRIEND, S. (1962) Substrates and inhibitors of dopamine-β-oxidase. *Biochim. biophys. Acta* **64**, 125–134.

CREVIER, M. and BÉLANGER, L. F. (1955) Simple method for histochemical detection of esterase activity. *Science, N.Y.* **122**, 556.

CROSSLAND, J. (1960) Chemical transmission in the central nervous system. *J. Pharm. Pharmac.* **12**, 1–36.

CROSSLAND, J. (1961) Biologic estimation of histamine. *Meth. med. Res.* **9**, 186–191.

CROSSLAND, J. and MITCHELL, J. F. (1956) The effect on the electrical activity of the cerebellum of a substance present in cerebellar extracts. *J. Physiol.* (*Lond.*) **132**, 391–405.

CSAPO, I. A. and KURIYAMA, H. A. (1963) Effects of ions and drugs on cell membrane activity and tension in the post-partum rat myometrium. *J. Physiol.* (*Lond.*) **165**, 575–592.

CSILLIK, B. and ERULKAR, H. (1964) Labile stores of monoamines in the central nervous system: a histochemical study. *J. Pharmac. exp. Ther.* **146**, 186–193.

CSILLIK, B., KALMAN, G. and KNYIHÁR, E. (1967) Adrenergic endings in the feline cervical superius ganglion. *Experientia* **23**, 477–478.

CSILLIK, B. and KÁSA, P. (1966) Localization of acetylcholinesterase in the guinea-pig cerebellar cortex. *Acta neurovegetativa* **29**, 289–296.

CURTIS, D. R. (1962) The action of 3-hydroxytyramine and some tryptamine derivatives upon spinal neurones. *Nature* (*Lond.*) **194**, 292.

CURTIS, D. R. (1964) Microelectrophoresis. In: *Physical Techniques in Biological Research*, vol. 5. Ed. W. L. Nastuk. New York: Academic Press.

CURTIS, D. R. (1965) The actions of amino acids upon mammalian neurones. In: *Studies in Physiology*, pp. 34–42. Ed. D. R. Curtis and A. K. McIntyre, Berlin: Springer.

CURTIS, D. R. and DAVIS, R. (1962) Pharmacological studies upon neurones of the lateral geniculate nucleus of the cat. *Br. J. Pharmac. Chemother.* **18**, 217–246.

CURTIS, D. R. and DAVIS, R. (1963) The excitation of lateral geniculate neurones by quaternary ammonium derivatives. *J. Physiol.* (*Lond.*) **165**, 62–82.

CURTIS, D. R., ECCLES, J. C. and ECCLES, R. M. (1955) Pharmacological studies on reflexes. *Am. J. Physiol.* **183**, 606.

CURTIS, D. R., ECCLES, J. C. and ECCLES, R. M. (1957) Pharmacological studies on spinal reflexes. *J. Physiol.* (*Lond.*) **136**, 420–434.

CURTIS, D. R. and ECCLES, R. M. (1958a) The excitation of Renshaw cells by pharmacological agents applied electrophoretically. *J. Physiol.* (*Lond.*) **141**, 435–445.

CURTIS, D. R. and ECCLES, R. M. (1958b) The effect of diffusional barriers upon the pharmacology of cells within the central nervous system. *J. Physiol.* (*Lond.*) **141**, 446–463.

CURTIS, D. R., HÖSLI, L. and JOHNSTON, G. A. R. (1967) Inhibition of spinal neurones by Glycine. *Nature* (*Lond.*) **215**, 1502–1503.

CURTIS, D. R., HÖSLI, L., JOHNSTON, G. A. R. and JOHNSTON, I. H. (1967) Glycine and spinal inhibition. *Brain Res.* **5**, 112–114.

304   THE PHARMACOLOGY OF SYNAPSES

Curtis, D. R., Hösli, L., Johnston, G. A. R. and Johnston, I. H. (1968) The hyper-polarization of spinal motoneurones by glycine and related amino acids. *Expl. Brain. Res.* 5, 235–258.

Curtis, D. R. and Koizumi, K. (1961) Chemical transmitter substances in brain stem of cat. *J. Neurophysiol.* 24, 80–90.

Curtis, D. R., Phillis, J. W. and Watkins, J. C. (1959) The depression of spinal neurones by γ-amino-n-butyric acid and β-alanine. *J. Physiol. (Lond).* 146, 185–203.

Curtis, D. R., Phillis, J. W. and Watkins, J. C. (1960) The chemical excitation of spinal neurones by certain acidic amino acids. *J. Physiol. (Lond.)* 150, 656–682.

Curtis, D. R., Phillis, J. W. and Watkins, J. C. (1961a) Cholinergic and non-cholinergic transmission in the mammalian spinal cord. *J. Physiol. (Lond.)* 158, 296–323.

Curtis, D. R., Phillis, J. W. and Watkins, J. C. (1961b) Actions of amino-acids on the isolated hemisected spinal cord of the toad. *Br. J. Pharmac. Chemother.* 16, 262–283.

Curtis, D. R. and Ryall, R. W. (1966a) The excitation of Renshaw cells by cholinomimetics. *Expl. Brain Res.* 2, 49–65.

Curtis, D. R. and Ryall, R. W. (1966b) The acetylcholine receptors of Renshaw cells. *Expl. Brain Res.* 2, 66–80.

Curtis, D. R. and Ryall, R. W. (1966c) The synaptic excitation of Renshaw cells. *Expl. Brain Res.* 2, 81–96.

Curtis, D. R. and Ryall, R. W. (1966d) Pharmacological studies upon presynaptic fibres. *Exp. Brain Res.* 1, 195–204.

Curtis, D. R., Ryall, R. W. and Watkins, J. C. (1966) The action of cholinomimetics on spinal interneurones. *Expl. Brain Res.* 2, 97–106.

Curtis, D. R. and Watkins, J. C. (1960a) The excitation and depression of spinal neurones by structurally related amino acids. *J. Neurochem.* 6, 117–141.

Curtis, D. R. and Watkins, J. C. (1960b) Investigations upon the possible synaptic transmitter function of gamma-aminobutyric acid and naturally occurring amino acids. In: *Inhibitions of the Nervous System and γ-Aminobutyric Acid*, pp. 424–444. Ed. E. Roberts, Oxford: Pergamon.

Curtis, D. R. and Watkins, J. C. (1963) Acidic amino acids with strong excitatory actions on mammalian neurones. *J. Physiol. (Lond.)* 166, 1–14.

Curtis, D. R. and Watkins, J. C. (1965) The pharmacology of amino acids related to gamma-aminobutyric acid. *Pharmac. Rev.* 17, 347–391.

Dagirmanjian, R., Laverty, R., Mantegazzini, P., Sharman, D. F. and Vogt, M. (1963) Chemical and physiological changes produced by arterial infusion of di-hydroxyphenylalanine into one cerebral hemisphere of the cat. *J. Neurochem.* 10, 177–182.

Dahl, E., Falck, B., Mecklenburg, C. von, and Myhrberg, H. (1963) The adrenergic nervous system in sea anemones. *Quart. J. micr. Sci.* 104, 531–534.

Dahl, E., Falck, B., Mecklenburg, C. von, Myhrberg, H. and Rosengren, E. (1966) Neuronal localization of dopamine and 5-hydroxytryptamine in some mollusca. *Z. Zellforsch. Mikrosk. Anat.* 71, 489–498.

Dahlström, A. and Fuxe, K. (1964a) Evidence for the existence of monoamine-containing neurons in the central nervous system. I. Demonstration of monoamines in the cell bodies of brain stem neurons. *Acta physiol. scand.* 62 suppl. 232, 1–55.

Dahlström, A. and Fuxe, K. (1964b) A method for the demonstration of monoamine-containing fibres in the central nervous system. *Acta physiol. scand.* 60, 293–294.

Dahlström, A. and Fuxe, K. (1965) Experimentally induced changes in the intra-neuronal amine levels of bulbospinal neurone systems. *Acta physiol. scand.* 64, suppl. 247, 5–36.

Dahlström, A., Fuxe, K. Olson, L. and Ungerstedt, U. (1965) On the distribution and possible function of monoamine nerve terminals in the olfactory bulb of the rabbit. *Life Sci. (Oxford)* **4,** 2071–2074.

DALE, H. H. (1914) The action of certain esters and ethers of choline, and their relation to muscarine. *J. Pharmac. exp. Ther.* **6,** 147–190.

DALE, H. H. (1935) Pharmacology and nerve endings. *Proc. R. Soc. Med.* **28,** 319–332.

DALE, H. H., FELDBERG, W. and VOGT, M. (1936) Release of acetylcholine at voluntary motor nerve endings. *J. Physiol. (Lond.)* **86,** 353–380.

DAMJANOVICH, S., FEHÉR, O., HALASZ, P. and MECHLER, F. (1960) The effect of alpha-amino acids on ganglionic transmission. *Acta physiol. hung.* **18,** 57–63.

DANIELS, E. G., HINMAN, J. W., LEACH, B. E. and MUIRHEAD, E. E. (1967) Identification of prostaglandin E2 as the principal vasodepressor lipid of rabbit renal medulla. *Nature (Lond.)* **215,** 1298–1299.

DAVID, J. P., MURAYAMA, S., MACHNE, X., and UNNA, K. R. (1963) Evidence supporting cholinergic transmission at the lateral geniculate body of the cat. *Int. J. Neuropharmac.* **2,** 113–125.

DAVIDOFF, R. A., GRAHAM, L. T., SHANK, R. P., WERMAN, R. and APRISON, M. H. (1967a) Changes in amino acid concentrations associated with loss of spinal interneurones. *J. Neurochem.* **14,** 1025–1031.

DAVIDOFF, R. A., SHANK, R. P., GRAHAM, L. T., APRISON, M. H. and WERMAN, R. (1967b) Is glycine a Neurotransmitter? Association of glycine with spinal interneurones. *Nature (Lond.)* **214,** 680–681.

DAVIS, R. and KOELLE, G. B. (1967) Electron microscopic localization of acetylcholinesterase and non-specific cholinesterase at the neuromuscular junction by the gold-thiocholine and gold-thiolacetic acid methods. *J. cell. Biol.* **34,** 157–171.

DAY, M. and VANE, J. R. (1963) An analysis of the direct and indirect actions of drugs on the isolated guinea-pig ileum. *Br. J. Pharmac. Chemother.* **20,** 150–170.

DEFFENU, G., BERTACCINI, G., and PEPEU, G. (1967) Acetylcholine and 5-hydroxytryptamine levels of the lateral geniculate bodies and superior colliculus of cats after visual deafferentation. *Expl. Neurol.* **17,** 203–209.

DE GROAT, W. C. (1966) The action of GABA and related amino acids on a sympathetic ganglion. Proc. Aust. Physiol. Soc., August 1966.

DE GROAT, W. C. and VOLLE, R. L. (1966a) The actions of the catecholamines on transmission in the superior cervical ganglion of the cat. *J. Pharmac. exp. Ther.* **154,** 1–13.

DE GROAT, W. C. and VOLLE, R. L. (1966b) Interactions between the catecholamines and ganglionic stimulating agents in sympathetic ganglia. *J. Pharmac. exp. Ther.* **154,** 200–215.

DE GROAT, W. C. and RYALL, R. W. (1967) An excitatory action of 5-hydroxytryptamine on sympathetic preganglionic neurones. *Expl. Brain Res.* **3,** 299–305.

DE LA LANDE, I. S., CANNELL, V. A. and WATERSON, J. G. (1966) The interaction of serotonin and noradrenaline on the perfused artery. *Br. J. Pharmac Chemother.* **28,** 255–272.

DE LA LANDE, I. S. and RAND, M. J. (1965) A simple isolated nerve-blood vessel preparation. *Aust. J. exp. Biol. med. Sci.* **43,** 639–656.

DEL CASTILLO, J. and ENGBAEK, L. (1954) The nature of the neuromuscular block produced by magnesium. *J. Physiol. (Lond.)* **124,** 370–384.

DEL CASTILLO, J. and KATZ, B. (1954a) Quantal components of the endplate potential. *J. Physiol. (Lond.)* **124,** 560–573.

DEL CASTILLO, J. and KATZ, B. (1954b) The membrane change produced by the neuromuscular transmitter. *J. Physiol. (Lond.)* **125,** 546–565.

DEL CASTILLO, J. and KATZ, B. (1955a) On the localization of acetylcholine receptors. *J. Physiol. (Lond.)* **128,** 157–181.

DEL CASTILLO, J. and KATZ, B. (1955b) Local activity at a depolarized nerve-muscle junction. *J. Physiol. (Lond.)* **128**, 396–411.

DEL CASTILLO, J. and KATZ, B. (1956) Biophysical aspects of neuromuscular transmission. *Prog. Biophys. biophys. Chem.* **6**, 121–170.

DEL CASTILLO, J. and KATZ, B. (1957a) I. Curare action studied by an electrical micromethod. *Proc. R. Soc. B.* **146**, 339–356.

DEL CASTILLO, J. and KATZ, B. (1957b) III. A comparison of acetylcholine and stable depolarizing agents. *Proc. R. soc. B.* **146**, 362–368.

DEL CASTILLO, J. and KATZ, B. (1957c) IV. Interaction at endplate receptors between different choline derivatives. *Proc. R. soc. B.* **146**, 369–381.

DELL, P. (1960) Intervention of an adrenergic mechanism during brain stem reticular activation. Ciba Symp. *Adrenergic Mechanisms*, pp. 393–409. London: J. & A. Churchill Ltd.

DE MOLINA, A. F., GRAY, J. A. B. and PALMER, J. F. (1958) Effects of acetylcholine on the activity of the lumbosacral cord of the cat. *J. Physiol. (Lond.)* **141**, 169–176.

DENGLER, H. J., MICHAELSON, I. A., SPEIGEL, H. E. and TITUS, E. (1962) The uptake of labelled norepinephrine by isolated brain and other tissues of the cat. *Int. J. Neuropharmac.* **1**, 23–38.

DENZ, F. A. (1953) On the histochemistry of the myoneural junction. *Br. J. exp. Path.* **34**, 329–339.

DE ROBERTIS, E. D. P. (1964) *Histophysiology of Synapses and Neurosecretion.* Oxford: Pergamon Press.

DE ROBERTIS, E. D. P., ARNAIZ, G. R. de L., SALGANICOFF, L., IRALDI, A. P. de and ZIEHER, L. M. (1963) Isolation of synaptic vesicles and structural organization of the acetylcholine system with brain nerve endings. *J. Neurochem.* **10**, 225–235.

DE ROBERTIS, E. D. P. and BENNETT, H. S. (1955) Some features of the submicroscopic morphology of synapses in frog and earthworm. *J. biophys. biochem. Cytol.* **1**, 47–58.

DE ROBERTIS, E. D. P. and FERREIRA, A. V. (1957) Submicroscopic changes of the nerve endings in the adrenal medulla after stimulation of the splanchnic nerve. *J. biophys. biochem. Cytol.* **3**, 611–614.

DE ROBERTIS, E. D. P. and FRANCHI, C. M. (1956) Electron microscope observations on synaptic vesicles in synapses of the retinal rods and cones. *J. biophys. biochem. Cytol.* **2**, 307–318.

DE ROBERTIS, E. D. P., IRALDI, A. P. DE, ARNAIZ, G. R. DE L. and SALGANICOFF, L., (1962) Cholinergic and non-cholinergic nerve endings in rat brain. I. Isolation and subcellular distribution of acetylcholine and acetylcholinesterase. *J. Neurochem.* **9**, 23–35.

DESMEDT, J. E. and LA GRUTTA, G. (1957) The effect of selective inhibition of pseudocholinesterase on the spontaneous and evoked activity of the cat's cerebral cortex. *J. Physiol. (Lond.)* **136**, 20–40.

DHAR, S. K. (1958) Cholinesterase in decentralized and axotomized sympathetic ganglia. *J. Physiol. (Lond.)* **144**, 27–28P.

DIAMOND, J. (1959) The effects of injecting acetylcholine into normal and regenerating nerves *J. Physiol. (Lond.)* **145**, 611–629.

DIAMOND, J. (1968) The activation and distribution of GABA and L-glutamate receptors on goldfish Mauthner neurones: an analysis of dendritic remote inhibition. *J. Physiol. (Lond.)* **194**, 669–723.

DIAMOND, J. and BRODY, T. M. (1966) Effect of catecholamines on smooth muscle mobility and phosphorylase activity. *J. Pharmac. exp. Ther.* **152**, 202–211.

DIKSHIT, B. B. (1938) Acetylcholine formation by tissues. *Quart. J. exp. Physiol.* **28** 243–251.

DIXON, W. E. (1906) Vagus inhibition. *Brit. med. J.* **2**, 1807.

DUCHARME, D. W. and WEEKS, J. R. (1967) Cardiovascular pharmacology of prostaglandin F2α, a unique pressor agent. In: *Nobel Symposium 2: Prostaglandins*, pp. 173–182. Ed. S. Bergström and B. Samuelsson. Stockholm: Almqvist & Wiksell.

DUDEL, J. (1963) Presynaptic inhibition of the excitatory nerve terminal in the neuromuscular junction of the crayfish. *Pflügers Arch. ges. Physiol.* **277**, 537–557.

DUDEL, J. (1965a) Facilitatory effects of 5-hydroxytryptamine on the crayfish neuromuscular junction. *Naunyn-Schmiedeberg's Arch. exp. Path. Pharmak.* **249**, 515–528.

DUDEL, J. (1965b) Presynaptic and postsynaptic effects of inhibitory drugs on the crayfish neuromuscular junction. *Pflügers Arch. ges. Physiol.* **283**, 104–118.

DUDEL, J. & KUFFLER, S. W. (1961) Presynaptic inhibition at the crayfish neuromuscular junction. *J. Physiol. (Lond.)* **155**, 543–562.

DOUGLAS, W. W. (1966) The mechanism of the release of catecholamines from the adrenal medulla. *Pharmac. Rev.* **18**, 471–480.

DOUGLAS, W. W. and LYWOOD, D. W. (1961) The stimulant action of TEA on acetylcholine from the superior cervical ganglion: comparison with barium. *Fed. Proc.* **20**, 324.

DOUGLAS, W. W., LYWOOD, D. W. and STRAUB, R. W. (1961) The stimulant effect of barium on the release of acetylcholine from the superior cervical ganglion. *J. Physiol. (Lond.)* **156**, 515–522.

DOUGLAS, W. W. and RUBIN, R. P. (1961) The role of calcium in the secretory response of the adrenal medulla to acetylcholine. *J. Physiol. (Lond.)* **159**, 40–57.

DUNCAN, C. J. (1964) Rhythmic activity in an isolated penis preparation from the freshwater snail *Limnaea stagnalis*. *Z. vergl. physiol.* **48**, 295–301.

ECCLES, J. C. (1935) Slow potential waves in the superior cervical ganglion. *J. Physiol. (Lond.)* **85**, 464–501.

ECCLES, J. C. (1957) *The Physiology of Nerve Cells*. Baltimore: Johns Hopkins Press.

ECCLES, J. C. (1964) *The Physiology of Synapses*. Berlin: Springer.

ECCLES, J. C., ECCLES, R. M. and FATT, P. (1956) Pharmacological investigations on a central synapse operated by acetylcholine. *J. Physiol. (Lond.)* **131**, 154–169.

ECCLES, J. C., FATT, P. and KOKETSU, K. (1954) Cholinergic and inhibitory synapses in a pathway from motor axon collaterals to motoneurones. *J. Physiol. (Lond.)* **126**, 524–562.

ECCLES, J. C., ITO, M. and SZENTÁGOTHAI, J. (1967) *The Cerebellum as a Neuronal Machine*. Berlin: Springer.

ECCLES, J. C. and JAEGER, J. C. (1958) The relationship between the mode of operation and the dimensions of the junctional regions at synapses and motor end-organs. *Proc. R. soc. B.* **148**, 38–56.

ECCLES, J. C., KATZ, B. and KUFFLER, S. W. (1942) Effect of eserine on neuromuscular transmission. *J. Neurophysiol.* **5**, 211–230.

ECCLES, J. C., LLINÁS, R. and SASAKI, K. (1966a) Parallel fibre stimulation and the responses induced thereby in the Purkinje cells of the cerebellum. *Expl. Brain Res.* **1**, 17–39.

ECCLES, J. C., LLINÁS, R. and SASAKI, K. (1966b) The excitatory synaptic action of climbing fibres on the Purkinje cells of the cerebellum. *J. Physiol. (Lond.)* **182**, 268–296.

ECCLES, J. C. and MALCOLM, J. L. (1946) Dorsal root potentials of the spinal cord. *J. Neurophysiol.* **9**, 139–160.

ECCLES, R. M. (1952) Responses of isolated curarized sympathetic ganglia. *J. Physiol. (Lond.)* **117**, 196–217.

ECCLES, R. M. (1955) Intracellular potentials recorded from a mammalian sympathetic ganglion. *J. Physiol. (Lond.)* **130**, 572–584.

ECCLES, R. M. (1963) Orthodromic activation of single ganglion cells. *J. Physiol. (Lond.)* **165**, 387–391.

ECCLES, R. M. and LIBET, B. (1961) Origin and blockade of the synaptic responses of curarized sympathetic ganglia. *J. Physiol. (Lond.)* **157**, 484–503.

EHINGER, B., FALCK, B. and SPORRONG, B. (1966) Adrenergic fibres to the heart and to peripheral vessels. *Biblthca. anat.* **8**, 35–45.

EHRENPREIS, S. (1960) Isolation and identification of the acetylcholine receptor protein of electric tissue. *Biochim. biophys. Acta* **44**, 561–577.

EHRENPREIS, S. (1962) Immunohistochemical localization of drug-binding protein in tissues of electric eel. *Nature (Lond.)* **194**, 586–587.

EIDELBERG, E., GOLDSTEIN, G. P. and DEZA, L. (1967) Evidence for serotonin as a possible inhibitory transmitter in some limbic structures. *Expl. Brain Res.* **4**, 73–80.

ELFVIN, L. G. (1963a) The ultrastructure of the superior cervical sympathetic ganglion of the cat. I. The structure of the ganglion cell processes as studied by serial sections. *J. Ultrastruct. Res.* **8**, 403–440.

ELFVIN, L. G. (1963b) The ultrastructure of the superior cervical sympathetic ganglion of the cat. II. The structure of the preganglionic end fibres and the synapses as studied by serial sections. *J. Ultrastruct. Res.* **8**, 441–476.

ELIASSON, R. (1959) Studies on prostaglandin; occurrence, formation and biological actions. *Acta physiol. scand.* **46**, Suppl. 158, 1–73.

ELIASSON, R. and POSSE, N. (1965) Rubin's test before and after intravaginal application of prostaglandin. *Int. J. Fert.* **10**, 373–377.

ELLAWAY, P. H. and PASCOE, J. E. (1968) Noradrenaline as a transmitter in the spinal cord. *J. Physiol. (Lond.)* **197**, 8–10P.

ELLIOT, K. A. C. (1958) γ-Aminobutyric acid and Factor I. *Rev. canad. Biol.* **17**, 367–388.

ELLIOT, K. A. C. and HENDERSON, N. (1951) Factors affecting acetylcholine found in excised rat brain. *Am. J. Physiol.* **165**, 365–374.

ELLIOTT, K. A. C., SWANK, R. L. and HENDERSON, N. (1950) Effects of anaesthetics and convulsants on acetylcholine content of brain. *Am. J. Physiol.* **162**, 469–474.

ELLIOTT, R. C. (1965) Centrally active drugs and transmission through the isolated superior cervical ganglion preparation of the rabbit when stimulated repetitively. *Br. J. Pharmac. Chemother.* **24**, 76–88.

ELLIOTT, T. R. (1904) On the action of adrenalin. *J. Physiol (Lond.)* **31**, XX–XXI.

ELLIS, C. H., THIENES, C. H. and WIERSMA, C. A. G. (1942) The influence of certain drugs on the crustacean nerve-muscle system. *Biol. Bull. mar. biol. Lab. Woods Hole* **83**, 334–352.

ELMQVIST, D. and FELDMAN, D. S. (1965) Calcium dependence of spontaneous acetylcholine release at mammalian motor nerve terminals. *J. Physiol. (Lond.)* **181**, 487–497.

ELMQVIST, D. and QUASTEL, D. M. J. (1965) Presynaptic action of hemicholinium at the neuromuscular junction. *J. Physiol. (Lond.)* **177**, 463–482.

ELOFSSON, R., KAURI, T., NIELSEN, S-O and STROMBERG, J.-O. (1966) Localization of monoaminergic neurons on the central nervous system of *Astacus astacus* LINNÉ (Crustacea) *Z. Zellforsch mikrosk. Anat.* **74**, 464–473.

EMMELIN, N. G. and MACINTOSH, F. C. (1956) The release of acetylcholine from perfused sympathetic ganglia and skeletal muscles. *J. Physiol. (Lond.)* **131**, 477–496.

ENGBERG, I., LUNDBERG, A. and RYALL, R. W. (1968) Reticulospinal inhibition of interneurones. *J. Physiol. (Lond.)* **194**, 225–236.

ENGBERG, I. and RYALL, R. W. (1966) The inhibitory action of noradrenaline and other monoamines on spinal neurones. *J. Physiol. (Lond.)* **185**, 298–322.

ERÄNKÖ, O. (1966) Demonstration of catecholamines and cholinesterases in the same section. *Pharmac. Rev.* **18**, 353–358.

ERÄNKÖ, O. and HÄRKÖNEN, M. (1965) Monoamine-containing small cells in the superior cervical ganglion of the rat and an organ composed of them. *Acta physiol. scand.* **63**, 511–512.

ERSPAMER, V. (1946) Presenza di enteramina o di una sostanza enteraminosimile negli estratti gastrointestinali & splenici dei pesci & negli estratti gastroenterici delle ascidie. *Experientia* **2**, 369–371.

ERSPAMER, V. (1948) Active substances in the posterior salivary glands of octopoda. I. Enteramine-like substance. *Acta pharmac. tox.* **4**, 213–223.

ERSPAMER, V. (1966) Peripheral physiological and pharmacological actions of indole-alkylamines. *Handb. exp. Pharmak.* **19**, 245–359.

ERSPAMER, V. and ASERO, B. (1952) Identification of enteramine, the specific hormone of the enterochromaffin cell system, as 5-hydroxytryptamine. *Nature (Lond.)* **169**, 800–801.

EULER, U. S. VON (1935) Über die spezifische Blutdrucksenkende Substanz des menschlichen Prostata- und Samen-blasensekretes. *Klin. Wschr.* **14**, 1182–1183.

EULER, U. S. VON (1936) On the specific vasodilating and plain muscle stimulating substances from accessory genital glands in man and certain animals (prostaglandin and vesiglandin). *J. Physiol. (Lond.)* **88**, 213–234.

EULER, U. S. VON (1946) A specific sympathomimetic ergone in adrenergic nerve fibres (sympathin) and its relations to adrenaline and noradrenaline. *Acta physiol. scand.* **12**, 73–97.

EULER, U. S. VON (1948) Preparation, purification and evaluation of noradrenaline and adrenaline in organ extracts. *Archs. int. Pharmacodyn. Thér.* **77**, 477–485.

EULER, U. S. VON (1949) Histamine as a specific constituent of certain autonomic nerve fibres. *Acta physiol. scand.* **19**, 85–93.

EULER, U. S. VON (1966) Relationship between histamine and the autonomic nervous system. *Handb. exp. Pharmak.* **18/1**, 318–333.

EULER, U. S. VON and PURKHOLD, A. (1951) Histamine in organs and its relation to the sympathetic nerve supply. *Acta physiol. scand.* **24**, 218–224.

EVANS, D. H. L., SCHILD, H. O. and THESLEFF, S. (1958) Effects of drugs on depolarized plain muscle. *J. Physiol. (Lond.)* **143**, 474–485.

EVARTS, E. V. (1958) Effects of a series of indoles on synaptic transmission in the lateral geniculate nucleus of the cat. In: *Progress in Neurobiology III—Psychopharmacology*, pp. 173–194. Ed. H. H. Pennes. New York: Hoeber-Harper.

EVARTS, E. V., LANDAU, W., FREYGANG, W. and MARSHALL, W. H. (1955) Some effects of lysergic acid diethylamide and bufotenine on electrical activity in the cat's visual system. *Am. J. Physiol.* **182**, 594–598.

FALCK, B. and OWMAN, C. (1965) A detailed methodological description of the fluorescence method for the cellular demonstration of biogenic monoamines. *Acta Univ. Lund. Sect. II, No. 7.*

FÄNGE, R. and MATTISSON, A. (1958) Studies on the physiology of the radula muscle of *Buccinum undatum. Acta zool.* **39**, 53–54.

FATT, P. and KATZ, B. (1951) An analysis of the endplate potential recorded with an intracellular electrode. *J. Physiol. (Lond.)* **115**, 320–370.

310   THE PHARMACOLOGY OF SYNAPSES

FATT, P. and KATZ, B. (1952) Spontaneous subthreshold activity at motor nerve endings. *J. Physiol. (Lond.)* **117**, 109–128.

FATT, P. and KATZ, B. (1953) The effect of inhibitory nerve impulses on a crustacean muscle fibre. *J. Physiol. (Lond.)* **121**, 374–389.

FELDBERG, W. (1945) Present views on the mode of action of acetylcholine in the central nervous system. *Physiol. Rev.* **25**, 596–642.

FELDBERG, W. (1957) Acetylcholine. In *Metabolism of the Nervous System*, pp. 493–509. Ed. D. Richter. London: Pergamon.

FELDBERG, W. (1963) *A Pharmacological Approach to the Brain from Its Inner and Outer Surface* (Evarts Graham Memorial Lectures, 1961). London: Arnold.

FELDBERG, W. and FLEISCHHAUER, K. (1965) A new experimental approach to the physiology and pharmacology of the brain. *Br. med. Bull.* **21**, 36–43.

FELDBERG, W. and GADDUM, J. H. (1934) The chemical transmitter at synapses in a sympathetic ganglion. *J. Physiol. (Lond.)* **81**, 305–319.

FELDBERG, W., GRAY, J. A. B. and PERRY, W. L. M. (1953) Effects of close arterial injections of acetylcholine on the activity of the cervical spinal cord of the cat. *J. Physiol. (Lond.)* **119**, 428–438.

FELDBERG, W. and LIN, R. C. Y. (1950) Synthesis of acetylcholine in the wall of the digestive tract. *J. Physiol. (Lond.)* **111**, 96–118.

FELDBERG, W., MALCOLM, J. L. and SHERWOOD, S. L. (1956) Some effects of tubocurarine on the electrical activity of the cat's brain. *J. Physiol. (Lond.)* **132**, 130–145.

FELDBERG, W. and MANN, T. (1946) Properties and distribution of the enzyme system which synthesises acetylcholine in nervous tissue. *J. Physiol. (Lond.)* **104**, 411–425.

FELDBERG, W. and MINZ, B. (1932) Die blutdrucksteigernde Wirkung des Azetylcholins au Katzen nach Entfernen der Nebennieren. *Naunyn-Schmiedeberg's Arch. exp. Path. Pharmak.* **165**, 261–290.

FELDBERG, W. and MYERS, R. D. (1966) Appearance of 5-hydroxytryptamine and an unidentified pharmacologically active lipid acid in effluent from perfused cerebral ventricles. *J. Physiol. (Lond.)* **184**, 837–855.

FELDBERG, W. and SHERWOOD, S. L. (1954) Injections of drugs into the lateral ventricle of the cat. *J. Physiol. (Lond.)* **123**, 148–167.

FELDBERG, W. and VARTIANEN, A. (1934) Further observations on the physiology and pharmacology of a sympathetic ganglion. *J. Physiol. (Lond.)* **83**, 103–128.

FELDBERG, W. and VOGT, M. (1948) Acetylcholine synthesis in different regions of the central nervous system. *J. Physiol. (Lond.)* **107**, 372–381.

FENG, T. P. and LI, T. H. (1941) Studies on the neuromuscular junction. XXIII. A new aspect of the phenomena of eserine potentiation and post-tetanic facilitation in mammalian muscles. *Chin. J. Physiol.* **16**, 37–50.

FERRY, C. B. (1966) Cholinergic link hypothesis in adrenergic neuroeffector transmission. *Physiol. Rev.* **46**, 420–456.

FERRY, C. B. (1967) The innervation of the vas deferens of the guinea-pig. *J. Physiol. (Lond.)* **192**, 463–478.

FLOREY, E. (1954) An inhibitory and an excitatory factor of mammalian central nervous system and their action on a single sensory neurone. *Archs. int. Physiol.* **62**, 33–53.

FLOREY, E. (1960) Studies on the nervous regulation of the heart beat in decapod crustacea. *J. gen. Physiol.* **43**, 1061–1081.

FLOREY, E. (1965) Comparative pharmacology: neurotropic and myotropic compounds. *A. Rev. Pharmac.* **5**, 357–382.

FLOREY, E. (1967) Cholinergic neurones in tunicates: an appraisal of the evidence. *Comp. Biochem. Physiol.* **22**, 617–627.

FLOREY, E. and BIEDERMAN, M. A. (1960) Studies on the distribution of Factor I and acetylcholine in crustacean peripheral nerve. *J. gen. Physiol.* **43**, 509–522.

FLOREY, E. and CHAPMAN, D. D. (1961) The non-identity of the transmitter substance of crustacean inhibitory neurons and gamma-aminobutyric acid. *Comp. Biochem. Physiol.* **3**, 92–98.

FLOREY, E. and FLOREY, E. (1965) Cholinergic neurons in the Onychophora: a comparative study. *Comp. Biochem. Physiol.* **15**, 125–136.

FOLDES, F. F. and FOLDES, V. M. (1965) Omega-amino fatty acid esters of choline: interaction with cholinesterases and neuromuscular activity in man. *J. Pharmac. exp. Ther.* **150**, 220–230.

FOURMAN, J. (1966) Cholinesterase in the mammalian kidney. *Nature (Lond.)* **209**, 812–813.

FOZZARD, H. A. and SLEATOR, W. (1967) Membrane ionic conductances during rest and activity in guinea-pig atrial muscle. *Am. J. Physiol.* **212**, 945–952.

FRANK, K. and TAUC, L. (1964) Voltage-clamp studies of molluscan neuron membrane properties. In: *The Cellular Function of Membrane Transport*, pp. 113–135. Ed. J. F. HOFFMAN, New Jersey: Prentice-Hall.

FRANZ, J., BOISSONNAS, R. A. and STÜRMER, E. (1961) Isolation of substance P from horse intestine and its chemical differentiation from bradykinin. *Helv. chim. Acta* **45**, 881–883.

FRIESEN, A. J. D., KEMP, J. W. and WOODBURY, D. M. (1965) The chemical and physical identification of acetylcholine obtained from sympathetic ganglia. *J. Pharmac. exp. Thér.* **148**, 312–319.

FRIGYESI, T. L. and PURPURA, D. P. (1966) Acetylcholine sensitivity of thalmic synaptic organisations activated by brachium conjunctivum stimulation. *Archs. int. Pharmacodyn. Thér.* **163**, 110–132.

FRONTALI, N. (1964) Brain glutamic acid decarboxylase and synthesis of gamma aminobutyric acid in vertebrate and invertebrate species. In: *Comparative Neurochemistry*, pp. 185–192. Ed. D. Richter. Oxford: Pergamon.

FRONTALI, N. and NORBERG, K. A. (1966) Catecholamine containing neurons in the cockroach brain. *Acta physiol. scand.* **66**, 243–244.

FRONTALI, N., WILLIAMS, L. and WELSH, J. H. (1967) Heart excitatory and inhibitory substances in molluscan ganglia. *Comp. Biochem. Physiol.* **22**, 833–841.

FUNAKI, S. and BOHR, D. F. (1964) Electrical and mechanical activity of isolated vascular smooth muscle of the rat. *Nature (Lond.)* **203**, 192–194.

FUNNELL, H. S. and OLIVER, W. T. (1965) Proposed physiological function for plasma cholinesterase. *Nature (Lond.)* **208**, 689–690.

FURCHGOTT, R. F. (1954) Dibenamine blockade in strips of rabbit aorta and its uses in differentiating receptors. *J. Pharmac. exp. Ther.* **111**, 265–284.

FURCHGOTT, R. F. (1955) The pharmacology of vascular smooth muscle. *Pharmac. Rev.* **7**, 183–265.

FURSHPAN, E. J. and POTTER, D. D. (1959) Transmission at the giant synapses of the crayfish. *J. Physiol. (Lond.)* **145**, 289–325.

FURUKAWA, T. and FURSHPAN, E. J. (1963) Two inhibitory mechanisms in the Mauthner neurons of goldfish. *J. Neurophysiol.* **26**, 140–176.

FURUKAWA, T. and FURUKAWA, A. (1959) Effects of methyl- and ethyl- derivatives of NH_4^+ on the neuromuscular junction. *Jap. J. Physiol.* **9**, 130–142.

FUXE, K. (1964) Cellular localization of monoamines in the median eminence and infundibular stem of some mammals. *Z. Zellforsch. mikrosk. Anat.* **61**, 710–724.

FUXE, K. (1965a) Evidence for the existence of monoamine neurons in the central nervous system. III. The monoamine nerve terminal. *Z. Zellforsch. mikrosk. Anat.* **65**, 573–596.

FUXE, K. (1965b) Evidence for the existence of monoamine neurons in the central nervous system. IV. Distribution of monoamine terminals in the central nervous system. *Acta physiol. scand.* **64**, Suppl. 247, 37–85.

FUXE, K. and SEDWALL, G. (1965) The distribution of adrenergic nerve fibres to the blood vessels in skeletal muscle. *Acta physiol. scand.* **64**, 75–86.

GADDUM, J. H. (1953) Tryptamine receptors. *J. Physiol. (Lond.)* **119**, 363–368.

GADDUM, J. H. (1957) Serotonin—LSD interactions. *Ann. N.Y. Acad. Sci.* **66**, 643–647.

GADDUM, J. H. and GIARMAN, N. J. (1956) Preliminary studies on the biosynthesis of 5-HT. *Br. J. Pharmac. Chemother.* **11**, 88–92.

GADDUM, J. H. and HAMEED, K. A. (1954) Drugs which antagonize 5-hydroxytryptamine. *Br. J. Pharmac. Chemother.* **9**, 240–248.

GADDUM, J. H. and PAASONEN, M. K. (1955) The use of some molluscan hearts for the estimation of 5-hydroxytryptamine. *Br. J. Pharmac. Chemother.* **10**, 474–483.

GADDUM, J. H. and PICARELLI, Z. P. (1957) Two kinds of tryptamine receptor. *Br. J. Pharmac. Chemother.* **12**, 323–328.

GAGE, P. W. and QUASTEL, D. M. J. (1966) Competition between sodium and calcium ions in transmitter release at a mammalian neuromuscular junction. *J. Physiol. (Lond.)* **185**, 95–123.

GAL, E. M., MORGAN, M., CHATTERJE, S. K. and MARSHALL, F. D. (1964) Hydroxylation of tryptophan by brain tissue *in vivo* and related aspects of 5-hydroxytryptamine metabolism. *Biochem. Pharmac.* **13**, 1639–1653.

GALINDO, A., KRNJEVIĆ, K. and SCHWARTZ, S. (1967) Micro-iontophoretic studies on neurones in the cuneate nucleus. *J. Physiol. (Lond.)* **192**, 359–377.

GAWECKA, I. and KOSTOWSKI, W. (1966) Studies on the effect of 5-hydroxytryptamine on neuromuscular conduction. *Acta physiol. polon.* **17**, 457–464.

GAY, W. S., RAND, M. J. and WILSON, J. (1967) Mechanism of the vasoconstrictor action of isoprenaline on an isolated artery preparation. *J. Pharm. Pharmac.* **19**, 468–473.

GEBBER, G. L. and VOLLE, R. L. (1965) Ganglionic stimulating properties of aliphatic esters of choline and thiocholine. *J. Pharmac. exp. Ther.* **150**, 67–74.

GEREBTZOFF, M. A. (1954) Appareil cholinestérasique a l'insertion tendineuse des fibres musculaires striées. *C.R. Soc. Biol. Paris* **148**, 632–634.

GEREBTZOFF, M. A. (1957) L'appareil cholinestérasique musculo-tendineux: Structure, développement, effet de la dénervation et de la ténotomie. *Acta physiol. pharm. néerl.* **5**, 419–427.

GEREBTZOFF, M. A. (1959) *Cholinesterases, a Histochemical Contribution to the Solution of Some Functional Problems.* London: Pergamon.

GEREBTZOFF, M. A., PHILIPPOT, E. and DALLEMAGNE, M. J. (1954) Recherche histochimiques sur les acétylcholine-, et choline-estérases. II. Activité enzymatique dens les muscles lents et rapides des mammifères et des oiseaux. *Acta anat.* **20**, 234–257.

GEROVÁ, M., GERO, J. and DOLEZEL, S. (1967) Mechanisms of sympathatic regulation of arterial smooth muscles. *Experientia* **23**, 639–640.

GERSCHENFELD, H. M. (1963) Observations on the ultrastructure of synapses in some pulmonate molluscs. *Z. Zellforsch. mikrosk. Anat.* **60**, 258–275.

GERSCHENFELD, H. M. (1964) A non-cholinergic synaptic inhibition in the central nervous system of a mollusc. *Nature (Lond.)* **203**, 415–416.

GERSCHENFELD, H. M., ASCHER, P. and TAUC, L. (1967) Two different excitatory transmitters acting on a single molluscan neurone. *Nature (Lond.)* **213**, 358–359.

GERSCHENFELD, H. M. and CHIARANDINI, D. J. (1965) Ionic mechanism associated with non-cholinergic synaptic inhibition on molluscan neurones. *J. Neurophysiol.* **28**, 710–723.

GERSCHENFELD, H. M. and LASANSKY, A. (1964) Action of glutamic acid and other naturally occurring amino acids on snail central neurones. *Int. J. Neuropharmac.* **3**, 301–314.

GERSCHENFELD, H. M. and STEFANI, E. (1966) An electrophysiological study of 5-hydroxytryptamine receptors of neurones in the molluscan nervous system. *J. Physiol. (Lond.)* **185**, 684–700.

GERSCHENFELD, H. M. and TAUC, L. (1961) Pharmacological specificities of neurons in an elementary nervous system. *Nature (Lond.)* **189**, 924–925.

GERSCHENFELD, H. M. and TAUC, L. (1964) Différents aspects de la pharmacologie des synapses dans le système nerveux central des Mollusques. *J. Physiol. (Paris)* **56**, 360–361.

GERTNER, S. B. (1955) The effect of compound 48/80 on ganglionic transmission. *Br. J. Pharmac. Chemother.* **10**, 103–109.

GERTNER, S. B. (1961) The effects of monoamine oxidase inhibitors on ganglionic transmission. *J. Pharmac. exp. Ther.* **131**, 223–230.

GERTNER, S. B. (1962) The effect of lowered calcium on the actions of acetylcholine (ACh) and 5-hydroxytryptamine (5HT) on the perfused superior cervical ganglion of the cat. *Pharmacologist* **4**, 174.

GERTNER, S. B. (1965) Histamine pools in sympathetic ganglia. *Pharmacologist* **7**, 153.

GERTNER, S. B. and KOHN, R. (1959) Effect of histamine on ganglionic transmission. *Br. J. Pharmac. Chemother.* **14**, 179–182.

GERTNER, S. B., PAASONEN, M. K. and GIARMAN, N. J. (1959) Studies concerning the presence of 5-hydroxytryptamine (serotonin) in the perfusate from the superior cervical ganglion. *J. Pharmac. exp. Ther.* **127**, 268–275.

GERTNER, S. B. and ROMANO, A. (1961) The effect of various amines on transmission through the superior cervical ganglion of the cat. *Biochem. Pharmac.* **8**, 19–20.

GESSA, G. L., COSTA, E., KUNTZMAN, R. and BRODIE, B. B. (1962) Evidence that the loss of brain catecholamine stores due to blockade of storage does not cause sedation. *Life Sci. (Oxford)* **9**, 441–452.

GIACHETTI, A. and SHORE, P. A. (1966) Studies *in vitro* of amine uptake mechanisms in heart. *Biochem. Pharmac.* **15**, 607–614.

GIACOBINI, E. and HOLMSTEDT, B. (1960) Cholinesterase in muscles: a histochemical and microgasometric study. *Acta pharmac. tox.* **17**, 94–105.

GIACOBINI, E., PALMBORG, B. and SJÖQVIST, F. (1967) Cholinesterase activity in innervated and denervated sympathetic ganglion cells of the cat. *Acta physiol. scand.* **69**, 355–361.

GIARMAN, N. J. and DAY, M. (1958) Presence of biogenic amines in the bovine pineal body. *Biochem. Pharmac.* **1**, 235.

GIARMAN, N. J. and PEPEU, G. (1964) The influence of centrally acting cholinolytic drugs on brain acetylcholine levels. *Br. J. Pharmac. Chemother.* **23**, 123–130.

GIBSON, I. M. and MCILWAIN, H. (1965) Continuous recording of changes in membrane potential in mammalian cerebral tissues *in vitro*; recovery after depolarization by added substances. *J. Physiol. (Lond.)* **176**, 261–283.

GINETZINSKY, A. G. and SHAMARINA, N. M. (1942) The tonomotor phenomenon in denervated muscle. *Usp. sovrem. Biol.* **15**, 283–294.

GINSBORG, B. L. (1965) The actions of McN-A-343, pilocarpine and acetyl-β-methyl-choline on sympathetic ganglion cells of the frog. *J. Pharmac. exp. Ther.* **150**, 216–219.

GLASSER, A. and MANTEGAZZINI, P. (1960) Action of 5-hydroxytryptamine and of 5-hydroxytryptophan on the cortical electrical activity of the midpontine pre-trigeminal preparation of the cat with and without mesencephalic hemisection. *Archs. ital. Biol.* **98**, 351–366.

GLOWINSKI, J. and AXELROD, J. (1965) Effects of drugs on the uptake, release and metabolism of H³ norepinephrine in the rat brain. *J. Pharmac. exp. Ther.* **149**, 43–49.

GLOWINSKI, J. and AXELROD, J. (1966) Effects of drugs on the disposition of H³ norepinephrine in the rat brain. *Pharmac. Rev.* **18**, 775–785.

GLOWINSKI, J., AXELROD, J. and IVERSEN, L. L. (1966) Regional studies of catecholamines in the rat brain. IV. Effects of drugs on the disposition and metabolism of H³-norepinephrine and H³-dopamine. *J. Pharmac. exp. Ther.* **153**, 30–41.

GLOWINSKI, J. and BALDESSARINI, R. J. (1966) Metabolism of norepinephrine in the central nervous system. *Pharmac. Rev.* **18**, 1201–1238.

GLOWINSKI, J. and IVERSEN, L. L. (1966a) Regional studies of catecholamines in the rat brain. I. Disposition of H³-norepinephrine, H³-dopamine and H³-DOPA in various regions of the brain. *J. Neurochem.* **13**, 655–669.

GLOWINSKI, J. and IVERSEN, L. L. (1966b) Regional studies of catecholamines in the rat brain. III. Subcellular distribution of endogenous and exogenous catecholamines in various brain regions. *Biochem. Pharmac.* **15**, 977–987.

GLOWINSKI, J., IVERSEN, L. L. and AXELROD, J. (1966) Storage and synthesis of norepinephrine in the reserpine treated rat brain. *J. Pharmac. exp. Ther.* **151**, 385–399.

GLOWINSKI, J., KOPIN, I. J. and AXELROD, J. (1965) Metabolism of H³-norepinephrine in the rat brain. *J. Neurochem.* **12**, 25–30.

GLOWINSKI, J., SNYDER, S. H. and AXELROD, J. (1966) Subcellular localization of H³-norepinephrine in the rat brain and the effects of drugs. *J. Pharmac. exp. Ther.* **152**, 282–292.

GOFFART, M. (1939) Acétylcholine tissulaire de tube digestif chez le chien. Influence de l'enervation. *Archs. int. Physiol.* **49**, 153–178.

GOLDBERG, A. M. and McCAMAN, R. E. (1967) A quantitative microchemical study of choline acetyltransferase and acetylcholinesterase in the cerebellum of several species. *Life Sci.* (*Oxford*) **6**, 1493–1500.

GOLDBLATT, M. W. (1935) Properties of human seminal plasma. *J. Physiol.* (*Lond.*) **84**, 208–218.

GOLDSTEIN, L., PFEIFFER, C. C. and MUNOZ, C. (1963) Quantitative EEG analysis of the stimulant properties of histamine and histamine derivatives. *Fed. Proc.* **22**, 424.

GOMORI, G. (1948) Histochemical demonstration of sites of choline esterase activity. *Proc. Soc. exp. Biol. Med.* (*N.Y.*) **68**, 354–358.

GORDON, P., HADDY, F. J. and LIPTON, M. A. (1958) Serotonin antagonism of noradrenaline *in vivo*. *Science, N.Y.* **128**, 531–532.

GORDON, P., HADDY, F. J. and LIPTON, M. A. (1959) Serotonin-adrenaline interaction *in vivo*. *Fed. Proc.* **18**, 397.

GRAHAM, L. T., WERMAN, R. and APRISON, M. H. (1965) Micro-determination of glutamate in single cat spinal roots. *Life Sci.* (*Oxford*) **4**, 1085–1090.

GRAHAME-SMITH, D. G. (1964) The enzymic conversion of tryptophan into 5-hydroxytryptophan by isolated brain tissue. *Biochem. J.* **92**, 52P.

GRAY, E. G. and WHITTAKER, V. P. (1962) The isolation of nerve endings from brain: an electron-microscopic study of cell fragments derived by homogenization and centrifugation. *J. Anat.* **96**, 79–88.

GREEN, H. and ERICKSON, R. W. (1960) Effect of trans-2-phenylcyclopropylamine upon norepinephrine concentration and monoamine oxidase activity of rat brain. *J. Pharmac. exp. Ther.* **129**, 237–242.

GREEN, H. and ERICKSON, R. W. (1964) Effect of some drugs upon rat brain histamine content. *Int. J. Neuropharmac.* **3**, 315–320.

GREEN, H., GREENBERG, S. M., ERICKSON, R. W., SAWYER, J. L. and ELLISON, T. (1962) Effect of dietary phenylalanine and tryptophan upon rat brain amine levels. *J. Pharmac. exp. Ther.* **136**, 174–178.

GREEN, H. and SAWYER, J. L. (1960) Intracellular distribution of norepinephrine. I. Effect of reserpine and the monoamine oxidase inhibitors trans-2-phenyl-cyclopropylamine and 1-isonicotinyl-2-isopropylhydrazine. *J. Pharmac. exp. Ther.* **129**, 243–249.

GREEN, J. D., MANCIA, M. and VON BAUMGARTEN, R. (1962) Recurrent inhibition in the olfactory bulb. I. Effects of antidromic stimulation of the lateral olfactory tract. *J. Neurophysiol.* **25**, 467–488.

GREEN, J. P. (1964) Histamine and the nervous system. *Fed. Proc.* **23**, 1095–1102.

GREENBERG, M. J. (1965) A compendium of responses of bivalve hearts to acetylcholine. *Comp. Biochem. Physiol.* **14**, 513–539.

GRILLO, M. A. (1966) Electron microscopy of sympathetic tissues. *Pharmac. Rev.* **18**, 387–399.

GRINNELL, A. D. (1966) A study of the interaction between motoneurones in the frog spinal cord. *J. Physiol.* (*Lond.*) **182**, 612–648.

GROMADZKI, C. G. and KOELLE, G. B. (1965) The effect of axotomy on the acetylcholinesterase of the superior cervical ganglion of the cat. *Biochem. Pharmac.* **14**, 1745–1754.

GROMAKOVSKAYA, M. M. (1962) On the problem of the mechanism of action of serotonin on the working capacity of the neuro-muscular apparatus. *Dokl. Akad. Nauk. S.S.S.R.* **144**, 578–581.

GRUNDFEST, H., REUBEN, J. P. and RICKLES, W. H. (1959) The electrophysiology and pharmacology of lobster neuromuscular synapses. *J. gen. Physiol.* **42**, 1301–1323.

GUROFF, G., KING, W. and UDENFRIEND, S. (1961) The uptake of tyrosine by rat brain in vitro. *J. biol. Chem.* **236**, 1773–1777.

GUTH, L., ALBERS, R. W. and BROWN, W. C. (1964) Quantitative changes in cholinesterase activity of denervated muscle fibers and sole plates. *Expl. Neurol.* **10**, 236–250.

GUTH, L. and BROWN, W. C. (1965) The sequence of changes in cholinesterase activity during reinnervation of muscle. *Expl. Neurol.* **12**, 329–336.

GWYN, D. G. and WOLSTENCROFT, J. H. (1966) Ascending and descending cholinergic fibers in cat spinal cord: histochemical evidence. *Science, N.Y.* **153**, 1543–1544.

GYERMEK, L. (1961) 5-Hydroxytryptamine antagonists. *Pharmac. Rev.* **13**, 399–439.

GYERMEK, L. (1962) Action of 5-hydroxytryptamine on the urinary bladder of the dog. *Archs. int. Pharmacodyn. Thér.* **137**, 137–144.

GYERMEK, L. and BINDLER, E. (1962a) Blockade of the ganglionic stimulant action of 5-hydroxytryptamine. *J. Pharmac. exp. Ther.* **135**, 344–348.

GYERMEK, L. and BINDLER, E. (1962b) Action of indole alkylamines and amidines on the inferior mesenteric ganglion of the cat. *J. Pharmac. exp. Ther.* **138**, 159–164.

HAEFELY, W. and HÜRLIMANN, A. (1962) Substance P, a highly active naturally occurring polypeptide. *Experientia* **18**, 297–303.

HAEFELY, W., HÜRLIMANN, A. and THOENEN, H. (1965) Effects of Bradykinin and Angiotensin on ganglionic transmission. *Biochem. Pharmac.* **14**, 1393.

HAGEN, P. B. and COHEN, L. H. (1966) Biosynthesis of indolealkylamines. Physiological release and transport of 5-hydroxytryptamine. *Handb. exp. Pharmak.* **14**, 182–211.

HÄGGENDAL, J. and LINDQVIST, M. (1964) Disclosure of labile monoamine fractions in brain and their correlation to behaviour. *Acta physiol. scand.* **60**, 351–357.

HAGIWARA, S., KUSANO, K. and SAITO, S. (1960) Membrane changes in crayfish stretch receptor neuron during synaptic inhibition and under action of gamma-aminobutyric acid. *J. Neurophysiol.* **23**, 505–515.

HAGIWARA, S. and MORITA, H. (1962) Electrotonic transmission between two nerve cells in leech ganglion. *J. Neurophysiol.* **25**, 721–731.

HALL, Z. W. and KRAVITZ, E. A. (1967) The metabolism of γ-aminobutyric acid (GABA) in the lobster nervous system—I. GABA-glutamate transaminase. *J. Neurochem.* **14**, 45–54.

HAMBERGER, B., NORBERG, K. A. (1965a) Studies on some systems of adrenergic synaptic terminals in the abdominal ganglia of the cat. *Acta physiol. scand.* **65**, 235–242.

HAMBERGER, B. and NORBERG, K. A. (1965b) Adrenergic synaptic terminals and nerve cells in bladder ganglia of the cat. *Int. J. Neuropharmac.* **4**, 41–45.

HAMBERGER, B., NORBERG, K. A. and SJÖQVIST, F. (1964) Evidence for adrenergic nerve terminals and synapses in sympathetic ganglia. *Int. J. Neuropharmac.* **2**, 279–282.

HAMBERGER, B., NORBERG, K. A. and UNGERSTEDT, U. (1965) Adrenergic synaptic terminals in autonomic ganglia. *Acta physiol. scand.* **64**, 285–286.

HANSON, A. S. and MAGILL, T. (1962) Effects of epinephrine and 5-hydroxytryptamine on strips of frog and turtle ventricle. *Proc. Soc. exp. Biol. Med. (N.Y.)* **109**, 329–333.

HÄRKÖNEN, M. (1964) Carboxylic esterases, oxidative enzymes and catecholamines in the superior cervical ganglion of the rat and the effect of pre- and post-ganglionic nerve division. *Acta physiol. scand.* **63**, Suppl. 237, 1–94.

HARLOW, P. A. (1958) The action of drugs on the nervous system of the locust (*Locusta migratoria*). *Ann. appl. Biol.* **46**, 55–73.

HARRIS, G. W., JACOBSOHN, D. and KAHLSON, G. (1952) The occurrence of histamine in cerebral regions related to the hypophysis. *Ciba Found. Colloq. Endocrin.* **4**, 186–194.

HARRY, J. (1962) Effect of cooling, local anaesthetic compounds and botulinum toxin on the responses of and the acetylcholine output from the electrically transmurally stimulated isolated guinea-pig ileum. *Br. J. Pharmac. Chemother.* **19**, 42–55.

HARRY, J. (1963) The action of drugs on the circular muscle strip from the guinea-pig isolated ileum. *Br. J. Pharmac. Chemother.* **20**, 399–417.

HART, E. R., RODRIGUEZ, J. M. and MARRAZZI, A. S. (1961) Carotid and vagal afferents and drug action on transcallosally evoked cortical potentials. *Science, N.Y.* **134**, 1696–1697.

HARVEY, A. M. and MACINTOSH, F. C. (1940) Calcium and synaptic transmission in a sympathetic ganglion. *J. Physiol. (Lond.)* **97**, 408–416.

HASSÓN, A. (1962) Interaction of quaternary ammonium bases with a purified acid polysaccharide and other macromolecules from the electric organ of the electric eel. *Biochim. biophys. Acta* **56**, 275–292.

HASSÓN, A. and CHAGAS, C. (1959) Selective capacity of components of the aqueous extract of the electric organ to bind curarizing quaternary ammonium derivatives. *Biochim. biophys. Acta* **36**, 301–308.

HASSÓN-VOLOCH, A. (1968) Curare and acetylcholine receptor substance. *Nature (Lond.)* **218**, 330–333.

HÄUSLER, H. F. (1953) On the central transmission of nervous impulses. Abst. XIX Int. Physiol. Congr. 443.

HÄUSLER, H. F. and STERZ, H. (1952) Zur Frage der Übertragung Sensibler Impulse Im Rückenmark des Frosches. *J. Mt. Sinai Hosp.* **19**, 121–130.

HAVERBACK, B. J. and WIRTSCHAFTLER, S. K. (1962) The gastrointestinal tract and naturally occurring pharmacologically active amines. *Advanc. Pharmac.* **1**, 309–348.

HAYASHI, T. (1959) The inhibitory action of β-hydroxy-γ-aminobutyric acid upon the seizure following stimulation of the motor cortex of the dog. *J. Physiol. (Lond.)* **145**, 570–578.

HAYASHI, T. and NAGAI, K. (1956) Action of ω-amino acids on the motor cortex of higher animals, especially γ-amino-β-oxybutyric acid as the real inhibitory principle in brain. Abstr. XX int. physiol. Congr. 410.

HAYES, A. H. and RIKER, W. F. (1963) Acetylcholine release at the neuromuscular junction. J. Pharmac. exp. Ther. 142, 200–205.

HEATH, R. G. and VERSTER, F. DE B. (1961) Effects of chemical stimulation to discrete brain areas. Am. J. Psychiat. 117, 980–989.

HEBB, C. O. (1957) Biochemical evidence for the neural function of acetylcholine. Physiol. Rev. 37, 196–220.

HEBB, C. O. (1963) Formation, storage and liberation of acetylcholine. Handb. exp. Pharmak. 15, 55–88.

HEBB, C. O. and SILVER, A. (1956) Choline acetylase in the central nervous system of man and some other mammals. J. Physiol. (Lond.) 134, 718–728.

HEBB, C. O. and SILVER, A. (1963) The effect of transection on the level of choline acetylase in the goat's sciatic nerve. J. Physiol. (Lond.) 169, 41–42P.

HEBB, C. O. and SMALLMAN, B. N. (1956) Intracellular distribution of choline acetylase. J. Physiol. (Lond.) 134, 385–392.

HEBB, C. O. and WAITES, G. M. H. (1956) Choline acetylase in antero- and retrograde degeneration of a cholinergic nerve. J. Physiol. (Lond.) 132, 667–671.

HELLER, A., HARVEY, J. A. and MOORE, R. Y. (1962) A demonstration of a fall in brain serotonin following central nervous lesions in the rat. Biochem. Pharmac. 11, 859–866.

HELLER, A. and MOORE, R. Y. (1965) Effect of central nervous system lesions on brain monoamines in the rat. J. Pharmac. exp. Ther. 150, 1–9.

HELLER, A., SEIDEN, L. S. and MOORE, R. Y. (1966) Regional effects of lateral hypothalamic lesions on brain norepinephrine in the cat. Int. J. Neuropharmac. 5, 91–101.

HELLER, A., SEIDEN, L. S., PORCHER, W. and MOORE, R. Y. (1966) Regional effects of lateral hypothalamic lesions on 5-hydroxytryptophan decarboxylase in the cat brain. J. Neurochem. 13, 967–974.

HENDERSON, V. E. and ROEPKE, M. H. (1937) Drugs affecting parasympathetic nerves. Physiol. Rev. 17, 373–407.

HERNANDEZ-PEON, R. (1965) Central neuro-humoral transmission in sleep and wakefulness. In: Sleep Mechanisms. Progress in Brain Research, vol. 18, pp. 96–117. Ed. K. Akert, C. Bally and J. P. Schadé Amsterdam: Elsevier.

HERNANDEZ-PEON, R. and CHAVEZ-IBARRA, G. (1963) Sleep induced by electrical or chemical stimulation of the forebrain. Electroen. Neurophysiol. Suppl. 24, 188–198.

HERNANDEZ-PEON, R., CHAVEZ-IBARRA, G., MORGAN, J. P. and TIMO-IARIA, C. (1963) Limbic cholinergic pathways involved in sleep and emotional behaviour. Expl. Neurol. 8, 93–111.

HERTTING, G., AXELROD, J. and PATRICK, R. W. (1962) Actions of bretylium and guanethidine on the uptake and release of [³H]-noradrenaline. Br. J. Pharmac. Chemother. 18, 161–166.

HERTTING, G., AXELROD, J. and WHITBY, L. G. (1961) Effect of drugs on the uptake and metabolism of H³-norepinephrine. J. Pharmac. exp. Ther. 134, 146–153.

HERTZLER, E. C. (1961) 5-Hydroxytryptamine and transmission in sympathetic ganglia. Br. J. Pharmac. Chemother. 17, 406–413.

HERZ, A. and NACIMIENTO, A. C. (1965) Über die Wirkung von Pharmaka auf neurone des Hippocampus nach mikroelektrophorefischer Verabfolgung. Naunyn-Schmiedeberg's Arch. exp. Path. Pharmak. 251, 295–314.

318 THE PHARMACOLOGY OF SYNAPSES

HERZ, A. and ZIEGELGÄNSBERGER, W. (1966) Synaptic excitation in the corpus striatum inhibited by microelectrophoretically administered dopamine. *Experientia* **22**, 839–840.

HESS, A. and PILAR, G. (1963) Slow fibres in the extraocular muscles of the cat. *J. Physiol. (Lond.)* **169**, 780–798.

HILL, R. B. (1958) The effects of certain neurohumours and the other drugs on the ventricle and radula protractor of *Busycon canaliculatum* and on the ventricle of *Strombus gigas*. *Biol. Bull. mar. biol. Lab. Woods Hole* **115**, 471–482.

HILLMAN, H. H. and McILWAIN, H. (1961) Membrane potentials in mammalian cerebral tissues *in vitro*: dependence on ionic environment. *J. Physiol. (Lond.)* **157**, 263–278.

HIMWICH, H. E. and HIMWICH, W. A. Eds. (1964) Biogenic amines. *Progr. Brain Res.* **8**, 1–250.

HIRSCH, H. E. and ROBINS, E. (1962) Distribution of γ-aminobutyric acid in the layers of the cerebral and cerebellar cortex. Implications for its physiological role. *J. Neurochem.* **9**, 63–70.

HOLMAN, M. E. and McLEAN, A. (1967) The innervation of sheep mesenteric veins. *J. Physiol. (Lond.)* **190**, 55–69.

HOLMES, S. W. and HORTON, E. W. (1967) The nature and distribution of prostaglandins in the central nervous system of the dog. *J. Physiol. (Lond.)* **191**, 134–135P.

HOLMES, S. W. and HORTON, E. W. (1968) The identification of four prostaglandins in dog brain and their regional distribution in the central nervous system. *J. Physiol. (Lond.)* **195**, 731–741.

HOLMSTEDT, B. and SJÖQVIST, F. (1959) Distribution of acetocholinesterase in the ganglion cells of various sympathetic ganglia. *Acta physiol. scand.* **47**, 284–296.

HOLTZ, P. (1950) Über die sympathicomimetische Wirksamkeit von Gehirn extrakten. *Acta physiol. scand.* **20**, 354–362.

HOLTZ, P. and SCHÜMANN, H. J. (1954) Butyrylcholin in Gehirnextrakten. *Naturwissenschaften.* **41**, 306.

HOLZBAUER, M. and VOGT, M. (1956) Depression by reserpine of the noradrenaline concentration in the hypothalamus of the cat. *J. Neurochem.* **1**, 8–11.

HONOUR, A. J. and McLENNAN, H. (1960) The effects of γ-aminobutyric acid and other compounds on structures of the mammalian nervous system which are inhibited by Factor I. *J. Physiol. (Lond.)* **150**, 306–318.

HOPKIN, J. M., HORTON, E. W. and WHITTAKER, V. P. (1967) Prostaglandin content of particulate and supernatant fractions of rat brain homogenates. *Nature (Lond.)* **217**, 71–72.

HORNYKIEWICZ, O. (1966) Dopamine (3-hydroxytyramine) and brain function. *Pharmac. Rev.* **18**, 925–964.

HORTON, E. W. (1963) Action of prostaglandin E₁ on tissues which respond to bradykinin. *Nature (Lond.)* **200**, 892–893.

HORTON, E. W. (1964) Actions of prostaglandins E₁, E₂ and E₃ on the central nervous system. *Br. J. Pharmac. Chemother.* **22**, 189–192.

HORTON, E. W. (1965) Biological activities of pure prostaglandins, *Experientia* **21**, 113–118.

HORTON, E. W. (1967) *Drugs of Animal Origin.* Inaugural Lecture by Wellcome Professor of Pharmacology at the University of London. London: Nelthropp.

HORTON, E. W. and MAIN, I. H. W. (1965) Differences in the effects of prostaglandins F2α, a constituent of cerebral tissue, and prostaglandin E₁ on conscious cats and chicks. *Int. J. Neuropharmac.* **4**, 65–69.

HORTON, E. W. and MAIN, I. H. M. (1967a) Identification of prostaglandins in central nervous tissues of the cat and chicken. *Br. J. Pharmac. Chemother.* **30**, 582–602.

HORTON, E. W. and MAIN, I. H. M. (1967b) Further observations on the central nervous actions of prostaglandins F2α and E₁. *Br. J. Pharmac. Chemother.* **30,** 568–581.

HORTON, E. W., MAIN, I. H. M. and THOMPSON, C. J. (1965) Effects of prostaglandins on the oviduct, studied in rabbits and ewes. *J. Physiol.* (*Lond.*) **180,** 514–528.

HOSEIN, E. A. and ORZECK, A. (1964) Some physiological and biochemical properties of acetyl-L-carnitine isolated from brain tissue extracts. *Int. J. Neuropharmac.* **3,** 71–76.

HOSEIN, E. A. and PROULX, L. (1965) Influence of electrical stimulation on the content of substances with acetylcholine-like activity in the superior cervical ganglion of the cat. *Archs. Biochem. Biophys.* **109,** 129–133.

HOSEIN, E. A., PROULX, P. and ARA, R. (1962) Substances with acetylcholine activity in normal rat brain. *Biochem. J.* **83,** 341–346.

HUBBARD, J. I. (1961) The effect of calcium and magnesium on the spontaneous release of transmitter from mammalian motor nerve endings. *J. Physiol.* (*Lond.*) **159,** 507–517.

HUBBARD, J. I. (1963) Repetitive stimulation at the mammalian neuromuscular junction, and the mobilization of transmitter. *J. Physiol.* (*Lond.*) **169,** 641–662.

HUBBARD, J. I. (1965) The origin and significance of antidromic activity in motor nerves. In: *Studies in Physiology,* pp. 85–92. Ed. D. R. Curtis and A. K. McIntyre Berlin: Springer-Verlag.

HUBBARD, J. I., JONES, S. F. and LANDAU, E. M. (1968) On the mechanism by which calcium and magnesium affect the spontaneous release of transmitter from mammalian motor nerve terminals. *J. Physiol.* (*Lond.*) **194,** 355–380.

HUBBARD, J. I. and KWANBUNBUMPEN, S. (1968) Evidence for the vesicle hypothesis. *J. Physiol.* (*Lond.*) **194,** 407–420.

HUBBARD, J. I., SCHMIDT, R. F. and YOKOTA, T. (1965) The effect of acetylcholine upon mammalian motor nerve terminals. *J. Physiol.* (*Lond.*) **181,** 810–829.

HUBBARD, J. I. and WILLIS, W. D. (1962) Hyperpolarization of mammalian motor nerve terminals. *J. Physiol.* (*Lond.*) **163,** 115–137.

HUGHES, G. M. and TAUC, L. (1965) A unitary biphasic post-synaptic potential (BPSP) in *Aplysia* "brain". *J. Physiol.* (*Lond.*) **179,** 27–28P.

HUGHES, J. and VANE, J. R. (1967) An analysis of the responses of the isolated portal vein of the rabbit to electrical stimulation and to drugs. *Br. J. Pharmac. Chemother.* **30,** 46–66.

HUKOVIĆ, S. (1961) Responses of the isolated sympathetic nerve-ductus deferens preparation of the guinea-pig. *Br. J. Pharmac. Chemother.* **16,** 188–194.

HUTTER, O. F. (1961) Ion movements during vagus inhibition of the heart. In: *Nervous Inhibition,* pp. 114–123. Ed. E. Florey. New York: Pergamon.

HUTTER, O. F. and KOSTIAL, K. (1954) Effect of magnesium and calcium ions on release of acetylcholine. *J. Physiol.* (*Lond.*) **124,** 234–241.

HUTTER, O. F. and LOEWENSTEIN, W. R. (1955) Nature of neuromuscular facilitation by sympathetic stimulation in the frog. *J. Physiol.* (*Lond.*) **130,** 559–571.

HUTTER, O. F. and TRAUTWEIN, W. (1956) Vagal and sympathetic effects on the pacemaker fibers in the sinus venosus of the heart. *J. gen. Physiol.* **39,** 715–733.

ICHIKAWA, S. and BOZLER, E. (1955) Monophasic and diphasic action potentials of the stomach. *Am. J. Physiol.* **182,** 92–96.

INNES, I. R. and NICKERSON, M. (1965) Drugs acting on postganglionic adrenergic nerve endings and structures innervated by them (Sympathomimetic Drugs). In: *The Pharmacological Basis of Therapeutics,* pp. 477–520. Ed. L. S. Goodman and A. Gilman. New York: Macmillan.

INOUYE, A. and KATAOKA, K. (1962) Sub-cellular distribution of the substance P in the nervous tissues. *Nature (Lond.)* **193**, 585.

INOUYE, A., KATAOKA, K. and SHINAGAWA, Y. (1963) Intracellular distribution of brain noradrenalin and De Robertis' non-cholinergic nerve endings. *Biochim. biophys. Acta* **71**, 491–493.

IRALDI, A. P. DE, DUGGAN, H. J. F. and DE ROBERTIS, E. D. P. (1963) Adrenergic synaptic vesicles in the anterior hypothalamus of the rat. *Anat. Rec.* **145**, 521–531.

ISRÄEL, M. and WHITTAKER, V. P. (1965) The isolation of mossy fibre endings from the granular layer of the cerebellar cortex. *Experientia* **21**, 325–326.

ITO, M., KOSTYUK, P. G. and OSHIMA, T. (1962) Further study on anion permeability in cat spinal motoneurones. *J. Physiol. (Lond.)* **164**, 150–156.

ITOH, T., KAJIKAWA, K., HASHIMOTO, Y., YOSHIDA, H. and IMAIZUMI, R. (1965) The uptake of catecholamine by subcellular granules in the brain stem. *Jap. J. Pharmac.* **15**, 335–338.

IVERSEN, L. L. (1967) *The Uptake and Storage of Noradrenaline in Sympathetic Nerves.* Cambridge: Cambridge University Press.

IWAMA, K. and JASPER, H. H. (1957) The action of gamma-aminobutyric acid upon cortical electrical activity in the cat. *J. Physiol. (Lond.)* **138**, 365–380.

IYATOMI, K. and KANESHINA, K. (1958) Localization of cholinesterase in the American cockroach. *Jap. J. appl. Ent. Zool.* **2**, 1–10.

JACOB, J. and POITE-BEVIERRE, M. (1960) Actions de la sérotonine et de la benzyl-l-diméthyl-2, 5- sérotonine sur le coeur isolé de lapin. *Archs. int. Pharmacodyn. Ther.* **127**, 11–26.

JACOBOWITZ, D. (1965) A method for the demonstration of both acetylcholinesterase and catecholamine in the same nerve trunk. *Life Sci. (Oxford)* **4**, 297–303.

JACOBOWITZ, D. and KOELLE, G. B. (1965) Histochemical correlations of acetylcholinesterase and catecholamines in postganglionic autonomic nerves of the cat, rabbit and guinea-pig. *J. Pharmac. exp. Ther.* **148**, 225–237.

JAEGER, C. P. (1961) Physiology of mollusca. I. Action of acetylcholine on the heart of *Strophocheilos oblongus. Comp. Biochem. Physiol.* **4**, 30–32.

JAEGER, C. P. (1962) Physiology of mollusca. III. Action of acetylcholine on the penis retractor muscle of *Strophocheilos oblongus. Comp. Biochem. Physiol.* **7**, 63–69.

JAEGER, C. P. (1966) Neuroendocrine regulation of cardiac activity in the snail *Strophocheilus oblongus. Comp. Biochem. Physiol.* **17**, 409–415.

JASPER, H. H. (1958) Reticular-cortical systems and theories of the integrative action of the brain. In: *Biological and Biochemical Bases of Behaviour*, pp. 37–61. Ed. H. F. Harlow and C. N. Woolsey Madison: University of Wisconsin Press.

JASPER, H. H., KHAN, R. T. and ELLIOTT, K. A. C. (1965) Amino acids released from cerebral cortex in relation to its state of activation. *Science, N.Y.* **147**, 1448–1449.

JASPER, H. H. and KOYAMA, I. (1968) Amino acids released from the cortical surface in cats following stimulation of the mesial thalamus and mid-brain reticular formation. *Electroen. Neurophysiol.* **24**, 292.

JENKINSON, D. H. (1960) The antagonism between tubocurarine and substances which depolarize the motor endplate. *J. Physiol. (Lond.)* **152**, 309–324.

JENKINSON, D. H. and MORTON, I. K. M. (1967a) The effect of noradrenaline on the permeability of depolarized intestinal smooth muscle to inorganic ions. *J. Physiol. (Lond.)* **188**, 373–386.

JENKINSON, D. H. and MORTON, I. K. M. (1967b) The role of α- and β-adrenergic receptors in some actions of catecholamines on intestinal smooth muscle. *J. Physiol. (Lond.)* **188**, 387–402.

JÉQUIER, E. (1965) Effet de la sérotonine sur la transmission synaptique dans les ganglion sympathique cervical isolé du rat. *Helv. physiol. pharmac. Acta* **23**, 163–179.

JÉQUIER, E., LOVENBERG, W. and SJOERDSMA, A. (1967) Tryptophan hydroxylase inhibition: the mechanism by which p-chlorophenylalanine depletes rat brain serotonin. *Molec. Pharmac.* **3**, 274–278.

JOHNSON, E. S. (1963) The origin of acetylcholine released spontaneously from the guinea-pig isolated intestine. *Br. J. Pharmac. Chemother.* **21**, 555–568.

JONASSON, J., ROSENGREN, E. and WALDECK, B. (1964) Effects of some pharmacologically active amines on the uptake of arylalkylamines by adrenal medullary granules. *Acta physiol. scand.* **60**, 136–140.

JONSON, B. and WHITE, T. (1964) Histamine metabolism in the brain of conscious cats. *Proc. Soc. Exptl. Biol. Med. N.Y.* **115**, 874–876.

JUHLIN, L. and SHELLEY, W. B. (1966) Detection of histamine by a new fluorescent O-phthalaldehyde stain. *J. Histochem Cytochem.* **14**, 525–528.

KAHLSON, G. and MACINTOSH, F. C. (1939) Acetylcholine synthesis in a sympathetic ganglion. *J. Physiol. (Lond.)* **96**, 277–292.

KAHLSON, G. and ROSENGREN, E. (1965) Histamine. *A. Rev. Pharmac.* **5**, 305–320.

KAKIMOTO, Y. and ARMSTRONG, M. D. (1962) On the identification of octopamine in mammals. *J. biol. Chem.* **237**, 422–427.

KANAI, T. and SZERB, J. C. (1965) Mesencephalic reticular activating system and cortical acetylcholine output. *Nature (Lond.)* **205**, 80–82.

KANDEL, E. R., FRAZIER, W. T., WAZIRI, R. and COGGESHALL, R. E. (1967) Direct and common connections among identified neurons in *Aplysia. J. Neurophysiol.* **30**, 1352–1376.

KAO, C. Y. and GRUNDFEST, H. (1957) Postsynaptic electrogenesis in septate giant axons. 1. Earthworm medium giant axon. *J. Neurophysiol.* **20**, 553–573.

KARCZMAR, A. G., KIM, K. C. and KOKETSU, K. (1961) Endplate effects and antagonism to d-tubocurarine and decamethonium of tetraethylammonium and of methoxyambenonium. *J. Pharmac. exp. Ther.* **134**, 199–205.

KARKI, N. T. and PAASONEN, M. K. (1959) Selective depletion of noradrenaline and 5-hydroxytryptamine from rat brain and intestine by Rauwolfia alkaloids. *J. Neurochem.* **3**, 352–357.

KÁSA, P. and CSERNOVSKY, E. (1967) Electron microscopic localization of acetylcholinesterase in the superior cervical ganglion of the rat. *Acta histochem.* **28**, 274–285.

KÁSA, P. and CSILLIK, B. (1965) Cholinergic excitation and inhibition in the cerebellar cortex. *Nature (Lond.)* **208**, 695–696.

KÁSA, P. and CSILLIK, B. (1966) Electron microscopic localization of cholinesterase by a copper-lead-thiocholine technique. *J. Neurochem.* **13**, 1345–1349.

KÁSA, P., CSILLIK, B., JOÓ, F. and KNYIHÁR, E. (1966) Histochemical and ultra-structural alterations in the isolated archicerebellum of the rat. *J. Neurochem.* **13**, 173–178.

KATAOKA, K. (1962) Subcellular distribution of 5-hydroxytryptamine in the rabbit brain. *Jap. J. Physiol.* **12**, 623–638.

KATAOKA, K. and DE ROBERTIS, E. (1967) Histamine in isolated small nerve endings and synaptic vesicles of rat brain cortex. *J. Pharmac. exp. Ther.* **156**, 114–125.

KATAOKA, K., RAMWELL, P. W. and JESSUP, S. (1967) Prostaglandins: localization in subcellular particles of rat cerebral cortex. *Science, N.Y.* **157**, 1187–1188.

KATO, J. (1960) Choline acetylase of human placenta. *J. Biochem.* **48**, 768–772.

KATZ, B. (1962) The transmission of impulses from nerve to muscle, and the subcellular unit of synaptic action. *Proc. R. Soc. B* **155**, 455–477.

322 THE PHARMACOLOGY OF SYNAPSES

KATZ, B. and MILEDI, R. (1963) A study of spontaneous miniature potentials in spinal motoneurones. *J. Physiol. (Lond.)* **168**, 389–422.

KATZ, B. and MILEDI, R. (1964a) Further observations on the distribution of acetyl-choline-reactive sites in skeletal muscle. *J. Physiol. (Lond.)* **170**, 379–388.

KATZ, B. and MILEDI, R. (1964b) The development of acetylcholine sensitivity in nerve-free segments of skeletal muscle. *J. Physiol. (Lond.)* **170**, 389–396.

KATZ, B. and MILEDI, R. (1965a) Propagation of electric activity in motor nerve terminals. *Proc. R. Soc. B* **161**, 453–482.

KATZ, B. and MILEDI, R. (1967) The timing of calcium action during neuromuscular transmission. *J. Physiol. (Lond.)* **189**, 535–544.

KAŽIĆ, T. and VARAGIĆ, V. M. (1968) Effect of increased intraluminal pressure on the release of acetylcholine from the isolated guinea-pig ileum. *Br. J. Pharmac. Chemother.* **32**, 185–192.

KEATINGE, W. R. (1964) Mechanism of adrenergic stimulation of mammalian arteries and its failure at low temperatures. *J. Physiol. (Lond.)* **174**, 184–205.

KEATINGE, W. R. (1966) Electrical and mechanical response of arteries to stimulation of sympathetic nerves. *J. Physiol. (Lond.)* **185**, 701–715.

KEHOE, J. (1967) Pharmacological characteristics and ionic bases of a two component postsynaptic inhibition. *Nature (Lond.)* **215**, 1503–1505.

KELLY, J. S., KRNJEVIĆ, K., MORRIS, M. E. and YIM, G. K. W. (1968) Anionic permeability of cortical neurones during inhibition. *J. Physiol. (Lond.)* **196**, 120–121P.

KENNARD, D. W. (1953) Local application of substances to the spinal cord. In: *The Spinal Cord*, pp. 214–221. Ciba Foundation Symposium. London: J. and A. Churchill Ltd.

KENNEDY, D. and EVOY, W. H. (1966) The distribution of pre- and postsynaptic inhibition at crustacean neuromuscular junctions. *J. gen. Physiol.* **49**, 457–468.

KERKUT, G. A. and LEAKE, L. D. (1966) The effect of drugs on the snail pharangeal retractor muscle. *Comp. Biochem. Physiol.* **17**, 623–633.

KERKUT, G. A., LEAKE, L. D., SHAPIRA, A., COWAN, S. and WALKER, R. J. (1965). The presence of glutamate in nerve-muscle perfusates of *Helix, Carcinus* and *Periplaneta. Comp. Biochem. Physiol.* **15**, 485–502.

KERKUT, G. A. and MEECH, R. W. (1966) The internal chloride concentration of H and D cells in the snail brain. *Comp. Biochem. Physiol.* **19**, 819–832.

KERKUT, G. A., SEDDEN, C. B. and WALKER, R. J. (1966) The effect of DOPA, α-methyl DOPA and reserpine on the dopamine content of the brain of the snail, *Helix aspersa. Comp. Biochem. Physiol.* **18**, 921–930.

KERKUT, G. A., SEDDEN, C. B. and WALKER, R. J. (1967a) Cellular localization of mono-amines by fluorescence microscopy in *Hirudo medicinalis* and *Lumbricus terrestris. Comp. Biochem. Physiol.* **21**, 687–690.

KERKUT, G. A., SEDDEN, C. B. and WALKER, R. J. (1967b) Uptake of DOPA and 5-hydroxytryptophan by monoamine-forming neurones in the brain of *Helix aspersa. Comp. Biochem. Physiol.* **23**, 159–162.

KERKUT, G. A., SHAPIRA, A. and WALKER, R. J. (1965) The effect of acetylcholine, glutamic acid and GABA on the contractions of the perfused cockroach leg. *Comp. Biochem. Physiol.* **16**, 37–48.

KERKUT, G. A. and THOMAS, R. C. (1964) The effect of anion injection and changes in the external potassium and chloride concentration on the reversal potentials of the IPSP and acetylcholine. *Comp. Biochem. Physiol.* **11**, 199–213.

KERKUT, G. A. and WALKER, R. J. (1961) The effects of drugs on the neurones of the snail, *Helix aspersa. Comp. Biochem. Physiol.* **3**, 143–160.

KERKUT, G. A. and WALKER, R. J. (1962) The specific chemical sensitivity of *Helix* nerve cells. *Comp. Biochem. Physiol.* 7, 277–288.

KERKUT, G. A. and WALKER, R. J. (1966) The effect of L-glutamate, acetylcholine and gamma-aminobutyric acid on the miniature endplate potentials and contractures of the coxal muscles of the cockroach, *Periplaneta americana. Comp. Biochem. Physiol.* 17, 435–454.

KERKUT, G. A., WALKER, R. J. and WOODRUFF, G. N. (1968) The effects of histamine and other naturally occurring imidazoles on neurones of *Helix aspersa. Br. J. Pharmac. Chemother.* 32, 241–252.

KEWENTER, J. (1965) The vagal control of the jejunal and ileal motility and blood flow. *Acta physiol. scand.* 65, Suppl. 251, 1–68.

KEWITZ, H. (1955) Über die Aktionssubstanz in sympathischen Ganglien. *Naunyn-Schmiedeberg's Arch. exp. Path. Pharmak.* 225, 111–114.

KHAIRALLAH, P. A., PAGE, I. H. and TURKER, R. K. (1967) Some properties of pro-staglandin E_1 action on muscle. *Archs. int. Pharmacodyn. Thér.* 169, 328–341.

KIM, K. C. and KARCZMAR, A. G. (1967) Adaptation of the neuromuscular junction to constant concentrations of ACh. *Int. J. Neuropharmac.* 6, 51–61.

KIRALY, J. K. and PHILLIS, J. W. (1961) The action of some drugs on the dorsal root potentials on the isolated toad spinal cord. *Br. J. Pharmac. Chemother.* 17, 224–231.

KIRSHNER, N., SAGE, H. J. and SMITH, W. J. (1967) Mechanism of secretion from the adrenal medulla. II. Release of catecholamines and storage vesicle protein in response to chemical stimulation. *Molec. Pharmac.* 3, 254–265.

KIRSHNER, N., SAGE, H. J., SMITH, W. J. and KIRSHNER, A. G. (1966) Release of cate-cholamines and specific protein from adrenal glands. *Science, N.Y.* 154, 529–531.

KISSEL, J. W. and DOMINO, E. F. (1959) The effects of some possible neurohumoral agents on spinal cord reflexes. *J. Pharmac. exp. Ther.* 125, 168–177.

KLAUS, W., LÜLLMANN, H. and MUSCHOLL, E. (1960) Potassium flux of normal and denervated rat diaphragm. *Pflügers Arch. ges. Physiol.* 271, 761–775.

KOBLICK, D. C. (1958) The characterization and localization of frog skin cholinesterase. *J. gen. Physiol.* 41, 1129–1134.

KOE, B. K. and WEISSMAN, A. (1966) p-Chlorophenylalanine: a specific depletor of brain serotonin. *J. Pharmac. exp. Ther.* 154, 499–516.

KOELLA, W. P. and CZICMAN, J. (1966) Mechanism of the EEG-synchronizing action of serotonin. *Am. J. Physiol.* 211, 926–934.

KOELLA, W. P., SMYTHIES, J. R., BULL, D. M. and LEVY, C. K. (1960) Physiological fractionation of the effect of serotonin on evoked potentials. *Am. J. Physiol.* 198, 205–212.

KOELLE, G. B. (1950) The histochemical differentiation of types of cholinesterases and their localizations in tissues of the cat. *J. Pharmac. exp. Ther.* 100, 158–179.

KOELLE, G. B. (1954) The histochemical localization of cholinesterases in the nervous system of the rat. *J. comp. Neurol.* 100, 211–235.

KOELLE, G. B. (1955) The histochemical identification of acetylcholinesterase in cholin-ergic, adrenergic and sensory neurons. *J. Pharmac. exp. Ther.* 114, 167–184.

KOELLE, G. B. (1962) A new general concept of the neurohumoral functions of acetyl-choline and acetylcholinesterase. *J. Pharm. Pharmac.* 14, 65–90.

KOELLE, G. B. (1963) Cytological distributions and physiological functions of cholinester-ases. *Handb. exp. Pharmak.* 15, 187–298.

KOELLE, G. B. and FOROGLOU-KERAMEOS, C. (1965) Electron microscopic localization of cholinesterases in a sympathetic ganglion by a gold-thiolacetic acid method. *Life Sci. (Oxford)* 4, 417–424.

KOELLE, G. B. and FRIEDENWALD, J. S. (1949) A histochemical method for localising cholinesterase activity. *Proc. Soc. exp. Biol. Med. N.Y.* **70**, 617–622.

KOELLE, W. A. and KOELLE, G. B. (1959) The localization of external or functional acetylcholinesterase at the synapses of autonomic ganglia. *J. Pharmac. exp. Ther.* **126**, 1–8.

KOENIG, E. and KOELLE, G. B. (1961) Mode of regeneration of acetylcholinesterase in cholinergic neurons following irreversible inactivation. *J. Neurochem.* **8**, 169–188.

KOHN, R. and MILLICHAP, J. G. (1958) Properties of seizures induced by histamine. *Proc. Soc. exp. Biol. Med. N.Y.* **99**, 623–628.

KOKETSU, K. (1956) Intracellular slow potential of dorsal root fibers. *Am. J. Physiol.* **184**, 338–344.

KOKETSU, K. (1958) Action of tetraethylammonium chloride on neuromuscular transmission in frogs. *Am. J. Physiol.* **193**, 213–218.

KOKETSU, K. and NISHI, S. (1959) Restoration of neuromuscular transmission in sodium-free hydrazinium solution. *J. Physiol. (Lond.)* **147**, 239–252.

KOKETSU, K. and NISHI, S. (1967) Characteristics of the slow inhibitory postsynaptic potential of bullfrog sympathetic ganglion cells. *Life Sci. (Oxford)* **6**, 1827–1836.

KONZETT, H. (1950) Sympathicomimetica und Sympathicolytica am isoliert durchströmten Ganglion cervicale superius der Katze. *Helv. physiol. pharmac. Acta* **8**, 245–258.

KONZETT, H. (1952) The effect of histamine on an isolated sympathetic ganglion. *J. Mt. Sinai Hosp.* **19**, 149–153.

KOPIN, I. J. (1964) Storage and metabolism of catecholamines: The role of monoamine oxidase. *Pharmac. Rev.* **16**, 179–191.

KOPIN, I. J. (1968) False adrenergic transmitters. *A. Rev. Pharmac.* **8**, 377–394.

KOPIN, I. J., FISCHER, J. E., MUSACCHIO, J. M. and HORST, W. D. (1964) Evidence for a false neurochemical transmitter as a mechanism for the hypotensive effect of monamine oxidase inhibitors. *Proc. natn. Acad. Sci. U.S.A.* **52**, 716–721.

KOPIN, I. J., FISCHER, J. E., MUSACCHIO, J. M., HORST, W. D. and WEISE, V. K. (1965) "False neurochemical transmitters" and the mechanism of sympathetic blockade by monamine oxidase inhibitors. *J. Pharmac. exp. Ther.* **147**, 186–193.

KOPPANYI, TH. (1932) Studies on the synergism and antagonism of drugs. I. The non-parasympathetic antagonism between atropine and the miotic alkaloids. *J. Pharmac. exp. Ther.* **46**, 395–405.

KOSTERLITZ, H. W., LEES, G. M. and WALLIS, D. I. (1968) Resting and action potentials recorded by the sucrose-gap method in the superior cervical ganglion of the rabbit. *J. Physiol. (Lond.)* **195**, 39–53.

KOTTEGODA, S. R. (1968) Are the excitatory nerves to the circular muscle of the guinea-pig ileum cholinergic? *J. Physiol. (Lond.)* **197**, 17–18P.

KRAVITZ, E. A., KUFFLER, S. W. and POTTER, D. D. (1963) Gamma-aminobutyric acid and other blocking compounds in Crustacea. III. Their relative concentrations in separated motor and inhibitory axons. *J. Neurophysiol.* **26**, 739–751.

KRAVITZ, E. A., KUFFLER, S. W., POTTER, D. D. and VAN GELDER, N. M. (1963) Gamma-aminobutyric acid and other blocking compounds in Crustacea. II. Peripheral nervous system. *J. Neurophysiol.* **26**, 729–738.

KRAVITZ, E. A., MOLINOFF, P. B. & HALL, Z. W. (1965) A comparison of the enzymes and substrates of gamma-aminobutyric acid metabolism in lobster excitatory and inhibitory axons. *Proc. natn. Acad. Sci. U.S.A.* **54**, 778–782.

KRIJGSMAN, B. J. (1952) Contractile and pacemaker mechanisms of the heart of arthropods. *Biol. Rev.* **27**, 320–346.

KRIJGSMAN, B. J. and DIVARIS, G. A. (1955) Contractile and pacemaker mechanisms of the heart of molluscs. *Biol. Rev.* **30**, 1–39.

KRNJEVIĆ, K. (1964) Micro-iontophoretic studies on cortical neurones. *Int. Rev. Neurobiol.* **7**, 41–98.

KRNJEVIĆ, K. (1965a) Action of drugs on single neurones in the cerebral cortex. *Br. med. Bull.* **21**, 10–14.

KRNJEVIĆ, K. (1965b). Cholinergic innervation of the cerebral cortex. In *Studies in Physiology*, pp. 144–151. Ed. D. R. Curtis and A. K. McIntyre Berlin: Springer.

KRNJEVIĆ, K. and MILEDI, R. (1958a) Acetylcholine in mammalian neuromuscular transmission. *Nature (Lond.)* **182**, 805–806.

KRNJEVIĆ, K. and MILEDI, R. (1958b) Some effects produced by adrenaline upon neuromuscular propagation in rats. *J. Physiol. (Lond.)* **141**, 291–304.

KRNJEVIĆ, K. and MILEDI, R. (1959) Presynaptic failure of neuromuscular propagation in rats. *J. Physiol. (Lond.)* **149**, 1–22.

KRNJEVIĆ, K. and MITCHELL, J. F. (1961) The release of acetylcholine in the isolated rat diaphragm. *J. Physiol. (Lond.)* **155**, 246–262.

KRNJEVIĆ, K. and PHILLIS, J. W. (1961) The action of certain amino acids on cortical neurones. *J. Physiol. (Lond.)* **159**, 62–63P.

KRNJEVIĆ, K. and PHILLIS, J. W. (1963a) Acetylcholine-sensitive cells in the cerebral cortex. *J. Physiol. (Lond.)* **166**, 296–327.

KRNJEVIĆ, K. and PHILLIS, J. W. (1963b) Pharmacological properties of acetylcholine-sensitive cells in the cerebral cortex. *J. Physiol. (Lond.)* **166**, 328–350.

KRNJEVIĆ, K. and PHILLIS, J. W. (1963c) Actions of certain amines on cerebral cortical neurones. *Br. J. Pharmac. Chemother.* **20**, 471–490.

KRNJEVIĆ, K. and PHILLIS, J. W. (1963d) Iontophoretic studies of neurones in the mammalian cerebral cortex. *J. Physiol. (Lond.)* **165**, 274–304.

KRNJEVIĆ, K., RANDIĆ, M. and STRAUGHAN, D. W. (1964) Unit responses and inhibition in the developing cortex. *J. Physiol. (Lond.)* **175**, 21–22P.

KRNJEVIĆ, K., RANDIĆ, M. and STRAUGHAN, D. W. (1966) Pharmacology of cortical inhibition. *J. Physiol. (Lond.)* **184**, 78–105.

KRNJEVIĆ, K. and SCHWARTZ, S. (1967a) Some properties of unresponsive cells in the cerebral cortex. *Expl. Brain Res.* **3**, 306–319.

KRNJEVIĆ, K. and SCHWARTZ, S. (1967b) The action of γ-aminobutyric acid on cortical neurones. *Expl. Brain Res.* **3**, 320–336.

KRNJEVIĆ, K. and SILVER, A. (1965) A histochemical study of cholinergic fibres in the cerebral cortex. *J. Anat.* **99**, 711–759.

KRNJEVIĆ, K. and SILVER, A. (1966) Acetylcholinesterase in the developing forebrain. *J. Anat.* **100**, 63–89.

KRNJEVIĆ, K. and STRAUGHAN, D. W. (1964) The release of acetylcholine from the denervated rat diaphragm. *J. Physiol. (Lond.)* **170**, 371–378.

KUBOTA, K. and BROOKHART, J. M. (1962) Recurrent facilitation of frog motoneurons. *Physiologist*, **5**, 170.

KUBOTA, K. and BROOKHART, J. M. (1963) Recurrent facilitation of frog motoneurones. *J. Neurophysiol.* **26**, 877–893.

KUFFLER, S. W. and EDWARDS, C. (1958) Mechanism of gamma-aminobutyric acid (GABA) action and its relation to synaptic inhibition. *J. Neurophysiol.* **21**, 589–610.

KUFFLER, S. W. and WILLIAMS, E. M. V. (1953a) Small nerve junctional potentials. The distribution of small motor nerves to frog skeletal muscle, and the membrane characteristics of the fibres they innervate. *J. Physiol. (Lond.)* **121**, 289–317.

KUFFLER, S. W. and WILLIAMS, E. M. V. (1953b) Properties of the "slow" skeletal muscle fibres of the frog. *J. Physiol. (Lond.)* **121**, 318–340.

KULKARNI, A. S. (1967) Effects on temperature of serotonin and epinephrine injected into the lateral cerebral ventricle of the cat. *J. Pharmac. exp. Ther.* **157**, 541–545.

KUNO, M. (1961) Site of action of systemc *gamma*-aminobutyric acid in the spinal cord. *Jap. J. Physiol.* **11**, 304–318.

KUNTZMAN, R., SHORE, P. A., BOGDANSKI, D. and BRODIE, B. B. (1961) Microanalytical procedures for fluorimetric assay of brain DOPA-5-HTP-decarboxylase, norepine-phrine and serotonin and a detailed mapping of decarboxylase activity in brain. *J. Neurochem.* **6**, 226–232.

KURIYAMA, H. (1963) Electrophysiological observations on the motor innervation of the smooth muscle cells in the guinea-pig vas deferens. *J. Physiol. (Lond.)* **169**, 213–228.

KURIYAMA, K., HABER, B., SISKEN, B. and ROBERTS, E. (1966) The γ-aminobutyric acid system in rabbit cerebellum. *Proc. natn. Acad. Sci. U.S.A.*, **55**, 846–852.

KURIYAMA, K., ROBERTS, E. and KAKEFUDA, T. (1968) Association of the γ-aminobutyric acid system with a synaptic vesicle fraction from mouse brain. *Brain Res.* **8**, 132–152.

KUSANO, K., LIVENGOOD, D. R. and WERMAN, R. (1967) Correlation of transmitter release with membrane properties of the presynaptic fiber of the squid giant synapse. *J. gen. Physiol.* **50**, 2579–2601.

KWANBUNBUMPEN, S. and JONES, S. F. (1968) The relationship of synaptic vesicles to acetylcholine storage and release. *Aust. J. exp. Biol. med. Sci.* **46**, 3P.

KWIATKOWSKI, H. (1943) Histamine in nervous tissue. *J. Physiol. (Lond.)* **102**, 32–41.

LANGLEY, J. N. (1891) On the course and connections of the secretory fibres supplying the sweat glands of the feet of the cat. *J. Physiol. (Lond.)* **12**, 347–374.

LANGLEY, J. N. (1893) Preliminary account of the arrangement of the sympathetic nervous system based chiefly on observations upon pilomotor nerves. *Proc. Roy Soc. (Lond.)* **52**, 547–556.

LANGLEY, J. N. and KATO, T. (1915) The physiological action of physostigmine and its action on denervated skeletal muscle. *J. Physiol. (Lond.)* **49**, 410–431.

LAPORTE, Y. and LORENTE DE NÓ (1950) Potential changes evoked in a curarized sympathetic ganglion by presynaptic volleys of impulses. *J. cell. comp. Physiol.* **35**, Suppl. 2, 61–106.

LAVERTY, R., MICHAELSON, I. A., SHARMAN, D. F. and WHITTAKER, V. P. (1963) The subcellular localization of dopamine and acetylcholine in the dog caudate nucleus. *Br. J. Pharmac. Chemother.* **21**, 482–490.

LAVERTY, R. and SHARMAN, D. F. (1965) The estimation of small quantities of 3,4-di-hydroxyphenylethylamine in tissues. *Br. J. Pharmac. Chemother.* **24**, 538–548.

LEE, J. B., COVINO, B. G., TAKMAN, B. H. and SMITH, E. R. (1965) Renomedullary vasodepressor substance, medullin: isolation, chemical characterization and physio-logical properties. *Circulation Res.* **17**, 57–77.

LEGGE, K. F., RANDIĆ, M. and STRAUGHAN, D. W. (1966) The pharmacology of neu-rones in the pyriform cortex, *Br. J. Pharmac. Chemother.* **26**, 87–107.

LEHRER, G. M. and ORNSTEIN, L. (1959) A diazo coupling method for the electron microscopic localization of cholinesterase. *J. biophys. biochem. Cytol.* **6**, 399–406.

LEIMDORFER, A. and METZNER, W. R. T. (1949) Analgesia and anaesthesia induced by epinephrine. *Am. J. Physiol.* **157**, 116–121.

LEMBECK, F. (1953) Zur Frage der zentralen Übertragung afferenter Impulse. III Mitteilung. Das Vorkommen und die Bedentung der Substanz P in den dorsaler wurzeln des Rückenmarks. *Naunyn-Schmiedeberg's Arch. exp. Path. Pharmak.* **219** 197–213.

LEMBECK, F. (1958) Die Beeinflussung der Darmmotilität durch Hydroxytryptamin *Pflügers Arch. ges. Physiol.* **265**, 567–574.

LEMBECK, F. and ZETLER, G. (1962) Substance P: A polypeptide of possible physiological significance, especially within the central nervous system. *Int. Rev. Neurobiol.* **4**, 159–215.

LEUSEN, I. and LACROIX, E. (1959) Influence of 5-hydroxytryptamine (serotonin) on the cat papillary muscle. *Archs. int. Physiol.* **67**, 93–96.

LEVI, R. and MAYNERT, E. W. (1964) The subcellular localization of brain-stem norepinephrine and 5-hydroxytryptamine in stressed rats. *Biochem. Pharmac.* **13**, 615–621.

LEVIN, E., LOVELL, R. A. and ELLIOTT, K. A. C. (1961) The relation of gamma-aminobutyric acid to Factor I in brain extracts. *J. Neurochem.* **7**, 147–154.

LEVITT, M., SPECTOR, S., SJOERDSMA, A. and UDENFRIEND, S. (1965) Elucidation of the rate-limiting step in norepinephrine biosynthesis in the perfused guinea-pig heart. *J. Pharmac. exp. Ther.* **148**, 1–8.

LÉVY, J. and MICHEL-BER, E. (1956) Contribution a l'action pharmacologique exercée par la sérotonine sur quelques organes isolés (intestin et oreillette). *J. Physiol. (Paris)* **48**, 1051–1084.

LEWIS, G. P. and REIT, E. (1965) The action of angiotensin and bradykinin on the superior cervical ganglion of the cat. *J. Physiol. (Lond.)* **179**, 538–553.

LEWIS, G. P. and REIT, E. (1966) Further studies on the actions of peptides on the superior cervical ganglion and suprarenal medulla. *Br. J. Pharmac. Chemother.* **26**, 444–460.

LEWIS, P. R. and SHUTE, C. C. D. (1967) The cholinergic limbic system: projection to hippocampal formation, medial cortex, nuclei of the ascending cholinergic reticular system, and the subfornical organ and supra-optic crest. *Brain* **90**, 521–540.

LEWIS, P. R., SHUTE, C. C. D. and SILVER, A. (1967) Confirmation from choline acetylase analyses of a massive cholinergic innervation to the rat hippocampus. *J. Physiol. (Lond.)* **191**, 215–224.

LEWIS, T. and MARVIN, H. M. (1927) Observations relating to vasodilatation arising from antidromic impulses, to herpes zoster and trophic effects. *Heart* **14**, 27–47.

LIBET, B. (1962) Slow excitatory and inhibitory synaptic responses in sympathetic ganglia. *Proc. XXII Int. Physiol. Congr.* vol. II, p. 809.

LIBET, B. (1964) Slow synaptic responses and excitatory changes in sympathetic ganglia. *J. Physiol. (Lond.)* **174**, 1–25.

LIBET, B. (1967) Long latent periods and further analysis of slow synaptic responses in sympathetic ganglia. *J. Neurophysiol.* **30**, 494–514.

LIBET, B. and TOSAKA, T. (1966) Slow postsynaptic potentials recorded intracellularly in sympathetic ganglia. *Fed. Proc.* **25**, 270.

LILEY, A. W. (1956) The quantal components of the mammalian endplate potential. *J. Physiol (Lond.)* **133**, 571–587.

LIPICKY, R. J., HERTZ, L. and SHANES, A. M. (1963) Ca^{45} transfer and acetylcholine release in the rabbit superior cervical ganglion. *J. cell. comp. Physiol.* **62**, 233–242.

LIPMANN, F. and KAPLAN, N. O. (1946) A common factor in the enzymatic acetylation of sulfanilamide and of choline. *J. biol. Chem.* **162**, 743–744.

LITTLE, K. D., DISTEFANO, V. and LEARY, D. E. (1957) LSD and serotonin effects on spinal reflexes in the cat. *J. Pharmac. exp. Ther.* **119**, 161.

LLOYD, D. P. C. (1942) Stimulation of peripheral nerve terminations by active muscle. *J. Neurophysiol.* **5**, 153–165.

LOEWI, O. (1921) Über humorale Übertragbarkeit der Herznervenwirkung. *Pflügers Arch. ges. Physiol.* **189**, 239–242.

LONG, J. P. (1963) Structure-activity relationships of the reversible anticholinesterase agents. *Handb. exp. Pharmak.* **15**, 374–427.

LONGO, V. G. (1962) *Rabbit Brain Research*, Vol. II. Electroencephalographic atlas for pharmacological research: effect of drugs on the electrical activity of the rabbit brain. Amsterdam: Elsevier.

LONGO, V. G. and SILVESTRINI, B. (1957) Effect of adrenergic and cholinergic drugs injected by intracarotid route on electrical activity of brain. Proc. Soc. exp. Biol. Med. (N.Y.) 95, 43–47.

LOVELAND, R. E. (1963) 5-hydroxytryptamine, the probable mediator of excitation in the heart of Mercenaria (Venus) mercenaria. Comp. Biochem. Physiol. 9, 95–104.

LOVENBERG, W., WEISSBACH, H. and UDENFRIEND, S. (1962) Aromatic L-amino acid decarboxylase. J. biol. Chem. 237, 89–93.

LOWE, I. P., ROBINS, E. and EYERMAN, G. S. (1958) The fluorimetric measurement of glutamic decarboxylase and its distribution in brain. J. Neurochem. 3, 8–18.

LUBINSKA, L. and ZELENÁ, J. (1967) Acetylcholinesterase at muscle-tendon junctions during postnatal development in rats. J. Anat. 101, 295–308.

LUNDBERG, A. (1965) Monoamines and spinal reflexes. In: Studies in Physiology, pp. 186–190. Ed. D. R. Curtis and A. K. McIntyre. Berlin: Springer.

LUX, H. D. and KLEE, M. R. (1962) Intracellulare Untersuchungen Über den Einfluss hemmender Potentiale im motorischen Cortex. I. Die Wirkung elektrischer Reizung unspezifisches Thalamuskerne. Arch. Psychiat. NervKrankh. 203, 648–666.

MACINTOSH, F. C. (1941) The distribution of acetylcholine in the peripheral and the central nervous system. J. Physiol. (Lond.) 99, 436–442.

MACINTOSH, F. C. (1961) Effect of HC-3 on acetylcholine turnover. Fed. Proc. 20, 562–568.

MACINTOSH, F. C., BIRKS, R. I. and SASTRY, P. B. (1956) Pharmacological inhibition of acetylcholine synthesis. Nature (Lond.) 178, 1181.

MACINTOSH, F. C. and OBORIN, P. E. (1953) Release of acetylcholine from intact cerebral cortex. Abstr. XIX int. Physiol. Congr. 580-581.

MACMILLAN, W. H. (1956) The effects of histamine on skeletal muscle contraction. Archs. int. Pharmacodyn. Ther. 108, 19–26.

McALLAN, J. W. and CHEFURKA, W. (1961) Some physiological aspects of glutamate-aspartate transamination in insects. Comp. Biochem. Physiol. 2, 290–299.

McCAMAN, R. E., ARNAIZ, G. R. DE L. and DE ROBERTIS, E. D. P. (1965) Species differences in subcellular distribution of choline acetylase in the C. N. S. A study of choline acetylase, acetylcholinesterase, 5-hydroxytryptophan decarboxylase and monoamine oxidase in four species. J. Neurochem. 12, 927–935.

McCANCE, I. and PHILLIS, J. W. (1964a) The action of acetylcholine on cells in cat cerebellar cortex. Experientia 20, 217–218.

McCANCE, I. and PHILLIS, J. W. (1964b) The discharge patterns of elements in cat cerebellar cortex and their responses to iontophoretically applied drugs. Nature (Lond.) 204, 844–846.

McCANCE, I. and PHILLIS, J. W. (1965) The location of microelectrode tips in nervous tissue. Experientia 21, 108–109.

McCANCE, I. and PHILLIS, J. W. (1968) Cholinergic mechanisms in the cerebellar cortex. Int. J. Neuropharmac. 7, 447–462.

McCANCE, I., PHILLIS, J. W., TEBÉCIS, A. K. and WESTERMAN, R. A. (1968) The pharmacology of ACh-excitation of thalamic neurones. Br. J. Pharmac. Chemother. 32, 652–662.

McCANCE, I., PHILLIS, J. W. and WESTERMAN, R. A. (1966) Responses of thalamic neurones to iontophoretically applied drugs. Nature (Lond.) 209, 715–716.

McCANCE, I., PHILLIS, J. W. and WESTERMAN, R. A. (1968a) Acetylcholine-sensitivity of thalamic neurones: its relationship to synaptic transmission. Br. J. Pharmac. Chemother. 32, 635–651.

McCance, I., Phillis, J. W. and Westerman, R. A. (1968b) Physiological and pharmacological studies on the cerebellar projections to the feline thalamus. *Expl. Neurol.* **21**, 257–269.

McCann, F. V. (1966) Curare as a neuromuscular blocking agent in insects. *Science, N.Y.* **152**, 225–226.

McCann, F. V. and Reece, R. W. (1967) Neuromuscular transmission in insects: effect of injected chemical agents. *Comp. biochem. Physiol.* **21**, 115–124.

McCawley, E. L., Leveque, P. E. and Dick, H. L. H. (1952) Certain actions of serotonin (5-hydroxytryptamine creatinine sulphate) on cardiac rhythm. *J. Pharmac. exp. Ther.* **106**, 406.

McCubbin, J. W., Kaneko, Y. and Page, I. H. (1962) Inhibition of neurogenic vasoconstriction by serotonin: vasodilator action of serotonin. *Circulation Res.* **11**, 74–83.

McDougal, M. D. and West, G. B. (1954) Inhibition of the peristaltic reflex by sympathomimetic amines. *Br. J. Pharmac. Chemother.* **9**, 131–137.

McGeer, E. G. and McGeer, P. L. (1962) Catecholamine content of spinal cord. *Can. J. Biochem. Physiol.* **40**, 1141–1151.

McGeer, P. L. (1964) The distribution of histamine in cat and human brain. In: *Comparative Neurochemistry*, pp. 387–391. Ed. D. Richter. London: Pergamon.

McGeer, P. L., Bagchi, S. P. and McGeer, E. G. (1965) Subcellular localization of tyrosine hydroxylase in beef caudate nucleus. *Life Sci. (Oxford)* **4**, 1859–1867.

McGeer, P. L., McGeer, E. G. and Wada, J. A. (1963) Central aromatic amine levels and behaviour. II. Serotonin and catecholamine levels in various cat brain areas following administration of psychoactive drugs or amine precursors. *Archs. Neurol. Psychiat. (Chicago)* **9**, 81–89.

McGregor, D. D. (1965) The effect of sympathetic nerve stimulation on vasoconstrictor responses in perfused mesenteric blood vessels of the rat. *J. Physiol. (Lond.)* **177**, 21–30.

McIntyre, A. R. (1959) Neuromuscular transmission and normal and denervated muscle-sensitivity to curare and acetylcholine. In: *International Symposium on Curare and Curare-like Agents*, pp 210–218. Ed. D. Bovet, F. Bovet-Nitti and G. B. Marini-Bettolo. Amsterdam: Elsevier.

McIsaac, R. J. and Koelle, G. B. (1959) Comparison of the effects of inhibition of external, internal, and total acetylcholinesterase upon ganglionic transmission. *J. Pharmac. exp. Ther.* **126**, 9–20.

McKinstry, D. N. and Koelle, G. B. (1967) Acetylcholine release from the cat superior cervical ganglion by carbachol. *J. Pharmac. exp. Ther.* **157**, 319–327.

McKinstry, D. N., Koenig, E., Koelle, W. A. and Koelle, G. B. (1963) The release of acetylcholine from a sympathetic ganglion by carbachol. *Can. J. Biochem. Physiol.* **41**, 2599–2609.

McLennan, H. (1961) The effect of some catecholamines upon a monosynaptic reflex pathway in the spinal cord. *J. Physiol. (Lond.)* **158**, 411–425.

McLennan, H. (1963) *Synaptic Transmission.* Philadelphia: W. B. Saunders.

McLennan, H. (1964) The release of acetylcholine and of 3-hydroxytyramine from the caudate nucleus. *J. Physiol. (Lond.)* **174**, 152–161.

McLennan, H., Curry, L. and Walker, R. (1963) The chromatographic behaviour of the acetylcholine activity of brain extracts. *Biochem. J.* **89**, 163–166.

McLennan, H. and York, D. H. (1966) Cholinergic mechanisms in the caudate nucleus. *J. Physiol. (Lond.)* **187**, 163–175.

McLennan, H. and York, D. H. (1967) The action of dopamine on neurones of the caudate nucleus. *J. Physiol. (Lond.)* **189**, 393–402.

MAGNUSSON, T. & ROSENGREN, E. (1963) Catecholamines of the spinal cord, normally and after transection. *Experientia* **19**, 229–230.

MAHNKE, J. H. and WARD, A. A. (1960) The effects of γ-aminobutyric acid on evoked potentials. *Expl. Neurol.* **2**, 311–323.

MAIN, I. H. M. (1964) The inhibitory actions of prostaglandins on respiratory smooth muscle. *Br. J. Pharmac. Chemother.* **22**, 511–519.

MAÎTRE, L. (1965) Presence of α-methyl dopa metabolites in heart and brain of guinea-pigs treated with α-methyl tyrosine. *Life Sci.* (*Oxford*) **4**, 2249–2256.

MALMÉJAC, J. (1955) Action of adrenaline on synaptic transmission and on adrenal medullary secretion. *J. Physiol.* (*Lond.*) **130**, 497–512.

MANN, P. J. G., TENNENBAUM, M. and QUASTEL, J. H. (1938) On the mechanism of acetylcholine formation in brain *in vitro*. *Biochem. J.* **32**, 243–261.

MANNARINO, E., KIRSHNER, N. and NASHOLD, B. S. (1963) The metabolism of C¹⁴ noradrenaline by cat brain *in vivo*. *J. Neurochem.* **10**, 373–379.

MANTEGAZZINI, P. (1957) Action of 5-hydroxytryptamine (enteramine) and acetylcholine on the electroencephalographic curve in cats. *Archs. int. pharmacodyn. Ther.* **112**, 199–211.

MANTEGAZZINI, P., POECK, K. and SANTIBANEZ, H. G. (1959) The action of adrenaline and noradrenaline on the cortical electrical activity of the "encéphale isolé" cat. *Archs. ital. Biol.* **97**, 222–242.

MARCHBANKS, R. M. (1968) Exchangeability of radioactive acetylcholine with the bound acetylcholine of synaptosomes and synaptic vesicles. *Biochem. J.* **106**, 87–95.

MARCZYNSKI, T. (1962) The pharmacological properties of several new derivatives of tryptamine. *Dissnes pharm. Warsz.* **14**, 247–258.

MARLEY, E. (1964) The adrenergic system and sympathomimetic amines. *Adv. Pharmac.* **3**, 167–266.

MARLEY, E. and VANE, J. R. (1967) Tryptamines and spinal cord reflexes in cats. *Br. J. Pharmac. Chemother.* **31**, 447–465.

MARNAY, A. and NACHMANSOHN, D. (1938) Choline esterase in voluntary muscle. *J. Physiol.* (*Lond.*) **92**, 37–47.

MARRAZZI, A. S. (1939) Electrical studies on the pharmacology of autonomic synapses. II. The action of a sympathomimetic drug (epinephrine) on sympathetic ganglia. *J. Pharmac. exp. Ther.* **65**, 395–404.

MARRAZZI, A. S. (1957) The effects of certain drugs on cerebral synapses. *Ann. N.Y. Acad. Sci.* **66**, 496–507.

MARRAZZI, A. S. (1961) Inhibition as a determinant of synaptic and behavioural patterns. *Ann. N.Y. Acad. Sci.* **92**, 990–1003.

MARRAZZI, A. S. and HART, E. R. (1955) Evoked cortical responses under the influence of hallucinogens and related drugs. *Electroen. Neurophysiol.* **7**, 146.

MARRAZZI, A. S., HART, E. R. and RODRIGUEZ, J. M. (1958) Action of blood-borne gamma-aminobutyric acid on central synapses. *Science, N.Y.* **127**, 284–285.

MARRAZZI, A. S. and MARRAZZI, R. N. (1947) Further localization and analysis of adrenergic synaptic inhibition. *J. Neurophysiol.* **10**, 165–178.

MARSHALL, J. M. (1959) Effects of estrogen and progesterone on single uterine muscle fibres in the rat. *Am. J. Physiol.* **197**, 935–942.

MARTIN, A. R. (1955) A further study of the statistical composition of the endplate potential. *J. Physiol.* (*Lond.*) **130**, 114–122.

MARTIN, A. R. (1966) Quantal nature of synaptic transmission. *Physiol. Rev.* **46**, 51–66.

MARTIN, A. R. and ORKAND, R. K. (1961) Postsynaptic effects of HC-3 at the neuromuscular junction of the frog. *Can. J. Biochem. Physiol.* **39**, 343–349.

MARTIN, A. R. and PILAR, G. (1963a) Dual mode of synaptic transmission in the avain ciliary ganglion. *J. Physiol. (Lond.)* **168**, 443–463.

MARTIN, A. R. and PILAR, G. (1963b) Transmission through the ciliary ganglion of the chick. *J. Physiol. (Lond.)* **168**, 464–475.

MARTIN, A. R. and VEALE, J. L. (1967) The nervous system at the cellular level. *Ann. Rev. Physiol.* **29**, 401–426.

MASLAND, R. L. and WIGTON, R. S. (1940) Nerve activity accompanying fasiculation produced by prostigmin. *J. Neurophysiol.* **3**, 269–275.

MASON, D. F. J. (1962) Depolarizing action of neostigmine at an autonomic ganglion. *Br. J. Pharmac. Chemother.* **18**, 572–587.

MASUOKA, D. T., SCHOTT, H. F. and PETRIELLO, L. (1963) Formation of catecholamines by various areas of cat brain. *J. Pharmac. exp. Ther.* **139**, 73–76.

MATSUOKA, M. (1964) Function and metabolism of catecholamines in the brain. *Jap. J. Pharmac.* **14**, 181–193.

MATSUOKA, M., YOSHIDA, H. and IMAIZUMI, R. (1964) Distribution of catecholamines and their metabolites in rabbit brain. *Biochim. biophys. Acta.* **82**, 439–441.

MATTHEWS, R. J. and ROBERTS, B. J. (1961) The effect of gamma-aminobutyric acid on synaptic transmission in autonomic ganglia. *J. Pharmac. exp. Ther.* **132**, 19–22.

MAYNERT, E. W. and KURIYAMA, K. (1964) Some observations on nerve ending particles and synaptic vesicles. *Life Sci. (Oxford)* **3**, 1067–1087.

MAYNERT, E. W., LEVI, R. and DE LORENZO, A. J. D. (1964) The presence of norepinephrine and 5-hydroxytryptamine in vesicles from disrupted nerve-ending particles. *J. Pharmac. exp. Ther.* **144**, 385–392.

MEAD, C. O. and VAN DER LOOS, H. (1964) Experimental synaptochemistry of the rat cerebellar glomerulus. *Anat. Rec.* **148**, 311.

MENDEL, B., MEYERS, D. K., UYLDERT, I. E., RUYS, A. C. and DE BRUYN, W. M. (1953) Ali-esterase inhibitors and growth. *Br. J. Pharmac. Chemother.* **8**, 217–224.

METCALF, R. L., WINTON, M. Y. and FUKUTO, T. R. (1964) The effects of cholinergic substances upon the isolated heart of *Periplaneta americana. J. insect. Physiol.* **10**, 353–361.

MEYER, M. (1965) Die wirkung von acetylcholin, L-glutaminsäure and dopamin auf neurone im gebiet der nuclei cuneatus und gracilis der katze. *Helv. physiol. pharmac. Acta.* **23**, 325–340.

MICHAELSON, I. A. and COFFMAN, P. Z. (1967) The association of histamine with nerve endings in the dog hypothalamus. *Pharmacologist* **9**, 348.

MICHAELSON, I. A. and DOWE, G. (1963) The subcellular distribution of histamine in brain tissue. *Biochem. Pharmac.* **12**, 949–956.

MICHAELSON, I. A. and WHITTAKER, V. P. (1963) The subcellular localization of 5-hydroxytryptamine in guinea-pig brain. *Biochem. Pharmac.* **12**, 203–211.

MILEDI, R. (1960a) The acetylcholine sensitivity of frog muscle fibres after complete or partial denervation. *J. Physiol. (Lond.)* **151**, 1–23.

MILEDI, R. (1960b) Junctional and extra-junctional acetylcholine receptors in skeletal muscle fibres. *J. Physiol. (Lond.)* **151**, 24–30.

MILEDI, R. (1966) Strontium as a substitute for calcium in the process of transmitter release at the neuromuscular junction. *Nature (Lond.)* **212**, 1233–1234.

MILEDI, R. and SLATER, C. R. (1966) The action of calcium on neuronal synapses in the squid. *J. Physiol. (Lond.)* **184**, 473–498.

MILHAUD, G. and GLOWINSKI, J. (1962) Metabolisme de la dopamine-C^{14} dans le cerveau du rat. Etude du monde d'administration. *C. R. Acad. Sci. (Paris)* **255**, 203–205.

MILHAUD, G. and GLOWINSKI, J. (1963) Metabolisme de la noradrénaline-C^{14} dans le cerveau du rat. *C. R. Acad. Sci. (Paris)* **256**, 1033–1035.

MITCHELL, J. F. (1963) The spontaneous and evoked release of acetylcholine from the cerebral cortex. *J. Physiol. (Lond.)* **165**, 98–116.

MITCHELL, J. F. and PHILLIS, J. W. (1962) Cholinergic transmission in the frog spinal cord. *Br. J. Pharmac. Chemother.* **19**, 534–543.

MITCHELL, J. F. and SILVER, A. (1963) The spontaneous release of acetylcholine from the denervated hemidiaphragm of the rat. *J. Physiol. (Lond.)* **165**, 117–129.

MITCHELL, J. F. and SZERB, J. C. (1962) The spontaneous and evoked release of acetylcholine from the caudate nucleus. Abstr. XXII int. physiol. Congr. 819.

MONNIER, M. and TISSOT, R. (1958) Action de la réserpine et de ses médiateurs (5-hydroxytryptophan-sérotonine et dopa-noradrenaline) sur le comportement et le cerveau du lapin. *Helv. physiol. pharmac. Acta* **16**, 255–267.

MOORE, R. Y., WONG, S. L. R. and HELLER, A. (1965) Regional effects of hypothalamic lesions on brain serotonin. *Archs. Neurol. Psychiat. (Chicago)* **13**, 346–354.

MORISON, R. S. and DEMPSEY, E. W. (1943) Mechanism of thalamocortical augmentation and repetition. *Am. J. Physiol.* **138**, 297–308.

MORLOCK, N. and WARD, A. A. (1961) The effects of curare on cortical activity. *Electroen. Neurophysiol.* **13**, 60–67.

MORRELL, R. M. (1959) Recurrent inhibition in cerebral cortex. *Nature (Lond.)* **183**, 979–980.

MUNEOKA, A. (1961) Depression and facilitation of spinal reflexes by systemic omega-amino acids. *Jap. J. Physiol.* **11**, 555–563.

MUNRO, A. F. (1933) Effect of adrenaline and noradrenaline on activity of isolated preparations of gut from foetal guinea-pig. *Br. J. Pharmac. Chemother.* **8**, 38–41.

MUSACHIO, J. M., KOPIN, I. J. and WEISE, V. K. (1965) Subcellular distribution of some sympathomimetic amines and their beta-hydroxylated derivatives in the rat heart. *J. Pharmac. exp. Ther.* **148**, 22–28.

MUSCHOLL, E. and MAÎTRE, L. (1963) Release by sympathetic stimulation of α-methyl-noradrenaline stored in the heart after administration of α-methyldopa. *Experientia* **19**, 658–659.

MYHRBERG, H. (1967) Monoaminergic mechanisms in the nervous system of *Lumbricus terrestris*. *Z. Zellforsch. mikrosk. Anat.* **81**, 311–343.

NACHMANSOHN, D. (1959) *Chemical and Molecular Basis of Nerve Activity*. New York: Academic Press.

NACHMANSOHN, D. (1963) Choline acetylase. *Handb. exp. Pharmak.* **15**, 40–54.

NACHMANSOHN, D. and BERMAN, M. (1946) Studies on choline acetylase. III. On the preparation of the coenzyme and its effect on the enzyme. *J. biol. Chem.* **165**, 551–563.

NACHMANSOHN, D. and MACHADO, A. L. (1943) The formation of acetylcholine. A new enzyme: "Choline acetylase". *J. Neurophysiol.* **6**, 397–403.

NACHMANSOHN, D. and ROTHENBURG, M. A. (1945) Studies on cholinesterase. On the specificity of the enzyme in nerve tissue. *J. biol. Chem.* **158**, 653–666.

NAESS, K. and SIRNES, T. (1953) A synergistic effect of adrenaline and d-tubocurarine on neuromuscular transmission. *Acta physiol. scand.* **29**, 293–306.

NAESS, K. and SIRNES, T. (1954) An antagonistic effect between adrenaline and neostigmine on striated muscle. *Acta pharmac. tox.* **10**, 14–29.

NAGATSU, T., LEVITT, M. and UDENFRIEND, S. (1964) Tyrosine hydroxylase. The initial step in norepinephrine biosynthesis. *J. biol. Chem.* **239**, 2910–2917.

NASTUK, W. L. (1953) The electrical activity of the muscle cell membrane at the neuromuscular junction. *J. cell. comp. Physiol.* **42**, 249–272.

NASTUK, W. L. (1959) Some ionic factors that influence the action of acetylcholine at the muscle endplate membrane. *Ann. N.Y. Acad. Sci.* **81**, 317–327.

NELSON, P. G. and FRANK, K. (1967) Anomalous rectification in cat spinal moto-neurones and effect of polarizing currents on excitatory postsynaptic potential. *J. Neurophysiol.* **30**, 1097–1113.

NICHOLLS, J. G. (1956) Electrical properties of denervated skeletal muscle. *J. Physiol. (Lond.)* **131**, 1–12.

NICKERSON, M. (1965) Drugs inhibiting adrenergic nerves and structures innervated by them. In: *The Pharmacological Basis of Therapeutics.* pp. 546–577. Ed. L. S. Goodman and A. Gilman. New York: Macmillan.

NISHI, S. and KOKETSU, K. (1960) Electrical properties and activities of single sympathe-tic neurons in frogs. *J. cell. comp. Physiol.* **55**, 15–30.

NISHI, S. and KOKETSU, K. (1966) Late afterdischarge of sympathetic postganglionic fibres. *Life Sc.i (Oxford)* **5**, 1991–1997.

NISHI, S. and KOKETSU, K. (1967) Origin of ganglionic inhibitory postsynaptic potential. *Life Sci. (Oxford)* **6**, 2049–2055.

NONOMURA, Y., HOTTA, Y. and OHASHI, H. (1966) Tetrodotoxin and manganese ions: Effects on electrical activity and tension in taenia coli of guinea-pig. *Science, N.Y.* **152**, 97–98.

NORBERG, K. A. (1964) Adrenergic innervation of the intestinal wall studied by fluor-escence microscopy. *Int. J. Neuropharmac.* **3**, 379–382.

NORBERG, K. A. and SJÖQVIST, F. (1966) New possibilities for adrenergic modulation of ganglionic transmission. *Pharmac. Rev.* **18**, 743–751.

OBATA, K., ITO, M., OCHI, R. and SATO, N. (1967) Pharmacological properties of the postsynaptic inhibition by Purkinje cell axons and the action of γ-aminobutyric acid on Deiters neurones. *Expl. Brain. Res.* **4**, 43–57.

OCHS, S., BOOKER, H. and APRISON, M. H. (1960) Serotonin on direct cortical responses. *Physiologist* **3**, 121.

OGAWA, T. (1963) Midbrain reticular influences upon single neurons in the lateral geniculate nucleus. *Science, N.Y.* **139**, 343–344.

OGSTON, A. G. (1955) Removal of acetylcholine from a limited volume by diffusion. *J. Physiol. (Lond.)* **128**, 222–223.

OOMURA, Y., OOYAMA, H. and SAWADA. M. (1965) Ionic basis of the effect of ACh on D and H neurons. 23rd Intern. Congr. Physiol. Sci. Tokyo, 913.

ORLOV, R. S. (1961) The intracellular potentials of smooth muscle during stimulation of excitor and inhibitor nerves. *Sechenov. Physiol. J. USSR* **47**, 552–556.

ORLOV, R. S. (1962) On impulse transmission from motor sympathetic nerve to smooth muscle. *Sechenov. Physiol. J. USSR* **48**, 342–348.

ORLOV, R. S. (1963) Transmission of inhibitory impulses from nerve to smooth muscle. *Sechenov. Physiol. J. USSR* **49**, 575–582.

ÖSTLUND, E. (1954) The distribution of catechol amines in lower animals and their effect on the heart. *Acta physiol. scand.* **31**, Suppl. 112, 1–67.

OTSUKA, M., ENDO, M. and NONOMURA, Y. (1962) Presynaptic nature of neuro-muscular depression. *Jap. J. Physiol.* **12**, 573–584.

OTSUKA, M., IVERSEN, L. L., HALL, Z. W. and KRAVITZ, E. A. (1966) Release of gamma-aminobutyric acid from inhibitory nerves of lobster. *Proc. Nat. Acad. Sci. U.S.* **56**, 1110–1115.

OTSUKA, M., KRAVITZ, E. A. and POTTER, D. D. (1967) Physiological and chemical architecture of a lobster ganglion with particular reference to gamma-amino-butyrate and glutamate. *J. Neurophysiol.* **30**, 725–752.

OZEKI, M. (1962) Effects of various drugs on the neuromuscular transmission in the retractor pharynx muscle of snail. *Kumamoto Med. J.* **15**, 159–165.

PAASONEN, M. K., MACLEAN, P. D. and GIARMAN, N. J. (1957) 5-Hydroxytryptamine (serotonin, enteramine) content of structures of the limbic system. *J. Neurochem.* **1**, 326–333.

PAGE, I. H. (1954) Certain aspects of neurogenic and humoral control of blood vessels. *Ciba Foundation Symposium on Hypertension*, pp. 3–30. London: J. and A. Churchill.

PAGE, I. H. and McCUBBIN, J. W. (1953) Variable arterial pressure response to serotonin in laboratory animals and man. *Circulation Res.* **1**, 354–362.

PALAIČ, D., PAGE, I. H. and KHAIRALLAH, P. A. (1967) Uptake and metabolism of ^{14}C serotonin in rat brain. *J. Neurochem.* **14**, 63–69.

PALAY, S. L. (1956) Synapses in the central nervous system. *J. biophys. biochem. Cytol.* **2**, Suppl. 2, 193–202.

PANISSET, J.-C., BIRON, P. and BEAULNES, A. (1966) Effects of Angiotensin on the superior cervical ganglion of the cat. *Experientia* **22**, 394–395.

PARDO, E. G., CATO, J., GIJÓN, E. and ALONSO DE FLORIDA, F. (1963) Influence of several adrenergic drugs on synaptic transmission through the superior cervical and the ciliary ganglia of the cat. *J. Pharmac. exp. Ther.* **139**, 296–303.

PARROT, J.-L. and THOUVENOT, J. (1966) Action de l'histamine sur les muscles lisses. *Handb. exp. Pharmak.* **18/1**, 202–224.

PATON, W. D. M. (1957) The action of morphine and related substances on contraction and on acetylcholine output of coaxially stimulated guinea-pig ileum. *Br. J. Pharmac. Chemother* **12**, 119–127.

PATON, W. D. M. and PERRY, W. L. M. (1953) Relationship between depolarization and block in cat's superior cervical ganglion. *J. Physiol. (Lond.)* **119**, 43–57.

PATON, W. D. M. and VANE, J. R. (1963) An analysis of the responses of the isolated stomach to electrical stimulation and to drugs. *J. Physiol. (Lond.)* **165**, 10–46.

PATON, W. D. M. and ZAIMIS, E. (1950) Actions and clinical assessment of drugs which produce neuromuscular block. *Lancet* **ii**, 568–570.

PATON, W. D. M. and ZAR, M. A. (1968) The origin of acetylcholine released from guinea-pig intestine and longitudinal muscle strips. *J. Physiol. (Lond.)* **194**, 13–33.

PÉCSI, T. (1968) Contributions to the innervation of the heart in the fresh-water mussel, *Anodonta cygnea*. *Acta. biol. Acad. Sci. (Hung.)* **19**, 1–10.

PEPEU, G., SCHMIDT, K. F. and GIARMAN, N. J. (1963) Identity with authentic acetylcholine of acetylcholine-like activity in extracts of rat brain. *Biochem. Pharmac.* **12**, 385–388.

PERNOW, B. (1953) Studies on substance P, purification, occurrence and biological actions. *Acta physiol. scand.* **29**, Suppl. 105, 1–90.

PERRY, W. L. M. (1953) Acetylcholine release in the cat's superior cervical ganglion. *J. Physiol. (Lond.)* **119**, 439–454.

PHILIPPOT, E. and DALLEMAGNE, M. J. (1956) L'action anti-curare de la 5-hydroxytryptamine. *Archs. int. Pharmacodyn. Ther.* **105**, 426–428.

PHILLIPS, C. G., POWELL, T. P. S. and SHEPHERD, G. M. (1963) Responses of mitral cells to stimulation of the lateral olfactory tract in the rabbit. *J. Physiol. (Lond.)* **168**, 65–88.

PHILLIS, J. W. (1965a) Cholinesterase in the cat cerebellar cortex, deep nuclei and peduncles. *Experientia* **21**, 266–268.

PHILLIS, J. W. (1965b) Cholinergic mechanisms in the cerebellum. *Br. med. Bull.* **21**, 26–29.

PHILLIS, J. W. (1966) Innervation and control of a molluscan (Tapes) heart. *Comp. Biochem. Physiol.* **17**, 719–739.

PHILLIS, J. W. (1968a) Acetylcholinesterase in the feline cerebellum. *J. Neurochem.* **15**, 691–704.

PHILLIS, J. W. (1968b) Acetylcholine release from the cerebral cortex: its role in cortical arousal. *Brain Res.* **7**, 378–389.

PHILLIS, J. W. and CHONG, G. C. (1965) Acetylcholine release from the cerebral and cerebellar cortices: its role in cortical arousal. *Nature (Lond.)* **207**, 1253–1255.

PHILLIS, J. W. and TEBĒCIS, A. K. (1967a) The effects of pentobarbitone sodium on acetylcholine excitation and noradrenaline inhibition of thalamic neurones. *Life Sci. (Oxford)* **6**, 1621–1625.

PHILLIS, J. W. and TEBĒCIS, A. K. (1967b) The responses of thalamic neurones to iontophoretically applied monoamines. *J. Physiol. (Lond.)* **192**, 715–745.

PHILLIS, J. W. and TEBĒCIS, A. K. (1968) Prostaglandins and toad spinal cord responses. *Nature (Lond.)* **217**, 1076–1077.

PHILLIS, J. W., TEBĒCIS, A. K. and YORK, D. H. (1967a) The inhibitory action of monoamines on lateral geniculate neurones. *J. Physiol. (Lond.)* **190**, 563–581.

PHILLIS, J. W., TEBĒCIS, A. K. and YORK, D. H. (1967b) A study of cholinoceptive cells in the lateral geniculate nucleus. *J. Physiol. (Lond.)* **192**, 695–713.

PHILLIS, J. W., TEBĒCIS, A. K. and YORK, D. H. (1968a) Histamine and some antihistamines: their actions on cerebral cortical neurones. *Br. J. Pharmac. Chemother.* **33**, 426–440.

PHILLIS, J. W., TEBĒCIS, A. K. and YORK, D. H. (1968b) Acetylcholine release from the feline thalamus. *J. Pharm. Pharmac.* **20**, 476–478.

PHILLIS, J. W., TEBĒCIS, A. K., YORK, D. H. (1968c) Depression of spinal motoneurones by noradrenaline, 5-hydroxytryptamine and histamine. *Ref. Europ. J. Pharmac.* **7**, 471–475.

PHILLIS, J. W. and YORK, D. H. (1967a) Cholinergic inhibition in the cerebral cortex. *Brain Res.* **5**, 517–520.

PHILLIS, J. W. and YORK, D. H. (1967b) Strychnine block of neural and drug induced inhibition in the cerebral cortex. *Nature (Lond.)* **216**, 922–923.

PHILLIS, J. W. and YORK, D. H. (1968a) An intracortical cholinergic inhibitory synapse. *Life Sci. (Oxford)* **7**, 65–69.

PHILLIS, J. W. and YORK, D. H. (1968b) Pharmacological studies on a cholinergic inhibition in the cerebral cortex. *Brain Res.* **10**, 297–306.

PICKLES, V. R. (1967) Prostaglandins. *Biol. Rev.* **42**, 614–652.

PISANO, J. J. (1968) Vasoactive peptides in venoms. *Fed. Proc.* **27**, 58–62.

PISANO, J. J. and UDENFRIEND, S. (1958) Formation of γ-guanidinobutyric and guanidinoacetic acids in brain. *Fed. Proc.* **17**, 403.

PLETSCHER, A. (1961) Monoaminoxydase-Hemmer. *Dt. med. Wschr.* **86**, 647–657.

PLETSCHER, A., BROSSI, A. and GEY, K. F. (1962) Benzoquinolizine derivatives: a new class of monoamine decreasing drugs with psychotropic action. *Int. Rev. Neurobiol.* **4**, 275–306.

PLETSCHER, A., SHORE, P. A. and BRODIE, B. B. (1956) Serotonin as a mediator of reserpine action in brain. *J. Pharmac. exp. Ther.* **116**, 84–89.

POIRIER, L. J., SINGH, P., BOUCHER, R., BOUVIER, G., OLIVIER, A. and LAROCHELLE, P. (1967) Effect of brain lesions on striatal monoamines in the cat. *Archs. Neurol. Psychiat., Chicago* **17**, 601–608.

POIRIER, L. J., and SOURKES, I. L. (1965) Influence of the substantia nigra on the catecholamine content of the striatum. *Brain* **88**, 181–192.

POLAK, R. L. and MEEUWS, M. M. (1966) The influence of atropine on the release and uptake of acetylcholine by the isolated cerebral cortex of the rat. *Biochem. Pharmac.* **15**, 989–992.

POLLEN, D. A. and AJMONE MARSAN, C. (1965) Cortical inhibitory postsynaptic potentials and strychninization. *J. Neurophysiol.* **28**, 342–356.

PORTER, C. C., WATSON, L. S., TITUS, D. C., TOTARO, J. A. and BYER, S. S. (1962) Inhibition of DOPA decarboxylase by the hydrazino analog of α-methyl-DOPA. *Biochem. Pharmac.* **11**, 1067–1077.

POTTER, L. T. and AXELROD, J. (1963a) Subcellular localization of catecholamines in tissues of the rat. *J. Pharmac. exp. Ther.* **142**, 291–298.

POTTER, L. T. and AXELROD, J. (1963b) Studies on the storage of norepinephrine and the effect of drugs. *J. Pharmac. exp. Ther.* **140**, 199–206.

PROSSER, C. L. (1940) Acetylcholine and nervous inhibition in the heart of *Venus mercenaria. Biol. Bull. mar. biol. Lab. (Woods Hole)* **78**, 92–102.

PROSSER, C. L., SMITH, C. E. and MELTON, C. E. (1955) Conduction of action potentials in the ureter of the rat. *Am. J. Physiol.* **181**, 651–660.

PSCHEIDT, G. R. and HIMWICH, H. R. (1963) Reserpine, monoamine oxidase inhibitors and distribution of biogenic amines in monkey brain. *Biochem. Pharmac.* **12**, 65–71.

PURPURA, D. P. (1957) Experimental analysis of the inhibitory action of lysergic acid diethylamide on cortical dendritic activity. *Ann. N.Y. Acad. Sci.* **66**, 515–536.

PURPURA, D. P., GIRADO, M. and GRUNDFEST, H. (1957) Selective blockade of excitatory synapses in the cat brain by γ-aminobutyric acid. *Science, N.Y.* **125**, 1200–1202.

PURPURA, D. P., GIRADO, M., SMITH, T. G. and GOMEZ, J. A. (1958). Effects of systemically administered ω-amino and guanidino acids on spontaneous and evoked cortical activity in regions of blood-brain barrier destruction. *Electroen. Neurophysiol.* **10**, 677–685.

PURPURA, D. P. and GRUNDFEST, H. (1957) Physiological and pharmacological consequences of different synaptic organisations in cerebral and cerebellar cortex of cat. *J. Neurophysiol.* **20**, 494–522.

RALL, W. (1967) Distinguishing theoretical synaptic potentials computed for different soma-dendritic distributions of synaptic input. *J. Neurophysiol.* **30**, 1138–1168.

RALL, W., BURKE, R. E., SMITH, T. G., NELSON, P. G. and FRANK, K. (1967) Dendritic location of synapses and possible mechanisms for the monosynaptic EPSP in motoneurons. *J. Neurophysiol.* **30**, 1169–1193.

RAMWELL, P. W. and SHAW, J. E. (1966) Spontaneous and evoked release of prostaglandins from the cerebral cortex of anaesthetised cats. *Am. J. Physiol.* **211**, 125–134.

RAMWELL, P. W., SHAW, J. E. and KUCHARSKI, J. (1965) Prostaglandin: release from the rat phrenic-nerve diaphragm preparation. *Science, N.Y.* **149**, 1390–1391.

RAMWELL, P. W., SHAW, J. E. and JESSUP, R. (1966) Spontaneous and evoked release of prostaglandins from frog spinal cord. *Am. J. Physiol.* **211**, 998–1004.

RANDIĆ, M., SIMINOFF, R. and STRAUGHAN, D. W. (1964) Acetylcholine depression of cortical neurons. *Expl. Neurol.* **9**, 236–242.

RANDIĆ, M. and STRAUGHAN, D. W. (1964) Antidromic activity in the rat phrenic nerve-diaphragm preparation. *J. Physiol. (Lond.)* **174**, 130–148.

RAPPORT, M. M., GREEN, A. A. and PAGE, I. H. (1948) Serum vasoconstrictor (serotonin). IV. Isolation and characterization. *J. biol. Chem.* **176**, 1243–1251.

RAPPORT, M. M. and KOELLE, G. B. (1953) The action of antihistaminics and atropine in blocking the spasmogenic activity of serotonin on the guinea-pig ileum. *Archs. int. Pharmacodyn. Ther.* **92**, 464–470.

RAY, J. W. (1964) The free amino acid pool of the cockroach (*Periplaneta americana*) central nervous system and the effect of insecticides. *J. Insect Physiol.* **10**, 587–597.

RECH, R. H. and DOMINO, E. F. (1960) Effects of *gamma*-aminobutyric acid on chemically- and electrically-evoked activity in the isolated cerebral cortex of the dog. *J. Pharmac. exp. Ther.* **130**, 59–67.

REGER, J. F. (1957) The ultrastructure of normal and denervated neuromuscular synapses in mouse gastrocnemius muscle. *Expl. Cell. Res.* **12**, 662–665.

REINHART, H. (1963) Role and origin of noradrenaline in the superior cervical ganglion. *J. Physiol. (Lond.)* **167**, 18–29.

REIVICH, M. and GLOWINSKI, J. (1966) An autoradiographic study of the distribution of C^{14}-norepinephrine in the brain of the rat. *Brain* **90**, 633–646.

RENSON, J., WEISSBACH, H. and UDENFRIEND, S. (1962) Hydroxylation of tryptophan by phenylalanine hydroxylase. *J. biol. Chem.* **237**, 2261–2264.

REVZIN, A. M. and COSTA, E. (1960) The effects of monoamine oxidase substrates on evoked potentials. *Fed. Proc.* **19**, 265.

RICHTER, D. and CROSSLAND, J. (1949) Variation in acetylcholine content of brain with physiologic state. *Am. J. Physiol.* **159**, 247–255.

RIKER, W. F. (1960) Pharmacologic considerations in a re-evaluation of the neuromuscular synapse. *Archs. Neurol. Psychiat. Chicago* **3**, 488–499.

RIKER, W. F., ROBERTS, J., STANDAERT, F. G. and FUJIMORI, H. (1957) The motor nerve terminals as the primary focus for drug-induced facilitation of neuromuscular transmission. *J. Pharmac. exp. Ther.* **121**, 286–312.

RIKER, W. F. and STANDAERT, F. G. (1966) The action of facilitatory drugs and acetylcholine on neuromuscular transmission. *Ann. N.Y. Acad. Sci.* **135**, 163–176.

RIKER, W. F., WERNER, G., ROBERTS, J. and KUPERMAN, A. (1959) Pharmacologic evidence for the existence of a presynaptic event in neuromuscular transmission. *J. Pharmac. exp. Ther.* **125**, 150–158.

RILEY, J. F. (1959) *The Mast Cells.* Edinburgh: S. Livingstone.

ROBBINS, J. (1959) The excitation and inhibition of crustacean muscle by amino acids. *J. Physiol. (Lond.)* **148**, 39–50.

ROBERTS, D. V. (1962) Neuromuscular activity of the triethyl analogue of choline in the frog. *J. Physiol. (Lond.)* **160**, 94–105.

ROBERTS, E. and EIDELBERG, E. (1960) Metabolic and neurophysiological roles of γ-aminobutyric acid. *Int. Rev. Neurobiol.* **2**, 279–332.

ROBERTS, E. and KURIYAMA, K. (1968) Biochemical-physiological correlations in studies of the γ-aminobutyric acid system. *Brain Res.* **8**, 1–35.

ROBERTS, M. H. T. and STRAUGHAN, D. W. (1967) Excitation and depression of cortical neurones by 5-hydroxytryptamine. *J. Physiol. (Lond.)* **193**, 269–294.

ROBERTS, M. H. T. and STRAUGHAN, D. W. (1968) Actions of noradrenaline and mescaline on cortical neurones. *Naunyn-Schmiedeberg's Arch. exp. Path. Pharmak.* **259**, 191–192.

ROBERTSON, J. D. (1956) The ultrastructure of a reptilian myoneural junction *J. biophys. biochem. Cytol.* **2**, 381–394.

ROBERTSON, P. A. (1953) An antagonism of 5-hydroxytryptamine by atropine. *J. Physiol. (Lond.)* **121**, 54–55P.

ROBERTSON, P. A. (1954) Potentiation of 5 HT by the true cholinesterase inhibitor 284 C 51. *J. Physiol. (Lond.)* **125**, 37P–38P.

ROBINSON, J. D. and GREEN, J. P. (1964) Presence of imidazoleacetic acid riboside and ribotide in rat tissues. *Nature (Lond.)* **203**, 1178–1179.

ROCHA E. SILVA, M. (1966) Action of Histamine on the smooth muscle. (On the nature of the receptors for histamine in the guinea-pig ileum). *Handb. exp. Pharmak.* **18/1**, 225–237.

ROCHA E. SILVA, M., VALLE, J. R. and PICARELLI, Z. P. (1953) A pharmacological analysis of the mode of action of serotonin (5-hydroxytryptamine) upon the guinea-pig ileum. *Br. J. Pharmac. Chemother.* **8**, 378–388.

RODDIE, I. C. (1962) Transmembrane potential changes associated with smooth muscle activity in turtle arteries and veins. *J. Physiol. (Lond.)* **163**, 138–150.

ROEDER, K. D. and WEIANT, E. A. (1950) The electrical and mechanical events of neuro-

THE PHARMACOLOGY OF SYNAPSES

muscular transmission in the cockroach, *Periplaneta americana*. *J. exp. Biol.* **27**, 1–13.

ROSELL, S., AXELROD, J. and KOPIN, I. J. (1964) Release of tritiated epinephrine following sympathetic nerve stimulation. *Nature (Lond.)* **201**, 301.

ROSS, S. B. and HALJASMAA, Ö. (1964a) Catechol-O-methyltransferase inhibitors. *In vitro* inhibition of the enzyme in mouse brain extract. *Acta pharmac. tox.* **21**, 205–214.

ROSS, S. B. and HALJASMAA, Ö. (1964b) Catechol-O-methyltransferase inhibitors. *In vivo* inhibition in mice. *Acta pharmac tox.* **21**, 215–225.

ROSZKOWSKI, A. P. (1961) An unusual type of sympathetic ganglionic stimulant. *J. Pharmac. exp. Ther.* **132**, 156–170.

ROTHBALLER, A. B. (1956) Studies on the adrenaline-sensitive component of the reticular activating system. *Electroen. Neurophysiol.* **8**, 603–621.

ROTHBALLER, A. B. (1959) The effects of catecholamines on the central nervous system. *Pharmac. Rev.* **11**, 494–547.

RUDE, S. (1967) Monoamine-containing neurons in the nerve cord and body wall of *Lumbricus terrestris*. *J. comp. Neurol.* **128**, 397–412.

RYALL, R. W. (1963) The identification of acetylcholine in presynaptic terminals isolated from brain. *Biochem. Pharmac.* **12**, 1055–1056.

RYALL, R. W. (1964) The subcellular distributions of acetylcholine, Substance P, 5-Hydroxytryptamine, γ-Aminobutyric acid and glutamic acid in brain homogenates. *J. Neurochem.* **11**, 131–145.

SAILER, S. and STUMPF, C. (1957) Beeinflußbarkeit der rhinencephalen Tätigkeit des Kaninchens. *Naunyn-Schmiedeberg's Arch. exp. Path. Pharmak.* **231**, 63–77.

SALA, E. and PERRIS, C. (1958) Ricerche sull'attività della 5-idrossitriptamina a livello della giunzione neuromuscolare. *Neurone (Mantova)* **6**, 127–136.

SALA Y PONS, C. (1892) Estructura de la medula espinal de los batracios. *Trab. Lab. Invest. biol. Univ. Barcelona*, 3–22.

SALMOIRAGHI, G. C., BLOOM, F. E. and COSTA, E. (1964) Adrenergic mechanisms in rabbit olfactory bulb. *Am. J. Physiol.* **207**, 1417–1424.

SALMOIRAGHI, G. C. and STEFANIS, C. N. (1965) Patterns of central neurons responses to suspected transmitters. *Archs. ital. Biol.* **103**, 705–724.

SALMOIRAGHI, G. C. and STEINER, F. A. (1963) Acetylcholine sensitivity of cat's medullary neurones. *J. Neurophysiol.* **26**, 581–597.

SAMUELSSON, B. (1964) Identification of a smooth muscle-stimulating factor in bovine brain. *Biochim. biophys. Acta* **84**, 218–219.

SAMUELSSON, B. (1965) The Prostaglandins. *Angew. Chem.* **4**, 410–416.

SANDBERG, F., INGELMANN-SUNDBERG, A. and RYDÉN, G. (1963) The effect of prostaglandin E_1 on the human uterus and the fallopian tubes *in vitro*. *Acta obst. gynec. scand.* **42**, 269–278.

SASAMORI, S. (1965) Isolation of prostaglandins from human seminal fluid and studies on their stimulating effects on the intestinal smooth muscle. *Sapporo med. J.* **28**, 286–299.

SATINSKY, D. (1967) Pharmacological responsiveness of lateral geniculate nucleus neurons. *Int. J. Neuropharmac.* **6**, 387–397.

SATO, M., AUSTIN, G., YAI, H. and MARUHASHI, J. (1968) The ionic permeability changes during acetylcholine-induced responses of *Aplysia* ganglion cells. *J. gen. Physiol.* **51**, 321–345.

SAVAY, G. and CSILLIK, B. (1956) The effect of denervation on the cholinesterase activity of motor endplates. *Acta morph. Acid. Sci. (Hung.)* **6**, 289–297.

SAWYER, C. H. (1955) Rhinencephalic involvement in pituitary activation by intraventricular histamine in the rabbit under nembutal anaesthesia. *Am. J. Physiol.* **180**, 37–46.

SAWYER, C. H., DAVENPORT, C. and ALEXANDER, L. M. (1950) Sites of cholinesterase activity in neuromuscular and ganglionic transmission. *Anat. Rec.* **106**, 287–288.

SAWYER, C. H. and HOLLINSHEAD, W. H. (1945) Cholinesterases in sympathetic fibres and ganglia. *J. Neurophysiol.* **8**, 137–153.

SCHAIN, R. J. (1961) Effects of 5-hydroxytryptamine on the dorsal muscle of the leech (*Hirudo medicinalis*). *Br. J. Pharmac. Chemother.* **16**, 257–261.

SCHAYER, R. W. (1952) Biogenesis of histamine. *J. biol. Chem.* **199**, 245–250.

SCHAYER, R. W. (1959) Catabolism of physiological quantities of histamine *in vivo*. *Physiol. Rev.* **39**, 116–126.

SCHENK, E. A. and ANDERSON, E. G. (1958) The effect of histamine on neuromyal block ing agents. *J. Pharmac. exp. Ther.* **122**, 234–238.

SCHILD, H. O. (1947) pA, a new scale for measurement of drug antagonism. *Br. J. Pharmac. Chemother.* **2**, 189–206.

SCHNEIDERMAN, N., MONNIER, M. and LEMBECK, F. (1965) Effects of sleep dialysate, Substance P and psychotropic drugs upon the thalamocortical evoked response. *Experientia* **21**, 596–598.

SCHREINER, G. L., BERGLUND, E., BORST, H. and MONROE, R. G. (1957) Effect of vagus stimulation and of acetylcholine on myocardial contractility, O_2 consumption and coronary flow in dogs. *Circulation Res.* **5**, 562–567.

SCHUBERTH, J. and SUNDWALL, A. (1967) Effects of some drugs on the uptake of acetylcholine in cortex slices of mouse brain. *J. Neurochem.* **14**, 807–812.

SCHUELER, F. W. (1960) The mechanism of action of the hemicholiniums. *Int. Rev. Neurobiol.* **2**, 77–97.

SCHWARZACHER, H. G. (1957) Der histochemisch nachweisbare cholinesterasegehalt in muskelenplatten nach Durchschneidung des motorischen Nerven. *Acta anat.* **31**, 507–521.

SCHWARZACHER, H. G. (1960) Untersuchungen über lokalisation und Funktion der Cholinesterase an der Skeletmuskel-Sehnenverbindung. *Naunyn-Schmiedeberg's Arch. exp. Path. Pharmak.* **238**, 48–49.

SCHWARZACHER, H. G. (1961) Acetylcholinesterase in mammalian myotendinous junction. *Bibl. anat.* **2**, 220–227.

SCHWEITZER, A. and WRIGHT, S. (1937) The action of adrenaline on the knee jerk. *J. Physiol.* (*Lond.*) **88**, 476–491.

SCUDDER, C. L., AKERS, T. K. and KARCZMAR, A. G. (1966) Effects of cholinergic drugs on tunicate smooth muscle. *Comp. Biochem. Physiol.* **17**, 559–567.

SHARMAN, D. F. and VOGT, M. (1965) The noradrenaline content of the caudate nucleus of the rabbit. *J. Neurochem.* **12**, 62.

SHAW, E. and WOOLLEY, D. W. (1953) Yohimbine and ergot alkaloids as naturally occurring antimetabolites of serotonin. *J. biol. Chem.* **203**, 979–989.

SHAW, E. and WOOLLEY, D. W. (1954) Pharmacological properties of some antimetabolites of serotonin having unusually high activity on isolated tissues. *J. Pharmac. exp. Ther.* **111**, 43–53.

SHORE, P. A. and COHN, V. H. (1960) Comparative effects of monoamine oxidase inhibitors on monoamine oxidase and diamine oxidase. *Biochem. Pharmac.* **5**, 91–95.

SHUTE, C. C. D. and LEWIS, P. R. (1961) The use of cholinesterase techniques combined with operative procedures to follow nervous pathways in the brain. *Biblthca anat.* **2**, 34–49.

SHUTE, C. C. D. and LEWIS, P. R. (1963) Cholinesterase-containing system of the brain of the rat. *Nature (Lond.)* **199**, 1160–1164.

SHUTE, C. C. D. and LEWIS, P. R. (1965) Cholinesterase-containing pathways of the hindbrain: afferent cerebellar and centrifugal cochlear fibres. *Nature (Lond.)* **205**, 242–246.

SHUTE, C. C. D. and LEWIS, P. R. (1967) The ascending cholinergic reticular system: neocortical, olfactory and subcortical projections. *Brain*, **90**, 497–520.

SIGG, E., OCHS, S. and GERARD, R. W. (1955) Effects of the medullary hormones on the somatic nervous system in the cat. *Am. J. Physiol.* **183**, 419–426.

SILVER, A. (1967) Cholinesterases of the central nervous system with special reference to the cerebellum. *Int. Rev. Neurobiol.* **10**, 57–109.

SILVER, M. S. (1942) Motoneurons of the spinal cord of the frog. *J. comp. Neurol.* **77**, 1–39.

SINGH, S. I. and MALHOTRA, G. L. (1962) Amino acid content of monkey brain—I. General pattern and quantitative value of glutamic acid/glutamine, γ-aminobutyric acid and aspartic acid. *J. Neurochem.* **9**, 37–42.

SINHA, Y. K. and WEST, G. B. (1953) The antagonism between local anaesthetic drugs and 5-hydroxytryptamine. *J. Pharm. Pharmac.* **5**, 370–374.

SJÖQVIST, F. (1963) Pharmacological analysis of acetylcholinesterase rich ganglion cells in the lumbosacral sympathetic system of the cat. *Acta physiol. scand.* **57**, 352–362.

SKOGLUND, C. R. (1961) Influence of noradrenaline on spinal interneurone activity. *Acta physiol. scand.* **51**, 142–149.

SLATER, I. H., DAVIS, K. H., LEARY, D. E. and BOYD, E. S. (1955) The action of serotonin and lysergic acid diethylamide on spinal reflexes. *J. Pharmac. exp. Ther.* **113**, 48–49.

SLEATOR, W., FURCHGOTT, R. F., GUBAREFF, T. DE and KRESPI, V. (1964) Action potentials of guinea-pig atria under conditions which alter contraction. *Am. J. Physiol.* **206**, 270–282.

SMALLEY, K. N. (1965) Adrenergic transmission in the light organ of the firefly. *Photinus pyralis. Comp. Biochem. Physiol.* **16**, 467–477.

SMITH, J. C. (1966) Observations on the selectivity of stimulant action of 4-(chlorophenylcarbamoyloxy)-2-butynyltrimethylammonium chloride on sympathetic ganglia. *J. Pharmac. exp. Ther.* **153**, 266–275.

SMITH, S. E. (1960) The pharmacological actions of 3,4-dihydroxyphenyl-α-methylalanine (α-methyldopa), an inhibitor of 5-hydroxytryptophan decarboxylase. *Br. J. Pharmac. Chemother.* **15**, 319–329.

SMITH, T. G., WUERKER, R. B. and FRANK, K. (1967) Membrane impedence changes during synaptic transmission in cat spinal motoneurones. *J. Neurophysiol.* **30**, 1072–1096.

SNELL, R. S. and MCINTYRE, N. (1956) Changes in the histochemical appearances of cholinesterase at the motor endplate following denervation. *Br. J. exp. Path.* **37**, 44–48.

SNYDER, S. H., GLOWINSKI, J. and AXELROD, J. (1965) The storage of norepinephrine and some of its derivatives in brain synaptosomes. *Life Sci. (Oxford)* **4**, 797–807.

SNYDER, S. H., GLOWINSKI, J. and AXELROD, J. (1966) The physiologic disposition of H³-histamine in the rat brain. *J. Pharmac. exp. Ther.* **153**, 8–14.

SOURKES, T. L. (1964) Actions of dopa and dopamine in relation to function of the central nervous system. In: *Biochemical and Neurophysiological Correlations of Centrally Acting Drugs*, Vol. 2, pp. 35–50. Ed. E. Trabucchi, R. Paoletti and N. Canal. Oxford: Pergamon Press.

SOURKES, T. L. (1965) Action of α-methyldopa in the brain. *Br. med. Bull.* **21**, 66–69.

SPECTOR, S., KUNTZMAN, R., SHORE, P. A. and BRODIE, B. B. (1960) Evidence for the release of brain amines by reserpine in the presence of monoamine oxidase inhibitors. Implications of monoamine oxidase in norepinephrine metabolism in brain. *J. Pharmac. exp. Ther.* **130**, 256–261.

SPECTOR, S., PROCKOP, D., SHORE, P. A. and BRODIE, B. B. (1958) Effect of iproniazid on brain levels of norepinephrine and serotonin. *Science, N.Y.* **127**, 704.

SPECTOR, S., SJOERDSMA, A. and UDENFRIEND, S. (1965) Blockade of endogenous norepinephrine synthesis by α-methyl-tyrosine, an inhibitor of tyrosine hydroxylase. *J. Pharmac. exp. Ther.* **147**, 86–95.

SPEHLMANN, R. (1963) Acetylcholine and prostigmine electrophoresis at visual cortex neurons. *J. Neurophysiol.* **26**, 127–139.

SPERELAKIS, N. and PROSSER, C. L. (1959) Mechanical and electrical activity in intestinal smooth muscle. *Am. J. Physiol.* **196**, 850–856.

SPERTI, L. and SPERTI, S. (1959a) Effects of chronic lesions of the peduncles on cerebellum cholinesterase activity, in the albino rat. *Experientia* **15**, 441.

SPERTI, L. and SPERTI, S. (1959b) Effects of midline cerebellar splitting and of lesions in cerebral cortex on cerebellum cholinesterase activity in the albino rat. *Experientia* **15**, 442.

S.-RÓZSA, K. and GRAUL, C. (1964) Is serotonin responsible for the stimulative effect of the extracardiac nerve in *Helix pomatia*? *Ann. Biol. Tihany* **31**, 85–96.

S.-RÓZSA, K. and ZS.-NAGY, I. (1967) Physiological and histochemical evidence for neuroendocrine regulation of heart activity in the snail *Lymnaea stagnalis* L. *Comp. Biochem. Physiol.* **23**, 373–382.

S.-RÓZSA, K. and PÉCSI, T. (1967) Comparative studies on the effect produced by biologically active agents on the isolated hearts of *Helix pomatia* L. and *Anodonta cygnea* L. *Ann. Biol. Tihany* **34**, 59–72.

S.-RÓZSA, K. and PERÉNYI, L. (1966) Chemical identification of the excitatory substance released in *Helix* heart during stimulation of the extracardial nerve. *Comp. Biochem. Physiol.* **19**, 105–113.

STANDAERT, F. G. (1963) Post-tetanic repetitive activity in the cat soleus nerve. Its origin, course and mechanism of generation. *J. gen. Physiol.* **47**, 53–70.

STANDAERT, F. G. (1964) The action of d-tubocurarine on the motor nerve terminal. *J. Pharmac. exp. Ther.* **143**, 181–186.

STANDAERT, F. G. and ADAMS, J. E. (1965) The actions of succinylcholine on the mammalian motor nerve terminal. *J. Pharmac. exp. Ther.* **149**, 113–123.

STAVRAKY, G. W. (1947) Action of adrenalin on spinal neurones. *Am. J. Physiol.* **150**, 37–45.

STEDMAN, E., STEDMAN, E. and EASSON, L. H. (1932) Choline-esterase. An enzyme present in the blood serum of the horse. *Biochem. J.* **26**, 2056–2066.

STEEDMAN, W. M. (1966) Micro-electrode studies on mammalian vascular muscle. *J. Physiol. (Lond.)* **186**, 382–400.

STEFANIS, C. (1964) Hippocampal neurons: their responsiveness to micro-electrophoretically administered endogenous amines. *Pharmacologist* **6**, 171.

STEINER, F. A. and MEYER, M. (1966) Actions of L-glutamate, acetylcholine and dopamine on single neurones on the nuclei cuneatus and gracilis of the cat. *Experientia* **22**, 58–59.

STEINER, F. A. and RUF, K. (1966) Excitatory effects of L-glutamic acid upon single unit activity in rat brain and their modification by thiosemicarbazide and pyridoxal-5'-phosphate. *Helv. physiol. acta* **24**, 181–192.

STERN, J. R., EGGLESTON, L. V., HEMS, R. and KREBS, H. A. (1949) Accumulation of glutamic acid in isolated brain tissue. *Biochem. J.* **44**, 410–418.

STERN, P., DOBRIĆ, V. and MITROVIĆ-KOCIĆ, D. (1957) Synergism of Substance P and mephenesin. *Archs. int. pharmacodyn. Ther.* **112**, 102–107.

STERN, P. and HUKOVIĆ, S. (1958) Inhibitory effect of substance P (a tranquilliser) on fighting fish, *Betta splendens*. *Naturwissenschaften* **45**, 626.

STERN, P. and MILIN, R. (1959) Tranquilizing effect of substance P. *Proc. Soc. exp. Biol. Med.* (*N.Y.*) **101**, 298–299.

STONE, C. A. and PORTER, C. C. (1967) Biochemistry and pharmacology of methyldopa and some related structures. *Adv. Drug. Res.* **4**, 71–93.

STRASBERG, P., KRNJEVIĆ, K., SCHWARTZ, S. and ELLIOTT, K. A. C. (1967) Penetration of blood-brain barrier by γ-aminobutyric acid at sites of freezing. *J. Neurochem.* **14**, 755–760.

STRAUGHAN, D. W. (1960) The release of acetylcholine from mammalian motor nerve endings. *Br. J. Pharmac. Chemother.* **15**, 417–424.

STRONG, C. G. and BOHR, D. F. (1967) Effects of prostaglandins E_1, E_2, A_1 and $F_{1\alpha}$ on isolated vascular smooth muscle. *Am. J. Physiol.* **213**, 725–733.

STUMPF, CH. (1965) Drug action on the electrical activity of the hippocampus. *Int. Rev. Neurobiol.* **8**, 77–138.

SUDEN, C. TUM, HART, E. R., LINDENBERG, R. and MARRAZZI, A. S. (1951) Pharmacologic and anatomic indications of adrenergic neurons participating in synapses at parasympathetic ganglia (ciliary). *J. Pharmac. exp. Ther.* **103**, 364–365.

SUDEN, C. TUM. and MARRAZZI, A. S. (1951) Synaptic inhibitory action of adrenaline at parasympathetic synapses. *Fed. Proc.* **10**, 138.

SULLIVAN, T. J. (1966) Response of the mammalian uterus to prostaglandins under differing hormonal conditions. *Br. J. Pharmac. Chemother.* **26**, 678–685.

SUTTER, M. C. (1965) The pharmacology of isolated veins. *Br. J. Pharmac. Chemother.* **24**, 742–751.

SUZUKI, H. and TUKAHARA, Y. (1963) Recurrent inhibition of the Betz cell. *Jap. J. Physiol.* **13**, 386–398.

SUZUKI, H. and TAIRA, N. (1961) Effect of reticular stimulation upon synaptic transmission in cat's lateral geniculate body. *Jap. J. Physiol.* **11**, 641–655.

SVENSMARK, O. (1965) Molecular properties of cholinesterases. *Acta physiol. scand.* **64**, Suppl. 245, 1–74.

SWEATMAN, W. J. F. and COLLIER, H. O. J. (1968) Effects of prostaglandins on human bronchial muscle. *Nature* (*Lond.*) **217**, 69.

SWEENEY, D. (1963) Dopamine: its occurrence in molluscan ganglia. *Science, N.Y.* **139**, 1051.

SZENTÁGOTHAI, J. and RAJKOVITS, K. (1959) Über den Ursprung der Kletterfasern des Kleinhirns. *Z. Anat. EtwGesch.* **121**, 130–141.

SZERB, J. C. (1958) Non-specific depressant effect of 5-hydroxytryptamine on guinea-pig ileum. *Fed. Proc.* **17**, 160.

SZERB, J. C. (1964) The effect of tertiary and quaternary atropine on cortical acetylcholine output and on the electroencephalogram in cats. *Can. J. Physiol. Pharmac.* **42**, 303–314.

TAKAGAKI, G., HIRANO, S., NAGATA, Y. (1959) Some observations on the effects of D-glutamate on the glucose metabolism and the accumulation of potassium ions in brain cortex slices. *J. Neurochem.* **4**, 124–134.

TAKESHIGE, C., PAPPANO, A. J., DE GROAT, W. C. and VOLLE, R. L. (1963) Ganglionic blockade produced in sympathetic ganglia by cholinomimetic drugs. *J. Pharmac. exp. Ther.* **141**, 333–342.

TAKESHIGE, C. and VOLLE, R. L. (1962) Bimodal response of sympathetic ganglia to acetylcholine following eserine or repetitive preganglionic stimulation. *J. Pharmac exp. Ther.* **138**, 66–73.

TAKESHIGE, C. and VOLLE, R. L. (1963a) Asynchronous postganglionic firing from the cat superior cervical sympathetic ganglion treated with neostigmine. *Br. J. Pharmac. Chemother.* **20**, 214–220.

TAKESHIGE, C. and VOLLE, R. L. (1963b) Cholinoceptive sites in denervated sympathetic ganglia. *J. Pharmac. exp. Ther.* **141**, 206–213.

TAKESHIGE, C. and VOLLE, R. L. (1964a) Modification of ganglionic responses to cholinomimetic drugs following preganglionic stimulation, anticholinesterase agents and pilocarpine. *J. Pharmac. exp. Ther.* **146**, 335–343.

TAKESHIGE, C. and VOLLE, R. L. (1964b) A comparison of the ganglion potentials and block produced by acetylcholine and tetramethylammonium. *Br. J. Pharmac. Chemother.* **23**, 80–89.

TAKEUCHI, A. and TAKEUCHI, N. (1959) Active phase of frog's endplate potential. *J. Neurophysiol.* **22**, 395–411.

TAKEUCHI, A. and TAKEUCHI, N. (1960a) On the permeability of endplate membrane during the action of the transmitter. *J. Physiol. (Lond.)* **154**, 52–67.

TAKEUCHI, A. and TAKEUCHI, N. (1960b) Further analysis of relationship between endplate potential and endplate current. *J. Neurophysiol.* **23**, 397–402.

TAKEUCHI, A. and TAKEUCHI, N. (1964) The effect on crayfish muscle of iontophoretically applied glutamate. *J. Physiol. (Lond.)* **170**, 296–317.

TAKEUCHI, A. and TAKEUCHI, N. (1965) Localized action of gamma-aminobutyric acid on the crayfish muscle. *J. Physiol. (Lond.)* **177**, 225–238.

TAKEUCHI, A. and TAKEUCHI, N. (1966a) A study of the inhibitory action of γ-aminobutyric acid on neuromuscular transmission in the crayfish. *J. Physiol. (Lond.)* **183**, 418–432.

TAKEUCHI, A. and TAKEUCHI, N. (1966b) On the permeability of the presynaptic terminal of the crayfish neuromuscular junction during synaptic inhibition and the action of γ-aminobutyric acid. *J. Physiol. (Lond.)* **183**, 433–449.

TAKEUCHI, N. (1963) Some properties of conductance changes at the endplate membrane during the action of acetylcholine. *J. Physiol. (Lond.)* **167**, 128–140.

TALLAN, H. H. (1962) A survey of amino acids and related compounds in nervous tissue. In: *Amino Acid Pools*, pp. 471–485. Ed. J. T. Holden. Amsterdam: Elsevier.

TALLAN, H. H., MOORE, S. and STEIN, W. H. (1954) Studies on the free amino acids and related compounds in the tissues of the cat. *J. biol. Chem.* **211**, 927–939.

TAUC, L. (1966) Physiology of the nervous system. In: *Physiology of Mollusca*, Vol. 2, pp. 387–454. Ed. K. M. Wilbur and C. M. Yonge. London: Academic Press.

TAUC, L. (1967) Transmission in invertebrate and vertebrate ganglia. *Physiol. Rev.* **47**, 521–593.

TAUC, L. and GERSCHENFELD, H. M. (1961) Cholinergic transmission mechanisms for both excitation and inhibition in molluscan central synapses. *Nature (Lond.)* **192**, 366–367.

TAUC, L. and GERSCHENFELD, H. M. (1962) A cholinergic mechanism of inhibitory synaptic transmission in a molluscan nervous system. *J. Neurophysiol.* **25**, 236–262.

TEBĒCIS, A. K. (1967) Are 5-hydroxytryptamine and noradrenaline inhibitory transmitters in the medial geniculate nucleus? *Brain Res.* **6**, 780–782.

TEBĒCIS, A. K. (1968) Acetylcholine and medial geniculate neurones. *Aust. J. exp. Biol. med. Sci.* **46**, 3P.

TEBĒCIS, A. K. and PHILLIS, J. W. (1967) The effects of topically applied biogenic monoamines on the isolated toad spinal cord. *Comp. Biochem. Physiol.* **23**, 553–563.

TEN CATE, J., BOELES, J. T. F. and BIERSTEKER, P. A. (1959) The action of adrenaline and noradrenaline on the knee jerk. *Arch. int. Physiol.* **67**, 468–488.

THESLEFF, S. (1955) The mode of neuromuscular block caused by acetylcholine, nicotine, decamethonium and succinylcholine. *Acta physiol. scand.* **34**, 218–231.

THESLEFF, S. (1958) A study of the interaction between neuromuscular blocking agents and acetylcholine at the mammalian motor endplate. *Acta anaesth. scand.* **2**, 69–79.

THESLEFF, S. (1959) Motor endplate desensitization by repetitive nerve stimuli. *J. Physiol. (Lond.)* **148**, 659–664.

THESLEFF, S. (1960) Supersensitivity of skeletal muscle produced by botulinum toxin. *J. Physiol. (Lond.)* **151**, 598–607.

THIES, R. E. (1965) Neuromuscular depression and apparent depletion of transmitter in mammalian muscle. *J. Neurophysiol.* **28**, 427–442.

THIES, R. E. and BROOKS, V. B., (1961) Postsynaptic neuromuscular block produced by hemicholinium, No. 3. *Fed. Proc.* **20**, 569–578.

THOMAS, R. C. and WILSON, V. J. (1965) Precise localization of Renshaw cells with a new marking technique. *Nature (Lond.)* **206**, 211–213.

TOBIAS, J. M., LIPTON, M. A. and LEPINAT, A. A. (1946) Effect of anaesthetics and convulsants on brain acetylcholine content. *Proc. Soc. exp. Biol. Med. (N.Y.)* **61**, 51–54.

TOSAKA, T. and LIBET, B. (1965) Slow postsynaptic potentials recorded intracellularly in sympathetic ganglia of frog. Abstr. XXIII Int. Physiol. Congr. 905.

TOSCHI, G. (1959) A biochemical study of brain microsomes. *Expl. Cell. Res.* **16**, 232–255.

TRAMS, E. and LAUTER, C. J. (1964) Properties of electroplax protein. *Biochim. Biophys. Acta* **83**, 296–304.

TRAUTWEIN, W. (1963) Generation and conduction of impulses in the heart as affected by drugs. *Pharmac. Rev.* **15**, 277–332.

TRAUTWEIN, W. and DUDEL, J. (1958a) Hemmende und erregende Wirkungen des Acetylcholin am Warmblüterherzen; Zur Frage der spontanen Errgeungsbildung. *Pflügers Arch. ges. Physiol.* **226**, 653–664.

TRAUTWEIN, W. and DUDEL, J. (1958b) Zum Mechanismus der Membranwirkung des Acetylcholin an der Herzmuskelfaser. *Pflügers Arch. ges. Physiol.* **266**, 324–334.

TRAUTWEIN, W., KUFFLER, S. W. and EDWARDS, C. (1956) Changes in membrane characteristics of heart muscle during inhibition. *J. gen. Physiol.* **40**, 135–145.

TRAUTWEIN, W. and SCHMIDT, R. F. (1960) Zur Membranwirkung des Adrenalin an der Herzmuskelfaser. *Pflügers Arch. des Physiol.* **271**, 715–726.

TREHERNE, J. E. (1966) *The Neurochemistry of Arthropods.* London: Cambridge University Press.

TRENDELENBURG, U. (1954) Action of histamine and pilocarpine on superior cervical ganglion and adrenal glands of the cat. *Br. J. Pharmac. Chemother.* **9**, 481–487.

TRENDELENBURG, U. (1955) The potentiation of ganglionic transmission by histamine and pilocarpine. *J. Physiol. (Lond.)* **129**, 337–351.

TRENDELENBURG, U. (1956a) The action 5-hydroxytryptamine on the nictitating membrane and on the superior cervical ganglion of the cat. *Br. J. Pharmac. Chemother.* **11**, 74–80.

TRENDELENBURG, U. (1956b) Modification of transmission through the superior cervical ganglion of the cat. *J. Physiol. (Lond.)* **132**, 529–541.

TRENDELENBURG, U. (1957) The action of histamine, pilocarpine and 5-HT on transmission through the superior cervical ganglion. *J. Physiol. (Lond.)* **135**, 66–72.

TRENDELENBURG, U. (1960) The action of histamine and 5-hydroxytryptamine on isolated mammalian atria. *J. Pharmac. exp. Ther.* **130**, 450–460.

TRENDELENBURG, U. (1967) Some aspects of the pharmacology of autonomic ganglion cells. *Ergebn. Physiol.* **59**, 1–85.

TSUKADA, Y., NAGATA, Y., HIRANO, S. and MATSUTANI, T. (1963) Active transport of amino acid into cerebral cortex slices. *J. Neurochem.* **10**, 241–256.

TUČEK, S. (1966) On subcellular localization and binding of choline acetyltransferase in the cholinergic nerve endings of the brain. *J. Neurochem.* **13**, 1317–1327.

TWAROG, B. M. (1954) Responses of a molluscan smooth muscle to acetylcholine and 5-hydroxytryptamine. *J. cell. comp. Physiol.* **44**, 141–164.

TWAROG, B. M. (1959) The pharmacology of a molluscan smooth muscle. *Br. J. Pharmac. Chemother.* **14**, 404–407.

TWAROG, B. (1960) Effects of acetylcholine and 5-hydroxytryptamine on the contraction of a molluscan smooth muscle. *J. Physiol. (Lond.)* **152**, 236–242.

TWAROG, B. M. (1967a) Excitation of *Mytilus* smooth muscle. *J. Physiol. (Lond.)* **192**, 857–868.

TWAROG, B. M. (1967b) The regulation of catch in molluscan muscle. *J. gen. Physiol.* **50**, 157–169.

TWAROG, B. M. and PAGE, I. H. (1953) Serotonin content of some mammalian tissues and urine and a method for its determination. *Am. J. Physiol.* **175**, 157–161.

TWAROG, B. M. and ROEDER, K. D. (1956) Properties of the connective tissue sheath of the cockroach nerve cord. *Biol. Bull. mar. biol. Lab. Woods Hole* **111**, 278–286.

UDENFRIEND, S., BOGDANSKI, D. F. and WEISSBACH, H. (1957) Biochemistry and metabolism of serotonin as it relates to the nervous system. In: *Metabolism of the Nervous System*, pp. 566–577. Ed. D. Richter. London: Pergamon Press.

UDENFRIEND, S., CLARK, C. T. and TITUS, E. (1953) 5-Hydroxytryptophan decarboxylase: a new route of metabolism of tryptophan. *J. Am. chem. Soc.* **75**, 501–502.

UDENFRIEND, S. and CREVELING, C. R. (1959) Localization of dopamine-β-oxidase in brain. *J. Neurochem.* **4**, 350–352.

UDENFRIEND, S., WEISSBACH, H. and BOGDANSKI, D. F. (1957) Biochemical findings relating to the action of serotonin. *Ann. N. Y. Acad. Sci.* **66**, 602–608.

UMRATH, K. (1961) The relation of Substance P to neurotransmitter substances. In: *Symposium on Substance P*, pp. 23–27. Ed. P. Stern. Sarajevo: Scientific Society of Bosnia & Herzegovina.

UNNA, K., KNIAZUK, J. G. and GRESLIN, J. G. (1944) Pharmacologic actions of erythrina alkaloids. I. β-Erythroidine and substances derived from it. *J. Pharmac. exp. Ther.* **80**, 39–52.

USHERWOOD, P. N. R. (1961) Spontaneous miniature potentials from insect muscle fibers. *Nature (Lond.)* **191**, 814–815.

USHERWOOD, P. N. R. and GRUNDFEST, H. (1965) Peripheral inhibition in skeletal muscle of insects. *J. Neurophysiol.* **28**, 497–518.

USHERWOOD, P. N. R. and MACHILI, P. (1966) Chemical transmission at the insect excitatory neuromuscular synapse. *Nature (Lond.)* **210**, 634–636.

UTLEY, J. D. (1966). Acetylcholinesterase and pseudocholinesterase in neural and non-neural tissue in the medial geniculate body of the cat. *Biochem. Pharmac.* **15**, 1–6.

VAN DER KLOOT, W. G. (1960) Factor S—a substance which excites crustacean muscle. *J. Neurochem.* **5**, 245–252.

VAN GELDER, N. M. (1965) The histochemical demonstration of γ-aminobutyric acid metabolism by reduction of a tetrazolium salt. *J. Neurochem.* **12**, 231–237.

VAN GELDER, N. M. and ELLIOTT, K. A. C. (1958) Disposition of γ-aminobutyric acid administered to animals. *J. Neurochem.* **3**, 139–143.

VAN HARREVELD, A. (1959) Compounds in brain extracts causing spreading depression of cerebral cortical activity and contraction of crustacean muscle. *J. Neurochem.* **3**, 300–315.

VAN HARREVELD, A. and KOOIMAN, M. (1965) Amino acid release from the cerebral cortex during spreading depression and asphyxiation. *J. Neurochem.* **12**, 431–439.

VAN HARREVELD, A. and MENDELSON, M. (1959) Glutamate-induced contractions in crustacean muscle. *J. cell comp. Physiol.* **54**, 85–94.

VANE, J. R., COLLIER, H. O. J., CORNE, S. J., MARLEY, E. and BRADLEY, P. B. (1961) Tryptamine receptors in the central nervous system. *Nature (Lond.)* **191**, 1068–1069.

VOGLER, K., HAEFELY, W., HÜRLIMANN, A., STUDER, R. O., LERGIER, W., STRÄSSLE, R. and BERNEIS, K. H. (1963) A new purification procedure and biological properties of substance P. *Ann. N.Y. Acad. Sci.* **104**, 378–389.

VOGT, M. (1954) Concentration of sympathin in different parts of the central nervous system under normal conditions and after the administration of drugs. *J. Physiol. (Lond.)* **123**, 451–481.

VOGT, M. (1965) Effect of drugs on metabolism of catecholamines in the brain. *Br. med. Bull.* **21**, 57–61.

VOLLE, R. L. (1962a) The actions of several ganglion blocking agents on the postganglionic discharge induced by di-iso-propylphosphofluoridate (DFP) in sympathetic ganglia. *J. Pharmac. exp. Ther.* **135**, 45–53.

VOLLE, R. L. (1962b) The responses to ganglionic stimulating and blocking drugs of cell groups within a sympathetic ganglion. *J. Pharmac. exp. Ther.* **135**, 54–61.

VOLLE, R. L. (1966) Modification by drugs of synaptic mechanisms in autonomic ganglia. *Pharmac. Rev.* **18**, 839–869.

VOLLE, R. L. and KOELLE, G. B. (1961) The physiological role of acetylcholinesterase (AChE) in sympathetic ganglia. *J. Pharmac. exp. Ther.* **133**, 223–240.

VON BAUMGARTEN, R., BLOOM, F. E., OLIVER, A. P. and SALMOIRAGHI, G. C. (1963) Response of individual olfactory nerve cells to microelectrophoretically administered chemical substances. *Pflügers Arch. ges. Physiol.* **277**, 125–140.

VOORHOEVE, P. E. (1960) Autochthonus activity of fusimotor neurones in the cat. *Acta Physiol. pharmac. néerl.* **9**, 1–43.

WACHTEL, H. and KANDEL, E. R. (1967) A direct synaptic connection mediating both excitation and inhibition. *Science, N.Y.* **158**, 1206–1208.

WAELSCH, H. (1957) Metabolism of proteins and amino acids. In: *Metabolism of the Nervous System*, pp. 431–447. Ed. D. Richter. London: Pergamon.

WALDRON, H. A. (1967) Cholinergic fibres in the spinal cord of the rat. *Brain Res.* **4**, 113–116.

WALKER, R. J., WOODRUFF, G. N., GLAIZNER, B., SEDDEN, C. B. and KERKUT, G. A. (1968) The pharmacology of *Helix* dopamine receptor of specific neurones in the snail, *Helix aspersa*. *Comp. Biochem. Physiol.* **24**, 455–469.

WALKER, R. J., WOODRUFF, G. N. and KERKUT, G. A. (1968) The effect of acetylcholine and 5-hydroxytryptamine on electrophysiological recordings from muscle fibres of the Leech, *Hirudo medicinalis*. *Comp. Biochem. Physiol.* **24**, 987–990.

WARE, F. and GRAHAM, G. D. (1967) Effects of acetylcholine on transmembrane potentials in frog ventricle. *Am. J. Physiol.* **212**, 451–455.

WASER, P. G. (1961) Chemistry and pharmacology of muscarine, muscarone and some related compounds. *Pharmac. Rev.* **13**, 465–515.

WASER, P. G. (1963) Nature of the cholinergic receptor. In: *Modern Concepts in the Relationship between Structure and Pharmacological Activity*, pp. 101–115. Ed. K. J. Brunings and P. Lindgren. Oxford: Pergamon.

WASHIZU, Y. (1960) Single spinal motoneurons excitable from two different antidromic pathways. *Jap. J. Physiol.* **10**, 121–131.

WEIDMANN, H. and CERLETTI, A. (1957) Die wirkung von D-Lysergsaüre—diäthylamid und 5-Hydroxytryptamin (serotonin) auf spinale Reflexe der Katze. *Helv. physiol. pharmac. Acta* **15**, 376–383.

WEIDMANN, H. and CERLETTI, A. (1960) Structure activity relationships of oxyindole derivatives with regard to their effect on the knee jerk of spinal cats. *Helv. physiol. pharmac. Acta* **18**, 174–182.

WEIGHT, F. F. and SALMOIRAGHI, G. C. (1966a) Responses of spinal cord interneurons to acetylcholine, norepinephrine and serotonin administered by microelectrophoresis. *J. Pharmac. exp. Ther.* **153**, 420–427.

WEIGHT, F. F. and SALMOIRAGHI, G. C. (1966b) Adrenergic responses of Renshaw cells. *J. Pharmac. exp. Ther.* **154**, 391–397.

WEIGHT, F. F. and SALMOIRAGHI, G. C. (1967) Motoneurone depression by norepinephrine. *Nature (Lond.)* **213**, 1229–1230.

WEIL-MALHERBE H., AXELROD, J. and TOMCHICK, R. (1959) Blood-brain barrier of adrenaline. *Science, N.Y.* **129**, 1226–1227.

WEIL-MALHERBE and BONE, A. D. (1957) Intracellular distribution of catecholamines in the brain. *Nature (Lond.)* **180**, 1050–1051.

WEIL-MALHERBE, H. and BONE, A. D. (1959) The effect of reserpine on the intracellular distribution of catecholamines in the brain stem of the rabbit. *J. Neurochem.* **4**, 251–263.

WEIL-MALHERBE, H., POSNER, H. S. and BOWLES, G. R. (1961) Changes in the concentration and intracellular distribution of brain catecholamines: the effects of reserpine, β-phenylisopropylhydrazine, pyrogallol and 3-4 dihydroxyphenylalanine, alone and in combination. *J. Pharmac. exp. Ther.* **132**, 278–286.

WEIL-MALHERBE, H., WHITBY, L. G. and AXELROD, J. (1961) The blood-brain barrier for catecholamines in different regions of the brain. In: *Regional Neurochemistry, The Regional Chemistry, Physiology and Pharmacology of the Nervous System*, pp. 284–291. Ed. S. S. Kety and J. Elkes. London: Pergamon.

WEIR, M. C. L. and MCLENNAN, H. (1963) The action of catecholamines in sympathetic ganglia. *Canad. J. Biochem. Physiol.* **41**, 2627–2636.

WEISS, P. (1947) Protoplasm synthesis and substance transfer in neurons. Abstr. XVII Int. Physiol. Congr. 101.

WEISS, P. and HISCOE, H. B. (1948) Experiments on the mechanism of nerve growth. *J. exp. Zool.* **107**, 315–395.

WEISSBACH, H., LOVENBERG, W., REDFIELD, B. G. and UDENFRIEND, S. (1961) *In vivo* metabolism of serotonin and tryptamine: effect of monoamine oxidase inhibition. *J. Pharmac. exp. Ther.* **131**, 26–30.

WEISSBACH, H., LOVENBERG, W. and UDENFRIEND, S. (1961) Characteristics of mammalian histidine decarboxylating enzymes. *Biochem. Biophys. Acta* **50**, 177–179.

WELSH, J. H. (1953) Excitation of the heart of *Venus mercenaria*. *Naunyn-Schmiedeberg's Arch. exp. Path. Pharmak.* **219**, 23–29.

WELSH, J. H. (1961) Neurohormones of mollusca. *Am. Zool.* **1**, 267–272.

WELSH, J. H. and MOORHEAD, M. (1959) The *in vivo* synthesis of 5-hydroxytryptamine from 5-hydroxytryptophan by nervous tissues of two species of molluscs. *Gunma J. Med. Sci.* **8**, 211–218.

WELSH, J. H. and MOORHEAD, M. (1960) The quantitative distribution of 5-hydroxytryptamine in the invertebrates, especially in their nervous systems. *J. Neurochem.* **6**, 146–169.

WELSH, J. H. and SLOCOMBE, A. G. (1962) The mechanism of action of acetylcholine on the *Venus* heart. *Biol. Bull. mar. biol. Lab. Woods Hole* **102**, 48–57.

WERLE, E. (1961) Hemmung der Histidin-Decarboxylase durch α-Methyldopa. *Natur-wissenschaften* **48**, 54–55.

WERLE, E. and PALM, u.D. (1950) Histamin in Nerven II. *Biochem. Z.* **320**, 322–334.

WERMAN, R. (1966) A Review—criteria for identification of a central nervous system transmitter. *Comp. Biochem. Physiol.* **18**, 745–766.

WERMAN, R., DAVIDOFF, R. A. and APRISON, M. H. (1967) Is Glycine a Neurotransmitter? Inhibition of motoneurones by iontophoresis of glycine. *Nature (Lond.)* **214**, 681–683.

WERMAN, R., DAVIDOFF, R. A. and APRISON, M. H. (1968) Inhibitory action of glycine on spinal neurons in the cat. *J. Neurophysiol.* **31**, 81–95.

WERNER, G. (1960) Neuromuscular facilitation and antidromic discharges in motor nerves: their relation to activity in motor nerve terminals. *J. Neurophysiol.* **23**, 171–187.

WERNER, G. (1961) Antidromic activity in motor nerves and its relation to a generator event in nerve terminals. *J. Neurophysiol.* **24**, 401–413.

WHEELER, D. D., BOYARSKI, L. L. and BROOKS, W. H. (1966) The release of amino-acids from nerve during stimulation. *J. cell. comp. Physiol.* **67**, 141–148.

WHITE, T. (1959) Formation and catabolism of histamine in brain tissue *in vitro. J. Physiol. (Lond.)* **149**, 34–42.

WHITE, T. (1960) Formation and catabolism of histamine in cat brain *in vivo. J. Physiol. (Lond.)* **152**, 299–308.

WHITE, T. (1966) Histamine and methylhistamine in cat brain and other tissues. *Br. J. Pharmac. Chemother.* **26**, 494–501.

WHITTAKER, V. P. (1958) A comparison of the distribution of lysosome enzymes and 5-hydroxytryptamine with that of acetylcholine in subcellular fractions of guinea-pig brain. *Biochem. Pharmac.* **1**, 351.

WHITTAKER, V. P. (1963) Identification of acetylcholine and related esters of biological origin. *Handb. exp. Pharmak.* **15**, 2–39.

WHITTAKER, V. P. (1964) Investigations on the storage sites of biogenic amines in the central nervous system. *Progr. Brain Res.* **8**, 90–117.

WHITTAKER, V. P. (1965) The application of subcellular fractionation techniques to the study of brain function. *Prog. Biophys. molec. Biol.* **15**, 39–96.

WHITTAKER, V. P., MICHAELSON, I. A. and KIRLAND, R. J. A. (1964) The separation of synaptic vesicles from nerve-ending particles ("synaptosomes"). *Biochem. J.* **90**, 293–303.

WHITTAKER, V. P. and SHERIDAN, M. N. (1965) The morphology and acetylcholine content of isolated cerebral cortical synaptic vesicles. *J. Neurochem.* **12**, 363–372.

WILLIAMS, J. D. and COOPER, J. R. (1965) Acetylcholine in bovine corneal epithelium. *Biochem. Pharmac.* **14**, 1286–1289.

WILLIAMS, T. H. W. (1967) Electron microscopic evidence for an autonomic interneuron. *Nature (Lond.)* **214**, 309–310.

WILSON, A. T. and WRIGHT, S. (1937) Anticurare action of potassium and other substances. *Quart. J. exp. Physiol.* **26**, 127–139.

WILSON, V. J. (1956) Effect of intra-arterial injection of adrenaline on spinal extensor and flexor reflexes. *Am. J. Physiol.* **186**, 491–496.

WINDER, A. F. (1967) The nature of substance P. *J. Physiol. (Lond.)* **189**, 66–67P.

WOOLLEY, D. W. and CAMPBELL, N. K. (1960) Serotonin receptors. II. Calcium transport by crude and purified receptor. *Biochem. biophys. Acta* **40**, 543–544.

WOOLLEY, D. W. and SHAW, E. N. (1954) A biochemical and pharmacological suggestion about certain mental disorders. *Proc. natn. Acad. Sci. U.S.A.* **40**, 228–231.

WOOLLEY, D. W. and SHAW, E. N. (1957) Evidence for the participation of serotonin in mental processes. *Ann. N.Y. Acad. Sci.* **66**, 649–665.

WRIGHT, A. M., MOORHEAD, M. and WELSH, J. H. (1962) Actions of derivatives of lysergic acid on the heart of *Venus mercenaria*. *Br. J. Pharmac. Chemother.* **18**, 440–450.

WURTMAN, R. J., AXELROD, J. and BARCHAS, J. D. (1964) Age and enzyme activity in the human pineal. *J. clin. Endocr. Metab.* **24**, 299–301.

YAMAGUCHI, N., LING, G. M. and MARCZYNSKI, T. J. (1964) The effects of chemical stimulation of the preoptic region, nucleus centralis medialis or brain stem reticular formation with regard to sleep and wakefulness. *Rec. Advanc. biol. Psychiat.* **6**, 9–20.

YAMAGUCHI, N., MARCZYNSKI, T. J. and LING, G. M. (1963) The effects of electrical and chemical stimulation of the preoptic region and some nonspecific thalamic nuclei in unrestrained, waking animals. *Electroen. Neurophysiol.* **15**, 154.

YAMAMOTO, C. (1967) Pharmacologic studies of norepinephrine, acetylcholine and related compounds on neurons in Deiters' nucleus and the cerebellum. *J. Pharmac. exp. Ther.* **156**, 39–47.

YORK, D. H. (1967) The inhibitory actions of dopamine on neurones of the caudate nucleus. *Brain Res.* **5**, 263–266.

YORK, D. H. (1968) A microiontophoretic study of neurones in the globus pallidus-putamen complex. *Aust. J. exp. Biol. med. Sci.* **46**, 3–4P.

YOSHIDA, H., NAMBA, J., KANIIKE, K. and IMAIZUMI, R. (1963) Studies on active transport of L-DOPA (dihydroxyphenylalanine) into brain slices. *Jap. J. Pharmac.* **13**, 1–9.

ZACKS, S. I., METZGER, J. F., SMITH, C. W. and BLUMBERG, J. M. (1962) Localization of ferritin-labelled botulinus toxin in the neuromuscular junction of the mouse. *J. Neuropath. exp. Neurol.* **21**, 610–633.

ZELLER, E. A. (ed.) (1959) Amine oxidase inhibitors. *Ann. N.Y. Acad. Sci.* **80**, 551–1046.

ZELLER, E. A. and BISSEGER, A. (1943) Influence of drugs and chemotherapy on enzyme reactions. III. Cholinesterases of brain and erythrocytes. *Helv. chim. Acta* **26**, 1619–1630.

ZETLER, G. (1956) Substanz P, ein Polypeptid aus Darm und Gehirn mit depressiven, hyperalgetischen und morphin-antagonistischen Wirkungen auf das zentralnerven-system. *Naunyn-Schmiedeberg's Arch. exp. Path. Pharmak.* **228**, 513–538.

ZIEHER, L. M. and DE ROBERTIS, E. D. P. (1963) Subcellular localization of 5-hydroxytryptamine in rat brain. *Biochem. Pharmac.* **12**, 596–598.

ZS.-NAGY, I., S-RÓZSA, K., SALÁNKI, J., FÖLDES, I., PERÉNYI, L. and DEMETER, M. (1965) Subcellular localization of 5-hydroxytryptamine in the central nervous system of lamellibranchiates. *J. Neurochem.* **12**, 245–251.

ZUBER, H. and JAQUES, R. (1962) Isolierung von Substanz P aus Rinderhirn. *Angew. Chem.* **74**, 216–217.

ŽUPANČIČ, A. C. (1953) The mode of action of acetylcholine. A theory extended to a hypothesis on the mode of action of other biologically active substances. *Acta physiol. scand.* **29**, 63–71.

INDEX

OTHER DIVISIONS IN THE SERIES IN
PURE AND APPLIED BIOLOGY

BIOCHEMISTRY

BOTANY

MODERN TRENDS
IN PHYSIOLOGICAL SCIENCES

PLANT PHYSIOLOGY